T0030700

Praise for THE FIGHT FOR HISTORY

"Cook [is] an indispensable war historian. . . . By exploring how Canadians arrived, after so long, at new ways of understanding World War II, Cook shows that even the most calcified historical perspectives can ultimately prove pliable. Anyone fighting for a better grasp of history—whether it's our constitutional roots, our colonial past, or our heroes and villains—should take heart."
—*Maclean's*

"[Cook] provides some insight into what has been driving this passion for the past and its stories. . . . What Cook makes clear is that the fight for history and the shaping of social memory is a process that never stops. Against the forces of apathy and indifference we must push back." —*Toronto Star*

Praise for THE SECRET HISTORY OF SOLDIERS

"Prof. Cook takes an unprecedented dive into . . . a rich and little-explored culture that developed among soldiers on the front lines." —*The Hill Times*

"Cook has revealed many of the secrets of the Great War's soldiers' lives. The veil of secrecy has been lifted and every chapter can be read over and over." —*Winnipeg Free Press*

Praise for VIMY

"Through this book, Cook . . . cements himself as the nation's premier military historian." —*Vancouver Sun*

"There is no one better equipped to retell the Vimy story than Cook." —*The Chronicle Herald*

Praise for THE MADMAN AND THE BUTCHER

"A triumph of the historian's craft, rich fare for both scholars and general readers. Confidently written and based on an impressive mastery of archival and secondary sources, it confirms Cook's stature as our leading military historian." —*The Walrus*

"[*The Madman and the Butcher*] is engagingly written, and for those inclined to the arcana of Canadian history, it will shed light on the making of reputations following the war." —*Quill & Quire*

Praise for SHOCK TROOPS

"Tremendous detail and almost unstoppable narrative momentum. . . . Through these stories of horror and heroism, what shines through most brilliantly is the complex humanity of the characters." —Charles Taylor Prize Jury, 2009

"An intimate and personal chronicle of the First World War." —CBC

Also by Tim Cook

No Place to Run:
The Canadian Corps and Gas Warfare
in the First World War

Clio's Warriors:
Canadian Historians and the
Writing of the World Wars

At the Sharp End:
Canadians Fighting the Great War,
1914–1916, Volume One

Shock Troops:
Canadians Fighting the Great War,
1917–1918, Volume Two

The Madman and the Butcher:
The Sensational Wars of Sam Hughes
and General Arthur Currie

Warlords: Borden, Mackenzie King,
and Canada's World Wars

The Necessary War:
Canadians Fighting the Second World War,
1939–1943, Volume One

Fight to the Finish:
Canadians in the Second World War,
1944–1945, Volume Two

Vimy: The Battle and the Legend

The Secret History of Soldiers:
How Canadians Survived the Great War

The Fight for History:
75 Years of Forgetting, Remembering,
and Remaking Canada's Second World War

LIFESAVERS AND BODY SNATCHERS

MEDICAL CARE AND THE STRUGGLE FOR SURVIVAL IN THE GREAT WAR

TIM COOK

PENGUIN

an imprint of Penguin Canada, a division of Penguin Random House Canada Limited

First published in Allen Lane hardcover by Penguin Canada, 2022

Published in this edition, 2023

1st Printing

Copyright © 2022 by Tim Cook

All rights reserved. Without limiting the rights under copyright reserved above,
no part of this publication may be reproduced, stored in or introduced into a retrieval system,
or transmitted in any form or by any means (electronic, mechanical, photocopying, recording
or otherwise), without the prior written permission of both the copyright owner and
the above publisher of this book.

Library and Archives Canada Cataloguing in Publication
Title: Lifesavers and body snatchers : medical care and the
struggle for survival in the Great War / Tim Cook.
Names: Cook, Tim, 1971- author.
Description: Includes bibliographical references and index.
Identifiers: Canadiana 20210395877 | ISBN 9780735242333 (softcover)
Subjects: LCSH: World War, 1914-1918—Medical care—Canada. |
LCSH: Body snatching—Canada—History—20th century. |
LCSH: Medicine, Military—Canada—History—20th century.
Classification: LCC D629.C2 C66 2023 | DDC 940.4/7571—dc23

Cover design by Matthew Flute
Cover images: (front) Canadian and German wounded help one another
through the mud during the Battle of Passchendaele, CWM 19930065-532,
(spine) Casualty Clearing Station - A nurse meeting wounded Canadians
with a dog brought out of the trenches, CWM 19920044-814, both from
the George Metcalf Archival Collection, © Canadian War Museum

Printed in the United States of America

www.penguinrandomhouse.ca

Penguin
Random House
PENGUIN CANADA

FOR SHARON, SARAH, CHLOE, EMMA,
PAIGE, AND BEAR, WITH LOVE.

CONTENTS

INTRODUCTION I

CHAPTER 1: The Canadian Medical Profession Goes to War 15

CHAPTER 2: Shot, Shell, and Poison Gas at Ypres, 1915 . . 39

CHAPTER 3: Preventative Care and the Hunt for
Malingerers. 61

CHAPTER 4: Vice and the Medical Corps 83

CHAPTER 5: Clearing the Wounded, 1916 103

CHAPTER 6: Saving Lives through Surgery 129

CHAPTER 7: Collecting Soldiers' Body Parts 151

CHAPTER 8: The Many Battles of the Mind 171

CHAPTER 9: The Canadian Army Medical Corps in Crisis .195

CHAPTER 10: Force Protection at Vimy Ridge, 1917. . . .217

CHAPTER 11: Care and Recovery 239

CHAPTER 12: A Toxic Plague 267

CHAPTER 13: Displaying Human Remains 287

CHAPTER 14: Medicine in the Mud, 1917. 309

CHAPTER 15: Adapting Medical Care in the War Zone,
1918 331

CHAPTER 16: Carnage in the Victory Campaign, 1918 353

CHAPTER 17: A Pandemic of Mass Death and an Epidemic of
Sexual Diseases 377

CHAPTER 18: Lessons and Legacies 397

CHAPTER 19: Memorializing the Medical War 421

CHAPTER 20: The Use and Misuse of Harvested Soldiers'
Organs 445

ENDNOTES 469
ACKNOWLEDGMENTS 521
CREDITS 525
INDEX 529

INTRODUCTION

At the Battle of Second Ypres in April 1915, Lieutenant-Colonel Walter Langmuir Watt wrote in his diary about the carnage at his medical aid station. It was "one never-ending stream which lasted all day and night for seven days without cessation: in all some five thousand two hundred cases passed through our hands. Wounds here, wounds there, wounds everywhere. Legs, feet, hands missing; bleeding stumps controlled by rough field tourniquets, large portions of the abdominal walls shot away; faces horribly mutilated; bones shattered to pieces; holes that you could put your clenched fist into, filled with dirt and mud, bits of equipment and clothing, until it all became like a hideous nightmare, as if we were living in the seventh hell of the damned."[1] Awful scenes like this were repeated time and time again in the large-scale battles along the Western Front, the smaller operations in between them, and the warfare in the trenches, where soldiers were killed, maimed, and forced from the line by illness and disease.

This is a story of the fighting Canadian soldiers and of those men and women in the Canadian Army Medical Corps (CAMC) who sought to save them from pestilence, injury, and death. It is a history of killing and curing—of the entwinement of the fighting units and the medical services. In response to the unimaginable wounds caused by this new industrialized war, medical treatment was undergoing a steady progression, from developing surgical techniques and diagnostics to using relatively new X-ray machines to engaging with mental injuries. New interventions through blood transfusions and facial reconstruction were radical departures from past treatment. While there were amputations for traumatic injuries or as a result of infection—a relentless killer of soldiers before the age of antibiotics—the surgeons were astonishingly good at saving lives. "Amongst all the misery of war and within easy distance of its relentless activities are found the more civilized and humane endeavors of humanity; the desire to alleviate suffering," observed one Canadian soldier, stressing the seeming contradictions of medicine and war. "On the one hand it is science straining every nerve to accomplish man's destruction, on the other hand it is science working overtime to save his life."[2] The battle for life was an ongoing struggle, braided with and inseparable from combat at the front.

Despite the extraordinary slaughter on the Western Front that was swept and saturated by the firepower of artillery, machine guns, and rifles, medical personnel also fought unseen adversaries in viruses and bacteria. "In every war the soldier faces two enemies," wrote CAMC lieutenant-colonel John W.S. McCullough. "The one is the armed forces of the foe, with their terrible engines of destruction, the other the silent and in the past the far greater foe, the grim purveyor of death, disease. The history of warfare for centuries has shown that of these two enemies the latter or silent enemy causes much the greater mortality."[3] During the

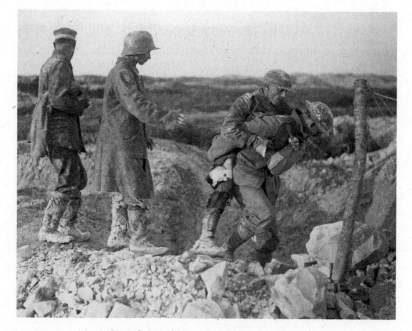

A Canadian soldier carrying his mate off the
battlefield, with two German prisoners.

American Civil War from 1861 to 1865, with its increased firepower and over 2,000 land battles, disease still killed five times as
many soldiers as conventional shot and shell.[4] And in almost every
war in human history, disease claimed more lives than human
weapons. Death by disease was a significant concern at the start
of the Great War, and the fact that the Canadian forces (and all
Allied or enemy armies) along the Western Front did not waste
away from the scourge of bacteria and viruses was a marvel of
preventative medical care.

Soldiering in conditions of dirt, deprivation, and hardship, the
medical forces also played a key role in sustaining morale. This
lesson had been learned by the time of the Great War, partially
because of the foul blight of the British army's neglect of the

wounded during the Crimean War of 1853–1856, which was a lasting cause of reproach. In that war far from Britain, the medical services had been overwhelmed, with hospitals filled with dying men left unattended. The abandonment of soldiers to perish in agony from festering infections was an appalling revelation that led to a far-reaching public scandal that shook faith in the military.[5] In response to that health disaster, widespread reforms in the medical support of armies and vast improvements in civilian medicine began in the mid-nineteenth century, so that by 1914 there was a firm belief in the need to offer the best care possible for the citizen-soldiers who enlisted to serve their country. Indeed, a social contract held sway between the state and the citizen-soldier in almost all armies, and those who enlisted had expectations that they would not be abandoned on the battlefield. While soldiers came to understand the high probability of death and maiming at the front, and generally accepted this or found ways to choke back the fear and continue in their duty, a well-functioning medical system was crucial to the war effort. This maintenance of morale through prevention and treatment was an acknowledged role of all doctors and nurses; at the same time, the high command relied on the medical services to keep their soldiers in the line, no matter the human cost. Individual suffering would be subsumed to the larger war effort. The medical practitioners were thus thrust into the role of ensuring that soldiers' motivation did not collapse, but also of acting as the gatekeepers who refused to let soldiers exit the front with all its horror and tragedy. These twin motivations—to repair the soldier and to keep him in the line—often pushed non-combatant doctors and nurses into agonizing ethical dilemmas.

Medical practitioners were forced to carry an emotional weight as they fought to save lives and bore witness to untold

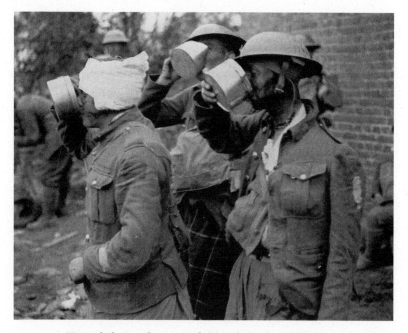

Wounded Canadians at a field ambulance medical unit.

misery. It was said that no one could understand war without first setting foot in a military hospital. The images of human bodies torn apart or eaten alive by infection imprinted themselves on the medical service personnel. These healers were deeply affected by their many interactions with wounded soldiers, who often had tremendous faith in the nurses and doctors that their flesh could be mended, that their nightmare-plagued minds could be restored, and that they would return safely to loved ones. And yet thousands still died of their wounds in the medical units. Private Ralph Watson, a Canadian CAMC orderly who was later a stretcher-bearer, shared a glimpse into the medical war when he wrote to his wife, "I have done things I never believed I could possibly do. I have seen wounds that you cannot bear to look at. . . . But I'm not going to tell you about all that."[6]

All of the Great War fighting services, from infantry and gunners to engineers and airmen, learned during the conflict, processing lessons through defeat as much as victory.[7] A clear trajectory of knowledge and professionalization was also evident within the medical services, including advancements in surgical techniques, preventative care, and public health awareness, all of which were brought back to Canada after the war. The unlimited war effort that demanded so much from Canadians over four long and costly years also conditioned the public to expect the state to provide aid to address postwar health challenges. Following victory, the medical practitioners who were now veterans were at the sharp end of new medical battles, and the legacy of treatment during the war profoundly shaped medicine and public health initiatives for decades to follow. "The war gave us a new social conscience," said one doctor after the war. "It taught us a new standard of generosity and impressed upon us the practical value of individual and community health."[8]

———

The Great War of 1914 to 1918 was a conflict of unprecedented scale and destruction. By war's end, over 9.4 million soldiers were killed, at least 21 million more were wounded in body, and countless millions would carry mental scars. From Canada, a country of not yet 8 million, at least 620,000 served or were conscripted, with about one in three adult males in uniform. A total of 2,845 nursing sisters also contributed to the war effort, and almost all of the men and women who formed the Canadian Expeditionary Force (CEF) were drawn from civilian life rather than the professional armed services. Coming from across the Dominion, from every city, town, and village, English, French, new Canadians, and Indigenous people came together in a common cause.[9]

Canada was not prepared for the Great War, with only 3,000 professional soldiers in uniform and a scarcity of modern weapons. The CAMC was no different, and it consisted of twenty officers in 1914. Attesting to their importance during the war, however, the medical services expanded to over 20,000 men and women, with about half of all Canadian doctors in uniform and about a third of the country's nurses.[10] There was no shortage of patients. Of the 424,589 Canadians who went overseas, around 140,000 were wounded at the front, and most of these injuries fell to the 345,000 Canadians who served in Europe along the Western Front.[11] And yet despite the long odds against the soldiers, nine out of ten wounded soldiers survived their injury if they were cared for by a medical practitioner, attesting to the skill of the

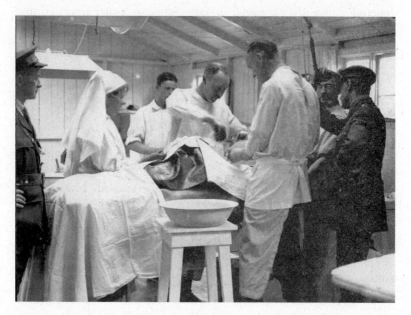

A Canadian surgical team operating on a soldier from the front.

doctors and nurses. That figure does not diminish the grievous losses at the front, where over 66,000 Canadians were killed during the war and in the immediate aftermath, although the butcher's bill would have been much higher without the medical services. Canada's doctors and nurses, noted an official 1919 report, came together to form a "great machine of healing."[12]

After the Great War, the Canadian medical services enlisted the aid of the country's most accomplished medical writer, Sir Andrew Macphail, to pen the services' official history, *The Medical Services* (1925).[13] Readers will see later in this book how the war veteran and McGill University professor excited much controversy, but *The Medical Services* remained the standard text for understanding Canada's medical war into the twenty-first century. Almost a hundred years later, and written in the midst of the coronavirus worldwide pandemic, *Lifesavers and Body Snatchers* draws together old and new research, connects it to other international historiographies, and offers a new way to understand the incredible challenges of this generation of Canadians who faced the Great War apocalypse. While this is a book about medical advances and failures, it is always centred on the experiences of soldiers, medical practitioners, and other eyewitnesses to history.

Combat and care are the focus in these pages, but the shocking story of the harvesting of human body parts, organs, and bones from slain Canadian soldiers will also be exposed. I have spent more than a decade investigating the story of Canadian doctors harvesting body parts of soldiers on the autopsy table and then using their brains, lungs, and other organs or bones for scientific study. While stretcher-bearers were sometimes described as body snatchers for their courage in carrying off the wounded from the battlefield under fire, this collection of body parts was another form of body snatching. This story has never been fully told, but my research into the nation's archives has revealed that almost 800 individual Canadian body parts, organs, and skeletal remains were extracted from Canadians killed at the front and sent to London, England, where they were stored, conserved, and put on display at the Royal College of Surgeons. Even more incredible, the first transfer of these Canadian body parts was sent to Montreal in 1918 to form a founding collection for a planned military medical museum that was to have been built in Ottawa. While little known at the time, this program of harvesting body parts was not a nefarious secret, and I have uncovered how the federal government even devoted significant funds in the immediate postwar years to the preservation of these organs and bones. This revelation is all the more surprising when one considers how Canadians after the war were seeking to make meaning of the nation's service and sacrifice by erecting memorials to the fallen in almost every community across Canada and overseas at former battlefields like Vimy Ridge. Riven with grief and hollowed out by sorrow, Canadians ennobled the fallen soldiers and they murmured "Lest We Forget." Few imagined that many of their loved ones who were slain overseas had been reduced to scientific specimens that would be transported back to Canada and put on display in jars as medical teaching tools and scientific oddities. This story, laid bare here for the first time in any book, is a wartime medical mystery that is startling and disturbing, calling into question what we know about the bodies of fallen soldiers.

The history of war and medicine presented here is different from other histories in another fundamental way. Medical studies of the war in Britain, the United States, France, and other countries have almost exclusively been written by medical historians. This is perhaps natural, but often the combat experience feels absent from these studies. Why is it important to include this experience in a medical history of war? First, combat and tactics, along with the weapons of war and the wounds they cause, all have an impact on medical treatment, especially through the changing nature of injuries. Second, given the medical services' essential role in supporting the morale of the fighting forces, and in ensuring that those forces did not wither away from disease, one is further struck by the absence in these histories of what was happening to

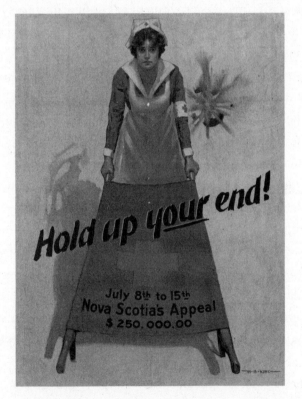

A recruiting poster from Nova Scotia featuring a nursing sister who implores the viewer to "hold up your end" and support the overseas men and women.

the fighting men. Finally, a medical history can and should reveal something of the human dimension of war—its effects on both caregivers and soldiers—and this is best understood through their tangled interactions. In the study of Canada's Great War, the tens of thousands of surviving letters, diary entries, and memoirs, not to mention material culture, photographs, and works of art, can disclose the complex interplay of people, circumstances, and events. An untapped additional source for understanding the medical war is the primary publication of the profession, the *Canadian Medical Association Journal (CMAJ)*. Established in 1911, and signalling the growing professionalization of physicians, the *CMAJ* holds a rich collection of contemporary wartime material, with many articles written by the Canadian doctors, surgeons, and other medical specialists in uniform. With the goal of improving care and saving lives, the physicians studied their patients and the nature of their injuries and diseases, writing about their experiences, providing eye-witness accounts, and describing the medical interventions to overcome the shattering effects of weapons on the body or to combat infection. Doctors were motivated to share their hard-won lessons with their colleagues, and in clinical or colourful language they admitted failure and documented successes. Moreover, the contemporary documents produced by the fighting and medical services, now stored at the Library Archives of Canada in Ottawa, are also important, with orders and reports revealing soldiers grappling with the evolving medical treatment for ailments ranging from rotting feet and decaying mouths to gaping wounds to the body and invisible injuries to the mind.

While this is a book that is grounded in the Great War and its aftermath, it is surprising how many of *Lifesavers and Body Snatchers'* subjects and themes resonate in contemporary Canada:

the public debate over inoculation; the lingering mental effects of war on veterans; the issue of providing aid to refugees in a war zone; questions of morality around battlefield triage; the links between the 1918–1919 pandemic that killed 55,000 Canadians and, 100 years later, the 2020–2022 coronavirus pandemic that has killed about two-thirds that number; the evolution of treatment and the processing of lessons in hard-pressed medical units overwhelmed by patients; the emotional load carried by practitioners and caregivers; and the impact of a cataclysmic event leading to changes in the approach to public health. And yet we must remember that the past was its own place and space, with its own historical actors who exerted agency and who did not have the benefit of hindsight to know how events would unfold. As a historian, I am more interested in understanding these actors and actions within the contours of their own time, rather than as characters to be studied, pitied, or condemned to score easy points in the context of present-day values and mores. However, I do not absolve past actors: criticisms and condemnation should be levelled where incompetence, immorality, and cruel actions were taken. At the core of *Lifesavers and Body Snatchers* is the narrative arc and authorial gaze that move from the national war effort to the chaos of combat to the bewildering front-line soldier's experience, and then to the medical system, with a focus on those who battled to save lives within it, and how they did it. After almost thirty years of study into the Great War, including reading thousands of books and articles and tens of thousands of pages from archival sources to draw out the history, I hope I have done so with empathy but also with a critical reading of the past.

———

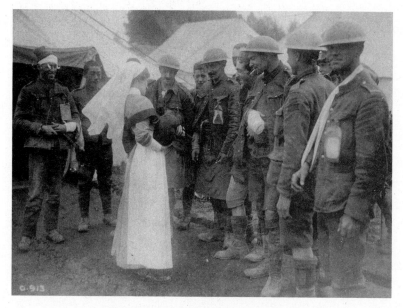

Wounded Canucks with a nursing sister.

The medical officers, practitioners, and nurses struggled in coming to grips with the violence inflicted on bodies during the war, but there were more victories than defeats, more success than failure. While not all patients could be saved, as Montreal surgeon George Armstrong, who served as a colonel in the CAMC, observed, "the burning desire to do one's best for those wounded on the field of battle comes to one and all with an intensity never before experienced."[14] These non-combatants engaged in a mission of care amid the bloody war of the trenches, and the war could not have been won without the full support and professionalism of the medical services.

CHAPTER I

THE CANADIAN MEDICAL PROFESSION GOES TO WAR

The war in Europe came with much warning. After the assassination of the archduke of Austria by a Serbian terrorist group on June 28, 1914, the once-great power of Austria-Hungary sought revenge even as it slipped further into decay and eventual dismemberment. A war, it was hoped, might hold together the collapsing parts of an empire that consisted of several dozen peoples and ethnic groups speaking different languages, and all bound by an ancient monarchy. On the empire's northwestern border was Germany, a rising power since the mid-nineteenth century. Under Kaiser Wilhelm II—erratic, juvenile, and impulsive—Germany had offered to support the Austrians in the war against Serbia. The conflict was expected to be short and decisive, except that Nicholas II—Russia's czar and Wilhelm II's first cousin—refused to let another Slavic nation be crushed. France was allied to Russia, seeking to revenge the festering shame over its inglorious defeat at the hands of the Germans in 1871, which included the loss of territory on its eastern border. This unlikely alliance system bound together the republic of France with the monarchy of Russia, and they were joined by the British Empire, which was anxious to prevent Germany from dominating Europe.[1] Weeks of sabre-rattling, reckless brinkmanship, and a failure of diplomacy ensured that decisions made and refused led Europe to war when the vast armies of citizens were mobilized.

Far from the European battlefields that saw German armies strike through Belgium on August 1, 1914, which brought Britain into the war on August 4, a great rippling was felt throughout the British Empire. When Britain was at war, the dominions and colonies were at arms too. That included the senior dominion, Canada, which by 1914 consisted of around eight million British subjects spread over an impossibly large land mass. Politicians in Ottawa, led by Prime Minister Sir Robert Borden, pledged a volunteer army, but they knew that it was up to Canadians to determine the nature of the commitment.

With about 3,000 soldiers, Canada's Permanent Force was pathetically small and ill-equipped for the fighting that was to come. But the unpredictable—some said unbalanced—minister of militia and defence, Sam Hughes, was not worried. An ardent militia officer, Hughes did not care for the professionals and instead put his faith in citizen-soldiers. The hardy people of Canada, shaped by their harsh land and frigid environment, were natural-born warriors, thought Hughes. He was not alone in this belief, and politicians and editors preached that this fighting formation of workers, farmers, students, and other civilian professions would need only minimal training to be forged into an army to defend Britain.[2]

A new Canadian Expeditionary Force (CEF) was created, consisting of infantry, artillery, engineers, cavalry, support units, and a medical service. The Canadian Army Medical Corps (CAMC) had been established in 1904, although physicians served with

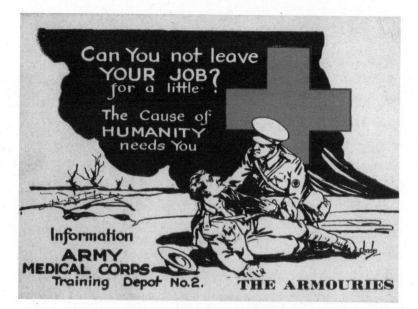

"The Cause of Humanity needs you,"
reads this recruiting poster for the medical corps.

units before that official date. While the CAMC was staffed by twenty Permanent Force officers, the corps was expected to expand by drawing upon civilian doctors, much like the larger CEF would seek soldiers within the country's 59,000 citizen-soldiers who formed militia units across the country. The CEF was also home to thousands of other men who had trained in the cadets or who had passed through the militia, including about 10 percent of all of the country's doctors who had served or were currently serving.[3] Thousands of men from across the country converged at Valcartier, near Quebec City, where they would train and then go overseas.

———

Following the more vigorous professionalization of medicine during the late nineteenth century, as doctors formed accredited organizations to denounce the many faith healers, cranks, and other practitioners of pseudo-medicine, men of medicine (and a few women who faced tremendous barriers based on their gender) had increasingly carved out respect, if not financial gain, in the emerging Canada.[4] At the universities, students learned about general medicine, obstetrics, pediatrics, and surgery, listening to lectures, dissecting cadavers, and studying organs removed from bodies. Fairly recent discoveries had shaped Canadian medical education and practice: Robert Koch's 1882 discovery of the bacillus that causes tuberculosis was a breakthrough in diagnosis and prevention, while Frederick Loffler's work on studying diphtheria offered new ways to understand the passing of disease through fecal matter and polluted water. Doctors and surgeons paid close attention to cleanliness and antiseptic conditions after Joseph Lister's lessons made it clear that keeping bacteria from open wounds saved lives. The discovery of the X-ray in 1895 by Wilhelm Roentgen allowed physicians and surgeons to use radiology for greater insight into the body, even if it was far more common to conduct the post-mortem autopsy where the dead were opened up and studied to uncover the secrets of life.[5] The great Canadian-born practitioner, scholar, and educator William Osler contributed to many fields of study, and he brought this new knowledge together in his widely read textbooks, including *The Principles and Practice of Medicine* (1892), which for decades was the most studied medical text in the English language. Instruction in medical schools was evolving and improving, even though the teaching of surgery still involved students most often viewing surgeons from an amphitheatre seat rather than carrying out the scalpel work themselves. As doctor H.L. Burns, a 1904 graduate of University of Toronto, recalled, "Our practical experience left something to be desired."[6]

Upon graduation, doctors had to start their own practices, running their own businesses for profit. There was no state-funded medicare, and each visit to the doctor required payment. Most Canadian physicians were generalists, although they encountered different injuries and illnesses depending on their rural or urban location. In this period, doctors charged a dollar or two for making a visit and writing prescriptions, with most of the practice devoted to setting broken bones, removing appendices and tonsils, delivering babies, and combatting colds that had progressed to pneumonia. In the age before the miracle drug of penicillin (made available during the Second World War), the doctor had few options at his disposal for treating patients and alleviating pain, with only about eighty pharmaceuticals in circulation. Most often doctors prescribed tonics for indigestion and coughs; aspirin, arsenic, and alcohol for pain relief; and the more powerful chloroform, ether, and morphine before surgery.[7]

Though the late nineteenth century saw an awakening to the value of proper sanitation and hygiene in preventing disease, it was a time of very few medical breakthroughs in treating disease, save for the introduction in 1894 of the diphtheria anti-toxin and, in 1910, of salvarsan, an anti-syphilitic to combat the sexually transmitted disease. Diabetes was a great killer of Canadians and there was no cure. The most common approach to treating it was to starve patients, forcing them to waste away before they slipped into a coma as their sugar-laced blood eventually destroyed organs. The other great threat was tuberculosis. It was regularly treated by specialists in sanatoriums where patients with wealth were ordered to rest. Those from the working class were not so lucky. Unable to stop earning money for their families, they continued in their jobs until their crimson-flecked coughs attracted attention and they were banished from the workplace to be cared for, and to infect, their families. The White Plague spread in the fetid cities and slums, and only isolation could lower the threat of tuberculosis passing through overcrowded communities. The occasional severe public health crisis, like the 1885 smallpox epidemic in Montreal that killed several thousand and brought terror, stimulated new reforms. Water sources were inspected and proper hygiene enforced in schools to help combat diseases that claimed shocking numbers of people, including in Montreal and Toronto, where, at the turn of the century, about one in five babies died before reaching the age of two.[8]

Given that more than half of the country was considered rural in the 1911 census, doctors were important members of their farming communities, with patients coming from afar to see them, and some doctors going even farther to care for the immobile.[9] Most general practitioners did not perform surgical operations other than appendectomies or emergencies such as the occasional mangled limb from farming, industrial, and rail accidents. As one doctor wrote, "few dared to open the body cavities, whether chest or abdomen, and certainly not the head, except in cases of extreme urgency."[10]

In the cities, some of the specialists were employed or attached to hospitals, which afforded them a steady if modest salary. Doctors in both urban and rural areas almost always provided free care to those who could not afford the rate, or they accepted a system of barter. Guelph-born John McCrae, a veteran of the South African War, a poet, and a respected doctor in Montreal, lived within his means, drawing a salary from the hospital, McGill University, and his own practice, which allowed him to provide free medical treatment to the needy. A country doctor, Robert J. Manion, who would serve in the Great War like McCrae, and would later have a successful political career, wrote that he and others frequently provided free treatment to the poor but levied heavier "fees upon those who can pay."[11] Most doctors found that their profession was no path to riches, even though they were respected members of their communities.

———

As thousands of soldiers began to filter into the new military camp at Valcartier in late August, the medical officers from the CAMC and the newly arriving physicians in uniform were instructed to prevent the looming sanitation disaster. Armies had died in the past from a single case of typhoid taking hold, as it transmitted rapidly in the close quarters. The American Civil War of 1861 to 1865 had seen disease fell an extraordinarily high number of combatants, with twenty-four sick to every one wounded by conventional weapons.[12] In the last major British Empire conflict, the war in South Africa from 1899 to 1902, typhoid fever had put more than 8,000 Empire soldiers in graves. Losses on the veldt to disease comprised about two thirds of the total fatalities in comparison to one third from Boer bullets and shells.[13]

The Canadian medical services had studied the problem of disease since the South African War, and the destruction of human and animal waste became a priority in preventing sickness and disease.[14] The many latrines at Valcartier were monitored to ensure proper sanitation, with horse manure piled at a distance

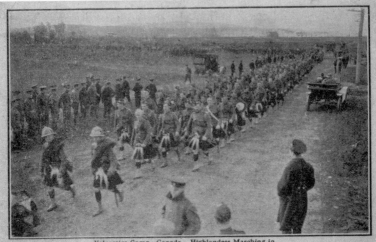

Valcartier Camp—Canada. Highlanders Marching in

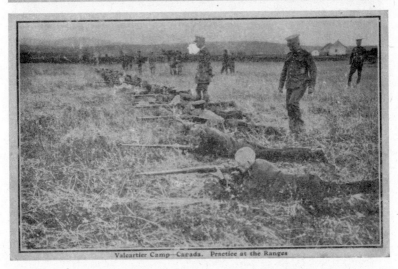

Valcartier Camp—Canada. Practice at the Ranges

Two 1914 postcards showing the Canadians
marching and shooting Ross rifles at Valcartier, Quebec.

from water sources and incinerated when possible. The water
pumped from the Saint-Charles River along new pipes was frequently tested for cleanliness and chlorinated.[15] If soldiering is
rarely glamorous—with drill, marching, and occasionally

shooting to enliven the drudgery—doctoring in such conditions was often equally mundane. The many foot blisters and weeping sores that were examined and treated sporadically broke the monotony, along with horse kicks and the occasional broken bone from some accident. A number of tubercular men were identified in the ranks and sent for hospital care in Quebec City, many of them in tears as they were denied going overseas. And while more than a few taunts were directed against the doctors, who were given nicknames like "Doc Feces" or "Lord of the Cough," the medical services' enforcement of public health regulations and isolation of sick men safeguarded against an epidemic spreading through the ranks. Such matters were not regularly top of mind for the harried senior officers, but an outbreak of cholera, typhus, or typhoid would have been devastating, and they listened to their medical officers.

With about 35,000 new soldiers converging on Valcartier, 10,000 beyond what the British had requested as part of the initial force, the medical officers there were instructed to begin a second round of health inspections in order to weed out the ill-suited and unfit, as well as those over forty-five or under nineteen. Thirty medical officers were assigned to the task, with long lines of soldiers snaking away from their examination tents. Like most men, Ernest Davis disliked the process, but although he described his discomfort at being poked and prodded "like so much meat," he was pleased to make it through.[16] Not all did, and men with flat feet or poor eyesight were often removed, as were those with more obvious ailments. Captain George Gibson wrote of encountering a man missing a hand who had spent days concealing his wrist in a pant pocket; another soldier, Andie Mack, had kept his wooden leg a secret until he was "told to take his trousers down."[17] Bad

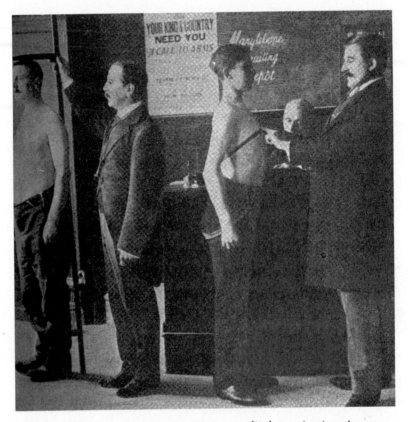

*Civilian doctors inspect new recruits in a medical examination. A young
man's chest is being measured while an older man's height is recorded.*

teeth led to some being sent home, even as gap-toothed men pro-
tested that they wanted to shoot the enemy, not bite him. Many of
the dentally challenged soldiers were accepted a year later when
standards were lowered and after military dentists were called in to
clear out the mess of broken and missing chompers in men's mouths.

Sunken chests and varicose veins in legs were surprisingly
common in many of the malformed recruits who were raised on
poor diets that included little dairy or vegetables and who had
endured extended bouts of malnourishment. In the first two years

of the war, non-white Canadians were usually denied service, as were Indigenous people, although records do not indicate that they were singled out in these examinations.[18] Throughout September, close to 5,000 soldiers were removed from the service, most for medical reasons, making them a part of the estimated 100,000 Canadian men who were rejected during the course of the war because they could not meet health requirements.[19] While this was not a fitness problem faced only by the Canadians, the shameful revelations of unhealthy men would be lamented by social reformers and then employed to launch a new crusade for reforms to aid the impoverished who had been too frail or sickly to serve their country as soldiers.

A few men were removed from service because of their refusal to accept inoculation against potential diseases. Fear of the needle, or what was in it, led to their dismissal. Fierce debates over vaccination had raged in Canada before the war, and opponents remained even after the 1885 smallpox outbreak in Montreal that killed thousands. Despite the horror of smallpox, one of the deadliest diseases in human history, those who railed against vaccination to prevent the contagious plague called it a hoax or a government conspiracy to poison children.[20] In this age of evolving medical advances, some Canadians had experienced severe anxiety about what was being injected into their bodies. But the deepening of state intervention through inoculation in the early twentieth century, especially in schools, saved lives, and an intense public health campaign was waged to spread positive information about the value of vaccination.

There had also been high-profile prewar discussions in Britain over whether to vaccinate soldiers in the British army against their will, which was reported in Canadian medical journals and

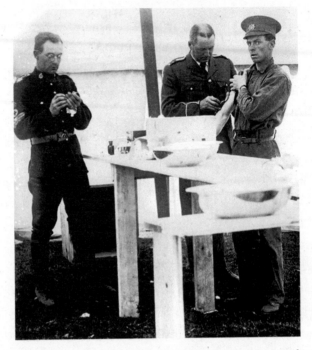

Rare photograph of a Canadian soldier being vaccinated.

newspapers. This opposition in Britain led the military authorities to make inoculation voluntary.[21] British soldiers who later campaigned in the Middle East and Gallipoli, with these regions' inhospitable environments, found clear-cut evidence for the value of vaccination in saving lives.[22] In Canada, Toronto doctor George Nasmith, who served on the Ontario Provincial Board of Health and was appointed as an officer of sanitation despite his diminutive size of four foot six, convinced Minister Hughes to accept the value of vaccination.[23] McGill University's Lieutenant-Colonel George Adami, one of the most respected doctors of his time, wrote that the soldier who declined the vaccination was to be removed from service: "He was not allowed to endanger the health of his comrades."[24]

Soldiers were eager to serve overseas, and so they took the prophylactic jab to protect against typhoid and smallpox. There was no shortage of written complaints by soldiers, especially regarding the not-so-gentle delivery mechanism of increasingly dull needles. Captain George Gibson, medical officer for the 7th Battalion, wrote about the "cold steel" shoved into arms (a reference to the soldiers' 17-inch steel bayonet) and how "it was remarkable to notice how nervous everyone was; men who afterwards faced every form of death from rifle bullet or shell quailed before this simple inoculation."[25] The vast majority of soldiers suffered no more than a sore arm, and their fears were alleviated by personal experience. The *Canadian Medical Association Journal*—the primary publication for the medical profession—took the opportunity to remind readers of the success of the mass vaccination at Valcartier, stating, "Never before has medical science been so well armed against the worst of our war pestilences."[26]

———

Colonel Guy Carleton Jones, the surgeon-general of the CAMC (its senior commanding officer), received his medical training at King's College in Britain, his military training at Aldershot, and his experience in battle during the South African War. While the Nova Scotian doctor was not well known to Canadians, those within the Permanent Force knew that he had a reputation of being a stickler for discipline, and he bore an unfortunate physical resemblance to Germany's Kaiser Wilhelm. He was, however, knowledgeable enough to turn to civilian practitioners to fill the ranks of the rapidly expanding CAMC.

The militia and civilian doctors arrived with their knowledge and understanding of medicine, but the small number of Permanent Force officers in the CAMC trained the new medical officers at Valcartier in the intricacies of military law, discipline, and their role of supporting a unit's morale through proper care of the soldiers' health.[27] Other medical men were attached directly to infantry, cavalry, or artillery units, and all were going through a transformation from civilian doctor to military officer. CAMC lieutenant-colonel John Taylor Fotheringham had described the challenge before the war, warning that "the duties of the Medical department of an Army must differ radically from those ordinarily associated in the public mind with the medical profession in civil life."[28] Instead of focusing solely on the patient, the military medical officer had also to ensure the needs of the army were met through the enforcing of discipline. The medical officer was part of the fighting machine as much as he was a physician to the sick or wounded.

Several militia field ambulances arrived at Valcartier from Montreal, Winnipeg, and Toronto, though they were without their full complement of officers and men. These field ambulances—mobile units meant to move with combat formations to care for the wounded and rapidly transport them to clearing stations and general hospitals further to the rear where they could be operated on in more antiseptic environments—consisted of motorized trucks, horse-drawn carriages, and medical equipment in large tents. Hastily assembled, the field ambulances were short of everything, and the recruits were, one doctor noted, "an un-military looking crowd."[29] Their officers set about grabbing the loose fish in the camp with any medical background, as well as many who had never been near a hospital. While doctors and nurses would form the core of medical units, privates more commonly carried out the more mundane tasks. It was not the doctors, for instance, who practised putting up the tents and setting up the medical equipment in faux training for the Western Front. Colonel Jones eventually sorted out the overseas medical force throughout August and September 1914, with the First Contingent having three field ambulances, a casualty clearing station, four hospitals, and a newly created sanitary section. When the Canadian Expeditionary Force went overseas in October 1914 with some 31,000 soldiers, the CAMC consisted of 63 medical officers and 951 other ranks.[30]

With the creation of hospitals came the need for nurses, and trained women stepped up immediately. Nurses had served in the North West campaign against Louis Riel and the Métis in 1885, and in the South African War, where twelve nurses had tried to save the Canadian and Imperial soldiers from the many diseases on the veldt. Now, at the start of the war, a new matron (commander of the service) was appointed, Major Margaret Macdonald. The Nova Scotian had prewar experience serving in British hospitals and had only two weeks to mobilize the nurses. Macdonald selected the 100 most eligible from over 1,000 applicants.[31] They were to be unmarried and experienced, and they wore the coveted blue uniforms with a white apron, CAMC buttons, and two stars on shoulder straps that earned them the affectionate nickname "Bluebirds." By war's end, 2,845 nurses would serve in the CEF, and almost all of them were professionally trained. Their average age at enlistment was 29.9, and they were significantly older than most soldiers, who were typically more than three years younger. They were also a very Canadian group, with 83 percent born in Canada, a far higher figure than in the rest of the CEF.[32] These Canadian nurses would carve out a key role for themselves within the medical system.

The doctors who enlisted faced a challenge with the hierarchy of rank, which did not easily map onto civilian expertise or medical hierarchy. Civilian doctors had their own standing based on positions in hospitals, universities, and high-profile practices. However, in the CAMC, the best doctors were not always the highest-ranking officers, with Permanent Force soldier-doctors often in command. It was odd to have world-class surgeons as captains along with newly minted doctors, and one solution was to allow universities to create their own hospital units. Within these newly formed hospitals that would follow after the First Contingent, the doctors self-policed their ranks, usually with the professors receiving a higher rank, although ultimately the medical officers tended to be captains, with a limited number of majors, a couple of lieutenant-colonels, and the commanding officer at the rank of colonel. Canada's nursing sisters were also commissioned as lieutenants—unlike in Britain, where they were not officers. As commissioned officers, the Canadian nurses could better carry out their duties within the military hierarchy, where influence was often linked to rank.

The universities saw most of the medical faculties enlist within the first two years of the war. McGill, Toronto, Laval, Queen's, Saskatchewan, Dalhousie, St. Francis Xavier, and Western all established overseas hospitals that were staffed largely by students and professors, with alumnae and local supporters raising large sums to provide medical supplies, X-ray machines, and even motorized ambulances.[33] For example, McGill's hospital drew from the university and the Montreal medical community, with all seventy-two nurses selected from the city's two primary hospitals, the Royal Victoria Hospital and Montreal General.[34] The Queen's University hospital in Kingston was formed in March 1915, with all officers being professors, eighty of the eighty-nine other ranks being students, and seven of them being doctors who were snuck in as privates.[35] And these were not small units. A single Canadian hospital, No. 10 Canadian Stationary from London, Ontario, packed over 90,000 individual items when it shipped across the Atlantic.[36] Furthermore, the hospitals all expanded during the war, with most having more than 1,000 beds and some double that number. As one doctor observed, "It is difficult for the civilian who has not been overseas to realize the size and extent of these base hospitals," with even the smallest one able to accommodate "more patients than any hospital in Canada."[37]

———

More than 31,000 Canadians sailed to England at the start of October 1914, on a tide of excitement as they were seen off by thousands of well-wishers and loved ones. "We were making history," wrote one Canadian medical officer. "The great epoch-making enterprise of our young country."[38] After a ten-day ocean crossing, the Canadians disembarked at Plymouth mid-month, met by celebrations, songs, and some curious gazes. The English came out to greet the supposed wild men of the Dominion; most were disappointed to find that the soldiers who had arrived from the northern land of ice did not consist entirely of Mounties and (in the language of the day) Indians. Mischievous soldiers played up their supposedly hard upbringing in igloos and snow drifts— reared with a rattle in one hand and a rifle in the other. In fact, about two thirds of the First Contingent was British-born, because many of them had military experience that was privileged by recruiting officers, although they were followed by increasingly more Canadian-born during the course of the war, until half of the Canadian Expeditionary Force was Dominion-born. Place of birth did not matter much, however, since most Anglo-Canadians were proud to be a part of the Empire. But a strand of Canadian identity was emerging, and what it meant to be Canadian was supercharged by the war effort as soldiers, politicians, and artists insisted on national recognition, as more Canadian units were formed and achieved victory on the battlefield, as Canadian officers took over senior commands, as Canadian symbols like the maple leaf and the beaver were worn on uniforms and became recognizable, and as Canadians demanded to be distinguished from other British and Dominion troops.[39]

Upon English soil, the Canadians moved by rail to the historic army training ground of Salisbury Plain, a desolate space 20 by 40 kilometres, located about 130 kilometres west of London. While ideal for manoeuvres of large groups of men, the thin soil was set atop a bedrock of chalk covered by clay, creating an impervious layer where water would collect. Over 1914–1915, the wettest winter in sixty years, the plain was reduced to a thick gruel of mud. The rain seemed to fall without pause, and it almost did—for 89 of the 124 days before the Canadians left for France in February 1915.[40] "It was the filthiest, dirtiest hole that men were ever expected to live in," remembered one Canadian. "Never take your clothes off, because it was much easier to get up in the morning damp wet than get up in the morning and try to put on cold damp clothes."[41] Bell tents that were not waterproof were pitched in the muck, and they initially had no wooden floor, forcing soldiers to lie directly on the ground save for what could be scrounged or stolen to create a makeshift tent floor. One Canuck riffed in poetry,

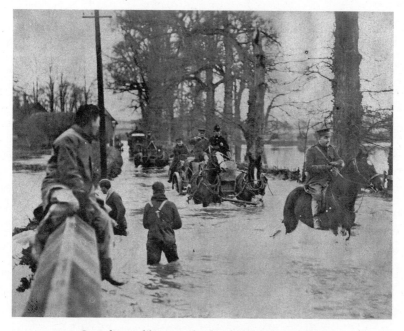

Canadian soldiers on the flooded Salisbury Plain.

"Mud, mud, damnable mud, / In mud we must wallow and mud we must swallow."[42] These conditions wore on morale and it was hard for officers and men to be motivated in the sludge that was, in places, knee deep.[43]

Private Peter A. Hughes of the 7th Battalion described the "veritable sea of mud" that contributed to a "great deal of sickness and a number of deaths."[44] From the early winter, the medical officers began to fight a new war against illness and disease. The tent living had been awful, and by November the Canadians began to erect little wooden huts, each with a small stove. As men huddled together to dry out, these sites became a breeding ground for illness. "A fearful lot of sickness here," wrote one Canadian diarist. "At night it sounds like hell with all those graveyard coughs."[45] Frederick Gault Finley of the CAMC, who enlisted as a medical officer at age fifty-two, was attached to No. 1 General Hospital, and rose to the rank of lieutenant-colonel, recounted how the influenza often progressed to bronchitis and then, in the unlucky ones, to broncho-pneumonia. These last cases were "of a severe and even fatal character. In a long hospital experience in Canada, I have not seen such virulent cases in young and robust adults."[46]

The medical war would be fought with skill, bravery, and no shortage of paper. Statistics were essential in this scientific battle, and from October 21, 1914 to February 12, 1915, the work at No. 1 General was tracked: doctors conducted 315 surgical operations, treated 1,132 soldiers for venereal disease, and carried out 1,196 dental operations.[47] At least sixty-three Canadians died on Salisbury Plain, but over 4,000 other soldiers who passed through the hospital were saved.[48] Those who succumbed to the virulent flu were often autopsied so that doctors had a better understanding of the war waged by bacteria, germs, and viruses. As one Canadian medical officer was later to write, "There was the long and endless offensive against dirt, which is the beginning of all that disease which ends in the destruction of armies."[49]

Most terrifyingly, the First Contingent also faced an outbreak of cerebro-spinal meningitis, an infection of the fluid and membranes around the brain and spinal cord. With victims suffering damage to the brain, the CAMC reacted rapidly by identifying carriers and isolating them in wards. Rumour spread of this terrible disease raging through the camp, and widespread distress erupted in the surrounding English villages. Recalling the outbreak, Arthur Hunt Chute, a lieutenant in the CAMC, felt "those were the saddest, bluest days that I experienced in my two and a half years of soldiering. Every day I could look out my tent into the melancholic blur of mist and rain and see the draped gun-carriage moving to the 'Dead March' from Saul, while one battalion or another slowly followed their comrade to the grave."[50] Soldiers felt that they were being picked off by an unseen enemy.

The Canadian medical officers and nurses received much praise when the contagious disease ran through the victims in isolation and burned itself out, although twenty-eight soldiers were eventually buried.[51] The outbreak of meningitis would have been far worse without the intervention of the medical services, and the epidemic was a harsh wake-up call, especially for officers who witnessed men dying in agony. The doctors had stopped the dreaded disease through observation, scientific medicine, and seclusion, but it was a lesson for the regimental officers and the Canadian high command on the impact of disease. "The epidemic," wrote CAMC sanitation officer George Nasmith, "proved to be a blessing in disguise, for it educated both combatant officers and men as to the necessity of observing certain simple precautions to prevent the spread of any contagious disease."[52]

While Salisbury was to have been a temporary billet, it was fast becoming permanent, with Christmas having come and gone and the soldiers grumbling about when they would get to the Western Front. After the last titanic battle of the British regular army around the Belgian city of Ypres—where, from October 19 to November 22, 1914, the rapid-firing Tommies defeated the mass of German forces in Belgium's Flanders region—the front had stalemated. With more than 54,000 British casualties and 80,000 Germans killed and wounded, the CAMC took note of the casualties along the Western Front—which would number over 1.5 million killed and wounded in the first four months of combat.[53] Canadian doctors also studied reports about the effects of typhus on French and German soldiers who were succumbing to disease in the late fall.[54] The French had done a poor job of inoculating their soldiers and they suffered 8,000 killed by disease in 1914.[55] It was nothing compared to the 200,000 Serbian civilians who died from typhus in the first six months of the war, but statistics like these gave Canadian medical officers a new understanding of the power of an uncontrolled disease like typhus to lay waste to armies and nations.[56]

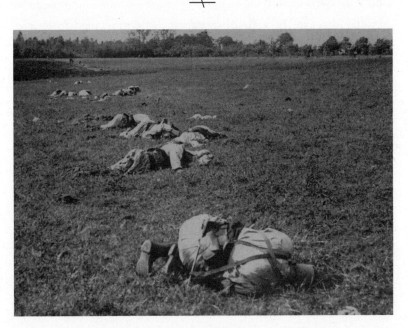

The lethality of the open battlefield is revealed through a row of dead soldiers cut down as they advanced.

The first Canadian formation sent to France was No. 2 Stationary Hospital, leaving on November 6, 1914, for Le Havre along the coast. The hospital's 320 beds opened to the rush of wounded from the Battle of First Ypres, making the staff—which included thirty-four nursing sisters—eligible for the coveted 1914 Star, a medal awarded to those who served in that first costly year of battle. The hospital was followed in early February 1915 by the Canadian Division of more than 18,000 soldiers, with the remaining men left behind as reinforcements. The hardening training process had helped to prepare the soldiers for trench warfare, as it did the medical services that were forced to confront how disease and illness could lay an army low. From the start of the war, doctors and nurses engaged in a force-protection role, studying bodies and selecting soldiers for service while enforcing vaccination to reduce disease. They also isolated the infected, applied scientific medical knowledge, cared for the accidentally injured, and above all conducted sanitation control and public health measures. Though these were often unglamorous roles, they were essential for the health and survival of an army of homeless soldiers living in cramped and closed quarters, and the Canadians' senior officers came to understand the value of the medical services in sustaining the combat power of the division.[57] "Lives lost in battle," wrote one doctor, "do not give an impression of useless sacrifice like those cut off by infectious disease."[58] Throughout the war the medical services would struggle against illness, sickness, and disease to ensure these enemies did not cut a swath through the Canadian forces. They were aided by the fighting officers, who had been frightened by the meningitis outbreak as well as impressed by the doctors' ability to overcome it. On the Western Front, the

CHAPTER 2

SHOT, SHELL, AND POISON GAS AT YPRES, 1915

In late February 1915 the Canadian Division of over 18,000 soldiers arrived on the Western Front, where the promise of open warfare had long been smashed by shellfire and snipers. Rapid-firing rifles and artillery, along with the machine guns that spewed hundreds of bullets a minute, had led to ghastly losses. To escape the scything firepower, soldiers dug holes in the ground. The holes became trenches, and eventually large underground cities emerged that ran through countries, extending 700 kilometres from Switzerland to the North Sea. The Germans and the Allied forces faced off against each other, and the only way to attack was in frontal assaults. In such conditions, the shovel was used every day, the rifle almost never, for the soldiers had nothing to shoot at as they burrowed deep. The back-breaking labour seemed a far cry from soldiering, and more than a few infantrymen scoffed that they seemed to be digging their own graves over and over again.

The trenches were usually four to six feet deep and built up several more feet with sandbags stuffed with soil, although in early

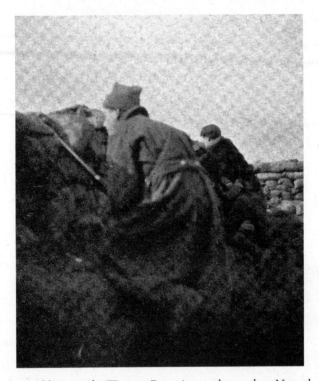

Canadian soldiers on the Western Front in rough trenches. Note the lack of a steel helmet, with the "tin hat" not introduced until early 1916.

1915 the trench system remained more shallow along parts of the front. Trailing back from the firing line that faced the enemy were communication trenches, narrow passageways with twists and turns that led to the rear and away from danger. Slippery wooden slats and boards were laid over the mud underfoot that occasionally oozed up, and in the winter months everyone felt the cold through their hobnailed boots. Lance-Corporal Edward Mockler of the 1st Battalion wrote jokingly in March 1915 that after a tour at the front he was "enclosed in a practically bullet-proof case of mud."[1] He would be killed two months later at age twenty-two by a bullet to the abdomen.

The Canadians took over the line from French soldiers in March 1915. It was a revolting mess. Every trench corner was filled with mounds of feces. Fighting to liberate their country, Gallic officers shrugged as the Canadians pointed out the mess and the likelihood of disease spreading from it. They dismissed the worries, saying that they did not expect to be in these trenches long, and that anything that suggested otherwise fostered a passive spirit.[2] But standing ankle deep in urine and feces and the occasional rotten German corpse was not good for the Canadian soldiers' morale. The officers set the men to shovel away the offending mounds, to dig proper latrines, and to douse the area with chloride of lime. To lose the sanitation war could have devastating effects, and word was spreading of Belgian soldiers—who, like the French, had poor hygiene discipline—dying of preventable illnesses in large numbers, with records later revealing that a third of the country's total 40,000 dead soldiers had succumbed to disease.[3]

Beyond the trenches lay the ground known ominously as No Man's Land, which typically ranged 200 to 300 metres across as it separated the two opposing trenches. Soldiers were warned not to sneak a peek, but many did, drawn by the zone's strange emptiness and by the hope of glimpsing the enemy. The vast sea of barbed wire that would characterize the battlefield in 1916 was not yet in place, although it was starting to emerge on the former farmers' fields as a strange iron harvest, meant to funnel potential attackers into kill grounds where enemy riflemen and machine-gunners waited. Any soldier who surveyed No Man's Land noticed a surprising amount of garbage—especially rusting tin cans that soldiers threw over their trench parapets—and many corpses lying half-submerged in water-filled craters. To look for too long, however, would be to invite a skull-smashing sniper's bullet. "Most of the trench injuries are of the head, and therefore there is a high proportion of killed in the daily warfare as opposed to an attack," wrote medical officer John McCrae to his mother.[4] As the Canadians were cycled into the trenches on four- to six-day tours, they steadily lost soldiers. From late February and March, 278 Canadians were killed and wounded, even though not a single attack was launched against the enemy.[5]

The CAMC's No. 1 Casualty Clearing Station was established behind the lines, staffed by surgeons, doctors, nurses, and orderlies to deal with the wreckage of the war. It was fed by the division's field ambulances—three mobile hospitals of around 190 doctors and privates, one for each of the infantry brigades of 4,000 soldiers. From the clearing station, the survivors were moved further to the rear when they could stand the strain of being transported in ambulances along rough roads, and Canada's No. 1 Stationary Hospital operated a 300-bed tent hospital at Wimereux along the coast, where it took in Canadian and other British Empire soldiers. The unit received its first patients on April 3, but along with several other Canadian hospitals, it would soon be confronted by an avalanche of wounded and dying men.

———

In April, the Canadians moved to the Ypres salient, which already had a reputation as one of the most dangerous spots on the Western Front. A semi-circle of trenches some 27 kilometres long and about 8 kilometres northwest from the Yser Canal protected the major road network leading into and out of the Belgian city of Ypres. The Battle of First Ypres saw the British and Belgians block a major German thrust to capture the city at a savage cost to all forces involved. The medical officer for the 5th Battalion, Captain William Malloch Hart, a thirty-three-year-old widower who was formerly head of the Saskatchewan Sanitorium for Consumptives, wrote in his diary about the terrible sights of the old battlefield. "The ground seemed so thickly sown with bodies which were barely below the surface that they were constantly cropping out when the surface soil was washed away by rain, and every attempt to enlarge a dug-out or dig a communication trench turned up a dead German. Unburied bodies lay in front of our trenches, while a listening post sent out at night reported some 200 German dead laying in a group of trees."[6] Hart was a specialist in tuberculosis, but he would be exposed to many other wounds, illnesses, and diseases on the Western Front.

With its once magnificent Gothic Cloth Hall now in ruins, Ypres symbolized the ravages of war and Belgium's plucky defence. To the east lay the battlefield where the Canadian units marched on April 14, taking over part of the trenches where they were flanked on the left by the French 45th Algerian Division and on the right by the 28th British Division. Elements of six Allied divisions were in the front lines of the salient that extended in a deep curve. The whole area was surrounded by the Germans, who had an advantage of five to one in the number of artillery pieces, along with superior observation points on Passchendaele Ridge, 2 kilometres to the east.[7] The Allies were shelled mercilessly.

The Germans had attacked in both the east and west in August 1914, hoping to defeat the French and Belgians before turning fully to the Russians. They had almost succeeded, and their great battles on the Eastern Front, especially at Tannenberg in late August 1914, had inflicted heavy losses on the lumbering Russian bear. While the Kaiser's senior generals hoped to finish off the

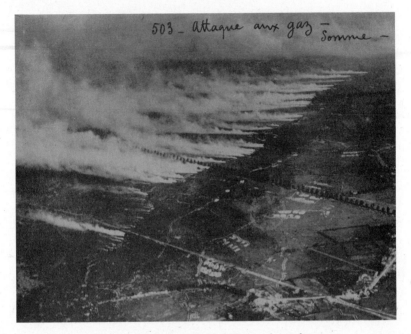

Chlorine gas being released along a large front.

Russians in 1915, they planned for a limited offensive in the west as a strategic diversion. On the Ypres front, the Germans had concentrated a strike force, although they also added a secret weapon to their arsenal. Scientists had weaponized lung-searing chlorine gas, and it was unleashed to start the Battle of Second Ypres on April 22.

The Canadians had four battalions in the forward trenches, with several additional infantry and artillery units behind them. At around 5 P.M., the soldiers of the 13th Canadian Infantry Battalion on the far left watched with concern as a 5-kilometre-long greenish-yellow cloud, some 30 metres high, rolled forward menacingly toward the Allied lines, passing through two divisions— the 45th Algerian and the 87th French Territorial. The Canadians could hear the muffled screams of the French troops as the tendrils of gas passed over them, eventually obscuring the trenches. In the face of this terror, many of the French soldiers threw away their rifles and fled in disorder. They did not get far as the death cloud caught them, leaving them choking and gasping and sinking to their knees before writhing on the ground. Major Andrew McNaughton, a Montreal engineer who emerged as one of Canada's most effective wartime gunners, described the sight of the Algerians, "their eyeballs showing white, and coughing their lungs out—they literally were coughing their lungs out."[8]

The German infantry advanced tentatively behind this lethal cloud, stepping through dead grass and over the corpses of small animals, hacking as they too breathed in the diluted vapours that still burned the throat. They encountered French soldiers, gasping through ruined lungs, while others lay still, eyes bulging, uniforms

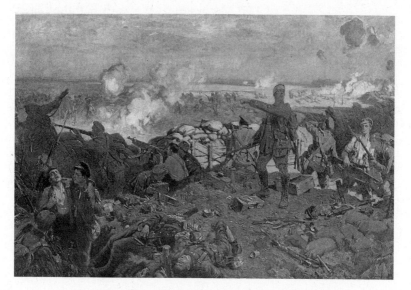

Artist Richard Jack depicted the Canadian stand at Ypres.
In this much-produced print, the Canadians withstand the
German assault but pay a high price.

covered in vomit. "The dead all lie on their backs with their fists clenched," wrote one German infantryman.[9] On the periphery of the cloud, the Canadians, straining through weeping eyes that felt like they had been rubbed raw with sandpaper, were lucky to miss the most toxic effects of the cloud, and they fired into the massed ranks of the Germans. The enemy went to ground but turned to face the Canadians. A firefight raged on all day.

The Canadians shifted to cover the gap in the French trenches and also gathered together a force—the 10th and 16th Battalions— to counterattack at midnight on the 22nd. It was an audacious operation and the first Canadian offensive action of the war.[10] The target was the German-held Kitcheners Wood, which they cleared in a 1,600-strong bayonet charge. The Canadians suffered heavy losses—of over two thirds of their force—although they drove the enemy back. Sergeant J.C. Matheson of the 10th Battalion later described holding the small copse of trees on April 23 in an exposed position: "All day long we had to stick to our posts in case of a counter attack, and believe me it was more nerve-racking than the bayonet charge itself, as all around us were the dead and wounded. . . . How I ever came through is a mystery to me."[11] Another Canadian, Captain H.A. Duncan of the 16th Battalion, remembered shooting and stabbing his way through the enemy. "Men blown out of a trench was a common occurrence, leaving nothing but possibly a boot." A single shell wounded three of his men. "One crawled out to the tall grass in the rear and made his way to the dressing station. Another who received eight wounds in one leg hopped across the open." The third, terribly injured, could only be carried, with a friend and his brother volunteering. With no stretcher, they dragged the bleeding man through tall grass, even as enemy riflemen fired without mercy. "A sniper got him," Duncan wrote.[12] Luckily his brother and mate survived. Duncan did too, although his luck ran out a year and a half later on the Somme, when he was killed in October 1916.

A second major Canadian attack on the 23rd against the enemy dug in on Mauser Ridge left dead and dying Canadians across the battlefield. Bloodied clumps of khaki-clad men lay unmoving, while the wounded hobbled or dragged themselves to the rear. "The machine gun fire was hellish," recounted Private Harold Peat of the 3rd Battalion. "A bullet would flash through the sleeve of a tunic, rip off the brim of a cap, bang against a water-bottle, bury itself in the mass of a knapsack. It seemed as though no one could live in such a hail of lead."[13] Many did not, and although Peat took a bullet through the chest and back, he survived the wounds. The remaining soldiers fought onward, the lingering effects of the gas revealed in their inflamed eyes and deep coughs. But still they backstopped the front, which appeared like it might collapse in the face of the overwhelming German forces and lethal gas.

———

Each infantry battalion of 1,000 men had its own regimental medical officer who travelled with the unit. When battalions were in the front lines or in immediate reserve, these men of medicine set up aid posts in key areas before the battle, usually in abandoned Belgian farms. As sites of care drew the walking wounded and those carried in by mates. Captain George Gibson, the medical officer of the 7th Battalion, wrote that the area in a farm where he cared for the injured "was filled with dying and badly wounded men; trampled straw and dirty dressings lay about in pools of blood."[14] Each of the medical officers also had sixteen stretcher-bearers under his command, although these bearers with the rank of private were utterly overwhelmed by the hundreds— and then thousands—of injured soldiers who were left bleeding on the battlefield. These were bewildering and traumatizing days, with almost all of the medical officers working continuously to deal with the rush of the broken and battered men.

Medical stations were also situated behind the Yser Canal, about 8 kilometres from the front lines. That was where Lieutenant-Colonel John McCrae had established a surgical station in a protected dugout. He was the medical officer for the 1st Artillery Brigade, Canadian Field Artillery, and the dugout was located in the reverse slope of an embankment to protect against shells. A professor of medicine at McGill and an artillery veteran of the South African War, McCrae wrote in his diary, which was penned in the form of a letter to his mother, "Of one's feelings all this night—of the asphyxiated French soldiers . . . I could write, but you can imagine."[15] Wounded men came in to the aid stations reeking of blood, chlorine gas, and feces, as many had defecated in their pants from the initial shock or as they lay unconscious. The chlorine impregnated the uniforms, and McCrae and other doctors found their eyes weeping from the strong fumes. "Gunfire and rifle fire never ceased 60 seconds," wrote McCrae, "and behind it all was the constant sights of the dead and wounded, the maimed and the terrible anxiety lest the line should give way."[16]

———

The Canadian medical services were spread across the front and echeloned to the rear. The assistant deputy medical services, Lieutenant-Colonel Gilbert Foster, the highest-ranking CAMC officer in Europe, had established his headquarters near that of the divisional commander, Lieutenant-General E.A.H. Alderson. It was some 3.5 kilometres northwest of Ypres at Brielen, and with telephone wires cut by enemy shelling, they were too far from the front to react to the dramatically fast-moving battle. Closer to the combat, No. 2 Canadian Field Ambulance was in the village of Wieltje, although it was almost 5 kilometres behind the front lines. With the 1st Canadian Infantry Brigade in reserve, its ambulance unit was there too, and so the epicentre of care was the advanced dressing station of No. 3 Canadian Field Ambulance, the primary medical formation for treating the wounded who washed in on a red tide. It had established a main dressing station at a girls'

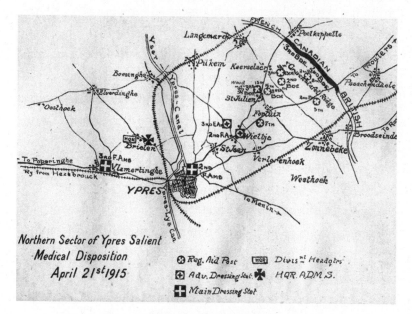

A map depicting the Canadian medical units during the Battle of Second Ypres. The 3rd and 2nd Canadian Infantry Brigades hold the front lines. Canadian medical units and regimental aid posts were spread over the battlefield.

school at Vlamertinghe, along the main Ypres–Poperinghe road, for easier evacuation, but its forward dressing station, at a farm that went by the name of Mouse Trap, was where most of the medical officers were stationed.[17]

"Some awful wounds were attended to, gashes large enough to put your fist in, many came with bullet wounds, many poor boys will have to have their arms or legs taken off," wrote Private Bert Goose of No. 3 Canadian Field Ambulance in his diary. "Other poor fellows will never live to tell the tale."[18] A doctor in the same unit, Captain P.G. Bell, took a few minutes on the third day of battle to jot into his personal diary, "'We have had all varieties of wounds—some bad fractures, etc. with shrapnel—relatively few heads, chests or abdomens—I suppose they haven't survived—most wounds in the limbs."[19] Indeed, the head and torso wounds were frequently fatal in these battlefield conditions, in part because of the trauma to the body, but also because, with so many casualties over such a short period, the medical officers were unable to devote significant attention to each patient. During a quiet time in the line, resulting in perhaps only one or two injured men, doctors were more able to spend the many hours necessary to try to save a soldier with a brain or gut wound. However, in this battle, with hundreds of wounded arriving each hour, these doomed men were studied and usually made comfortable with morphine until they succumbed to their injuries so that others could be saved.

It was a scene of bedlam at the dressing stations and field ambulances, and No. 3 Canadian Field Ambulance processed a staggering 5,200 patients throughout the week of battle.[20] Wounded soldiers arrived with bodies opened red and raw. "The number of wounded pouring in is frightful," wrote CAMC surgeon William

Boyd in his diary. "All the talk about the glory and glamour of war is rather apt to stick in one's throat." Boyd believed that the generals and politicians who started the war "ought to be made to spend a few hours in a dressing station."[21] The horror there would be enough for any sane person to demand peace.

Further behind the lines, No. 1 Casualty Clearing Station took hundreds of these stretcher cases who began to arrive on the night of the 22nd, and this became the site where surgery was most often performed, with only the most desperate cases treated at the field ambulances and by the regimental medical officers nearest the front lines. Canon Frederick Scott, a much-respected poet and man of faith, sought to offer comfort and last rites to many who were close to death. "Ghastly sights were disclosed when the stretcher bearers ripped off the blood-stained clothes and laid bare the hideous wounds." Those who had a fighting chance were rushed into the operating rooms. Canon Scott looked in on one, wondering if he might help, but saw it was a "veritable shambles," with soiled bandages lying in heaps around the table. "The doctor had his shirt sleeves rolled up and his hands and arms were covered with blood."[22]

———

The Canadians had been pushed back slightly on the 22nd and 23rd, even as they had fought resolutely and bought time for the British to rush forward reinforcements. Before dawn on the 24th, the Germans tried to break the Canadian lines again, unleashing a second, smaller but denser chlorine cloud, directed to pass through the 8th and 15th Battalions in the front lines. The Canadians were still without proper respirators, although officers and men in the ranks with an education in chemistry had seen their brass buttons tarnished green two days earlier and warned their comrades that the discolouration was likely caused by chlorine. Wetted rags with water or urine offered some protection. As infantryman George Bell recounted, "'Piss on your handkerchiefs and tie them over you faces,' yells our lieutenant. There are some who do not make this precaution. They roll about gasping for breath."[23]

Heavier than air, the chlorine gas pooled in the low depressions of the ground. Most of the infantrymen climbed out of the trenches—although this made them more vulnerable to shot and shell; however, those who sheltered deeper in the ground were often killed by the dense gas. Among the most vulnerable were the many wounded men who had taken refuge in shell craters and trenches, especially those who were unconscious or unable to rise above the vapours due to their blood loss and pain.

Through hacking lungs, the Canadians held off the Germans, but the second gas attack drove back the two forward battalions, who were trapped in the swirling cloud. Hundreds of infantrymen fought on despite damaged lungs and debilitating coughs, some to the last bullet, before being killed or captured, especially since the Canadian-made Ross rifle jammed repeatedly during rapid fire. While the mass-produced British ammunition was often the culprit for the jams, it happened too frequently to blame it only on ammunition. Frustrated and furious Canadians used boots, bleeding hands, and even shovels to pry open the Ross rifle's breech, often to no avail as they were killed or captured by the Germans advancing on helpless soldiers whose rifles did not fire.[24]

———

Slight, unassuming, and bespectacled, Francis Scrimger seemed an unlikely hero. Born in Montreal on February 7, 1880, he grew up there, attending McGill University, where he studied under John McCrae. Scrim, as his friends called him, went overseas with the First Contingent as a regimental medical officer to the 14th Battalion, which was composed of men primarily drawn from Montreal. Throughout the battle at Ypres, Scrimger was near the front lines, caring for gunshot and shrapnel-peppered soldiers. "There were some bad wounds—legs and arms crushed and heads torn open," Scrimger penned in his diary during a brief interlude.[25] On April 24, his third continuous day with no sleep, he learned that the limited number of stretcher-bearers had been overwhelmed by the hundreds of wounded men, who now lay bleeding and unattended in forward positions. They could not be moved and so Scrimger ran towards them—and into the fierce fighting.

Even as the Canadians were being driven back on the 24th by the second gas attack, Scrimger set up a dressing station at a farm near the front, which was surrounded by a small moat. On the morning of the 25th, he had over thirty patients under his care. Many of his brave "body snatchers," as the stretcher-bearers were sometimes called, had already been hit by bullets or shrapnel while carrying the wounded over the open ground, and the situation grew steadily worse as German shells detonated near the farm. Most of the Canadian infantry were now behind the aid post, and with enemy shells ranging closer in the late afternoon on the 25th, Scrimger organized the evacuation of the wounded. The injured helped each other, gritting their teeth through the pain, realizing that they had to move or be captured. Only a single Canadian soldier, Captain H.F. McDonald, who had a terrible gash to his head and an eye ripped out, could not be transported. Scrimger continued to work on McDonald until early evening, when shells began to rain down on the farm, igniting stored ammunition that started to cook off in all directions when the building was set ablaze. The slight five-foot-seven doctor, who weighed only 148 pounds, carried McDonald out of the death trap and, after evading German patrols, brought his patient back to a dressing station at Wieltje. McDonald survived and later testified that each time the shells exploded around them, "Captain Scrimger curled himself round my wounded head and shoulder to protect me from the heavy shell fire, at obvious peril to his life."[26] The thirty-four-year-old Scrimger became one of four Canadians during the battle to receive the Victoria Cross, the Empire's highest award for bravery, the first for the CAMC.[27] Scrim served throughout the war in a number of medical capacities, both near the front lines and in rear hospitals, eventually rising to become chief surgeon at No. 3 Canadian General Hospital.

Many of the medical officers were no less brave than Scrimger in the face of enemy fire. On the 25th, as the lines collapsed, Captain William Hart ordered stretcher-bearers to carry out those who could not walk from his aid post, but he stayed behind with some of the wounded who could not be moved. Within the apocalyptic landscape of eviscerated horses and dead men, Hart was eventually captured. The medical officer of the 3rd Battalion, Captain A.K. Haywood, was in a similar situation, treating the soldiers in his care when a bombardment of shells crashed down. One of his patients broke under the strain, tearing off his clothes and running towards the German lines. Haywood raced after him, tackling the soldier amid sweeping bullet fire and bringing him back to his dugout before starting surgery anew. He only stopped when a shell smashed his aid post, burning it to the ground.[28] Haywood received the Military Cross for his gallant work, and Hart should have as well, although he did not have to spend the war in a prison camp since, through an exchange program in June of 1915, he was returned to England, where he cared for Canadian tubercular soldiers. The soldiers' and doctors' mettle had been tested and they had not been found wanting.

———

Canadian engineer William Johnson survived the battle, writing to his wife, "I have had an awful time this last ten days. . . . I got . . . about six hours sleep in a week. I was in the hottest part of it . . . and never expected to get out alive. I've missed death by inches."[29] By the end of the 25th, most of the surviving Canadian infantrymen limped off the battlefield, uniforms stiff with sweat and sometimes fouled with blood. They did not know the full cost of their gallant stand, although it was clear to all that a heavy price had been paid. For John Armstrong of the 3rd Canadian Field Artillery, the horror was brought home by a lone horse that limped over the battlefield "with just the lower part of a man's body in the saddle. From the waist up there was nothing."[30] Dead and dying soldiers lay across the pitted farmers' fields, and it was later determined that 6,036 Canadians had been killed, wounded, and taken prisoner.[31] The figures for casualties included those wounded and rendered sick, as well as other forms of losses, and generally the military tried to distinguish the dead, the wounded, the ill, the missing (presumed killed with no known grave), and the prisoners of war. Due to the chaos at Ypres, the separation of the types of losses was not possible, but over the course of the war, British medical statistics revealed that one in four battle casualties in France and Flanders resulted in death.[32]

Most Canadians were killed or wounded by bullet or shell. The poison gas nonetheless made a deep impression on all who witnessed the poisoned victims who writhed in pain as they slowly suffocated through corrupted lungs. "I was seized with a spasm of coughing," recounted one gassed Canadian who was destined to survive, "as my lungs suddenly seemed filled with red-hot needles."[33] While the conventional wounds were equally distressing, Captain James Stewart Walker of the CAMC was drawn to observe the gassed patients with their unnaturally coloured skin the shade of sickly avocado. Many of the patients seemed beyond care, he said, as they underwent the "slow process of drowning."[34] It was an ugly death as the chlorine destroyed the lung's alveoli and led to the impairment of oxygen exchange. Fluid in the lungs was vomited up repeatedly in between rasping coughs, and, according to one doctor, the sputum looked like "greenish slime."[35] As breath rattled in despoiled lungs, men whispered for mercy. Morphine was administered for the pain, but the stocks ran out rapidly. Some died over several agonizing hours, conscious almost to the end.

Despite many being taken by this horrible death, most of the gassed men survived, although few returned to the front, suffering from burnt-out lungs for the rest of their shortened lives. The total figure of gassed soldiers was impossible to count and almost everyone at the front breathed a dose of chlorine. The official figures ranged anywhere from 122 admitted to hospital for gas treatment to 1,556 men evacuated for sickness, of which a very high proportion were gassed.[36] Many of the dead had also been gassed while they lived, although they were uncounted as gas victims because they succumbed to their wounds in No Man's Land or were buried by the Germans who had pushed back the Allied lines.

Ypres was the Canadians' trial-by-fire battle. The Canucks had stood against crushing German forces, artillery, and the first massed use of chemical agents. The Dominion soldiers' defence at Ypres was lauded throughout the British Empire and the Canadians' stand forged their reputation as dependable, tough soldiers, which would only be furthered in future battles at Vimy, Hill 70, Passchendaele, and during the final series of battles in late 1918 known as the Hundred Days campaign.

———

Lieutenant-Colonel John McCrae of Montreal spent almost two weeks operating on the wounded from his makeshift dugout on the opposite side of the Yser canal, long after the Canadian infantry were cycled into reserve. It had been a ghastly period as men arrived ripped open by shell and bullet, with the doctor performing emergency surgery in his dark, narrow dugout. Hands soaked in blood, McCrae worked himself into near delirium. During the occasional breaks, he left the abattoir, with its stench of body fluid and burned flesh, and went outside to watch the shelling and a steadily expanding nearby cemetery of simple white crosses. Above this violent battlefield, he could occasionally hear the larks singing as they soared through the air. Returning to his terrible task of cutting, suturing, and bandaging, he composed poetry in his head to take his thoughts away from the bodies on his operating table. The death

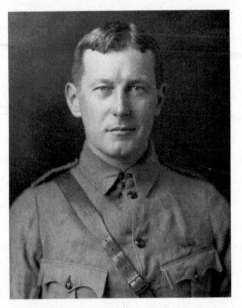

Medical officer and poet John McCrae.

of so many of his comrades and countrymen haunted him, and he felt that "the general impression in my mind is of a nightmare."[37]

On May 2, spent and exhausted, McCrae heard about the death of a friend, Alexis Helmer, who had been hit by a high explosive shell and blown apart. McCrae insisted on officiating over a short funeral, where parts of the dismembered body were buried. The next day, deep in grief and expecting his own death, he wrote a draft of his poem "In Flanders Fields." The fifteen-line poem struck a chord with a few friends who read it, and they encouraged him to submit it for publication and not to throw it away as he was inclined to do. It was rejected by the English magazine *The Spectator*, but the poet-gunner-surgeon resubmitted it to *Punch*, a widely read satirical magazine. It was published there on December 8, 1915, and "In Flanders Fields" rapidly became the most famous English-language poem of the war.

In Flanders fields the poppies blow
Between the crosses, row on row,
That mark our place; and in the sky
The larks, still bravely singing, fly
Scarce heard amid the guns below.

We are the Dead. Short days ago
We lived, felt dawn, saw sunset glow,
Loved and were loved, and now we lie
In Flanders fields.

Take up our quarrel with the foe:
To you from failing hands we throw
The torch; be yours to hold it high.
If ye break faith with us who die
We shall not sleep, though poppies grow
In Flanders fields.

His words were a plea from the fallen soldiers—McCrae's comrades who died in the gas attack, succumbed to the hail of bullets, or were shredded by the blast of shells. They called on the living to keep up the fight against the enemy. The poem was used in recruiting drives, in appeals to civilians to purchase Victory Bonds, and in election campaigns.[38] While the verse's popularity grew, McCrae, who survived the battle but suffered from mental trauma, found little solace in his poem, taking comfort instead from the medical expertise that he applied over the next three years to save soldiers' lives in bleak hospital wards where the desperate battle for survival played out day after day.

CHAPTER 3

PREVENTATIVE CARE AND THE HUNT FOR MALINGERERS

Half a dozen wretchedly ill soldiers could typically be found lined up outside the regimental medical officer's dugout in the front lines every day. They were sniffling and coughing, leaning heavily against the trench walls, or even collapsed and curled up in the fetal position. This "sick parade" was a trying part of the day for most medical officers, for they were charged with determining who was legitimately unwell and who was faking it to get out of the line. The inspection encapsulated the struggle for medical officers: the desire to follow the Hippocratic oath of doing no harm to patients and the challenge of squaring that with the officers' oath to the army that they would do their duty, which often included keeping sick soldiers in the line to continue to serve against the enemy.

The medical officer had a critical role in taking care of the 1,000 or so soldiers in the infantry regiment. They were, in effect, like a general practitioner in civilian life, with a wide knowledge of ailments rather than a specialization. The ratio of the single medical officer to soldiers was much more favourable than that of doctors to civilians at home, although the murder rate at the front was of course much higher. Each of the twelve infantry battalions had a doctor, with another five assigned to other combat units or roving from group to group. Ten more medical officers served in each of the three field ambulances, along with a few others temporarily posted to the unit, to form about fifty in total for each 20,000-strong infantry division (as these formations would expand to by 1916). Further Canadian Army Medical Corps officers were stationed to the rear, at the various medical formations, including the field ambulance, casualty clearing station, and hospitals in France and England.

Preventative medicine was a primary duty of the regimental medical officer. In all armies, health care was intimately tied to sustaining morale and bolstering fighting efficiency. Though these doctors were tasked with ensuring the men in their battalion did not waste away from the many diseases at the front, they were also charged with assisting in the enforcement of discipline. Few of the physicians drawn from civilian practice seemed to like this aspect of soldiering, as they were instructed to be harsh in carrying out the army's rules that no physically fit man be allowed to leave the unit through the funnel of the medical system. But given the hostile conditions at the front, with death and brutality at every turn, not to mention the dirt, rats, lice, and sleep deprivation, all of the fighting men were susceptible to breaking down. One of the medical officers remarked that he was often expected, in the name of "King and country," to "convince a sick man that he is not sick."[1]

———

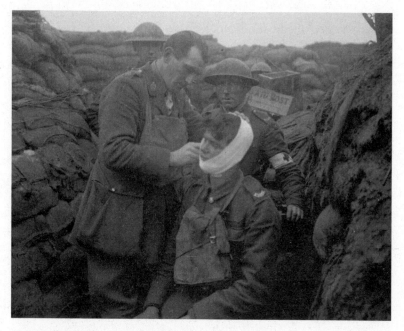

A medical officer at an aid post cares for a soldier with a head wound.

The Canadians licked their wounds after Second Ypres, having shown tremendous courage and resilience, but also having lost a third of the division. New recruits arrived from England and were acclimatized to the infantry battalions that had taken the heaviest losses. Another forlorn battle took place in May at Festubert, a blind battering of the enemy trenches with insufficient artillery support, inaccurate maps, and much callous slaughter of the infantry, which suffered 2,605 casualties.[2] However, after those terrible losses, the summer of 1915 was relatively quiet, although shells and snipers took their toll on the soldiers who lived in the underground cities of the Western Front.

"If I am to be engaged in war work at all," wrote CAMC Captain Harold McGill, "I want to be at least near enough the fighting line to hear a gun now and then."[3] Indeed, not only did the regimental medical officers hear the guns, they worked under artillery fire. They moved in and out of the line with their unit, and medical officers like Captain McGill set up an aid post close to the front, usually in the second line of defences of a trench system. With the firing line the most dangerous place and subject to enemy raids or even large-scale attacks, it made sense to have the doctor a few hundred metres to the rear.

The hard life of the medical officer at the front demanded that they be young and fit. These generalists remained as part of the CAMC, although they were often attached to a battalion or artillery brigade for many months—and some for years—before cycling back to a field ambulance. While some of the medical officers could not find their footing within the battalion's closed society, most did, becoming good and learned comrades to the officers, even as they remained men of medicine in a band of warriors. They also had to interact with the privates who formed the vast majority of a battalion. "In time he became the friend of every man," observed a medical officer about the position of doctor in the unit. He "knew their names and faces, and the ultimate history of their lives. He knew the hardy soldier who suffered in silence as well as the man who made the most of his ailment."[4] As Lieutenant-Colonel A. Mackenzie Forbes, commander of No. 1 Canadian General Hospital, enthused about the medical officer in the front lines, "to them is deservedly given the greatest credit of all, because from them is expected the greatest self-sacrifice. They must be characterized by strength, both physical and moral, courage, resource and faith in their high ideal of service."[5]

When in the front lines, the medical officer made his office in the regimental aid post, which was usually a well-protected dugout of good size to accommodate an operating room, a station for

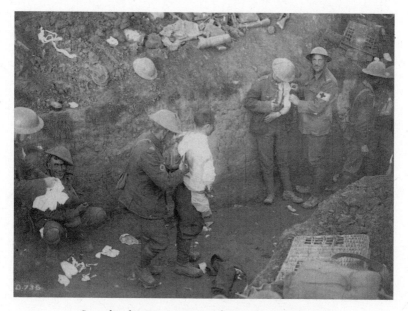

Stretcher-bearers engage in forward medical care.
Note the bloodied bandages littering the trench floor.

examination and bandaging, medical supplies, and space for several stretchers near a stove. As battalions cycled through the front lines, the medical supplies were tracked and left for the next doctor, much like other provisions in the trenches—be it shovels or barbed wire or wood. Doctors had their own personal medical items—surgical tools like scalpels, saws, and needles usually stored in a roll-up sleeve—often carried in leather medical bags like in civilian life. The nearest field ambulance supported the medical officer with supplies and extra stretcher-bearers before battle.

This was forward care that could hardly be more "forward," as the regimental medical officer was in range of shot and shell. Every tour of the front lines, usually lasting from four to six days, would result in a number of wounded soldiers. When a shell exploded, or shrapnel rained down in a deadly hail of steel, or a sniper's bullet found its mark, a call for aid went up. "The grind, grind, grind" of trench work was hard on all men, wrote Private Ralph Watson, a Canadian stretcher-bearer who was a veteran of the South African War, "and always the casualties—always them."[6] When the shout for assistance rang out, the medical officer might go racing down the maze of sunken alleyways to offer immediate care for an injured soldier, but most experienced doctors knew that it was better to wait for the patient to be carried to the aid post, which had proper lighting, a supply of medicine, and a more antiseptic environment.

The wounds were of every size and nature. Some bullets passed straight through the body, leaving minor entry and exit wounds, while others struck and shattered bone, leaving the body in a burst of gore and creating a wound the size of a small dinner plate. More irregularly shaped shell splinters from high explosive shells tumbled through the body, ripping internal organs and breaking bone. Flesh was lacerated and contused, body parts were torn away and crushed, and bits of dirty uniform were dragged into the wound, leading to festering infections. With these traumatic injuries, the medical officer might be called upon to perform emergency surgery, but more often, in the words of one medical officer, "Very little is attempted in dressing wounds where the missile has penetrated."[7] The conditions in the regimental aid post, while better than a filthy trench, were far from antiseptic, and therefore the goal was to stabilize a man and get him to the field ambulance unit as rapidly as possible, where he could be treated before being sent further on to the clearing station for surgery. And so at the aid post the wounds were most often simply cleaned and bandaged, with rum and morphine administered for the pain, depending on what was available.

The will to keep fighting is crucial in any army. In the face of unbelievable hardship and a high probability of death or maiming, soldiers stayed in the line and did their duty for a constellation of reasons. Good leaders who shared the danger and led by example; minor rewards of leave, rum, or the chance for a medal; a belief in the cause; and standing by one's comrades were all factors in supporting both individual and collective morale. But so too was the soldiers' knowledge that if they were sick or injured they would receive care. The morale of a unit was a fragile thing, and a long period of service at the front, with casualties, inevitably damaged the fighting spirit of the men. It was the medical officer, usually known as the "doc" or "croaker," who was there for the men. Captain Andrew Macphail of the CAMC noted, "A powerful element in morale is the certainty in the soldiers' mind that they will be cared for if they fall; the presence of the medical officer at the advance is a sign that relief is always at hand."[8] Another Canadian medical officer observed that soldiers feared being left to bleed to death on the battlefield, and the knowledge that trained doctors were on hand to offer expert care was a source of comfort that "did much to allay the perfectly justifiable apprehension."[9] Reflecting on the rank and file, Captain P.G. Bell, who served in a field ambulance for much of the war, felt that the medical officer "should take a genuine interest in their progress and welfare," so that the soldiers "will trust him through thick and thin."[10]

———

As the fighting degenerated into a siege war of monumental proportions, the Western Front became the perfect Petri dish for inculcating disease. In almost every war in human history up to this point, far more soldiers had been killed by disease than by sharpened steel, especially in static sieges. Cholera, dysentery, malaria, typhoid: these and other diseases were the great reaper of soldiers in long campaigns. The astonishing success of the medical services in all the fighting forces of the Great War was in preventing disease from wreaking havoc with armies. One set of casualty statistics reveals that 51,678 Canadian soldiers died of wounds sustained in battle, while another 4,960 succumbed to disease.[11] These figures do not account for soldiers who died from infected wounds—which would number in the thousands and would be included in the larger figure—but disease never destroyed the fighting efficiency of Allied or enemy forces.

This was not by chance. An active campaign was waged to prevent sickness from taking hold in the closely packed soldiers in the trenches, behind the lines, and in the training camps. Its success was not inevitable, however, as soldiers had to accept the new medical science or be forced to follow these stringent rules. The issue of sanitation was central in disease control. A unit's medical officer was responsible for advising the commanding officer "in all matters appertaining to the health of the troops and to the sanitary state of the area they may be occupying."[12] And his advice was almost always heeded.

Soldiers' latrines were a key area for the transmission of disease. A battalion of 1,000 men produces a huge mound of waste per day. At the front and in rear trenches, the building and monitoring of latrines was crucial to public health.[13] These were sites of potential disease, and uncontrolled defecation was both disgusting—giving new meaning to the phrase "shitting where you sleep"—and very likely to lead to an outbreak of disease among the closely packed soldiers. Within the battalion, the medical officer worked with the sanitary non-commissioned officer (NCO)—often known as the "shit wallah"—so that latrines did not became a vector for disease.[14] By the end of 1915, the units had mobile laboratories and official sanitation sections that oversaw much of the work to ensure the availability of clean water as well as the means to dispose of human and animal waste.[15] "The water in the wagon was chlorinated and was safe, if not pleasant to drink," wrote a miffed Canadian infantryman Lance-Corporal Charles Savage, a prewar schoolmaster. "Whoever chlorinated the water apparently went on the theory that if twenty chlorine tablets made it safe, then fifty would make it even safer."[16] The importance of tea and rum to the soldiers was partially a result of the water tasting like chemical swill.

An added horror was the unburied corpses of soldiers slain and left to rot on the battlefield. Stepping on the dead was like sinking into the mud, except it was usually accompanied by an eruption of maggots and putrid flesh spilling over the boots. Men retched at the smell, made the sign of the cross, and tried to rebury the monstrous sight. But sometimes a forward sap or new trench junction had to pass through an old grave, and in such cases the dirty work of digging up a skeleton in mouldy uniform and pieces of flesh could only be done with a firm order and the promise of a double shot of rum as a reward to the unlucky man who was handed the shovel. Ernest Black, a Canadian gunner who enlisted while attending law school in Toronto, shuddered at the protruding bones of the dead: in his mind, a man could not see such things "without being coarsened and brutalized."[17]

The rats liked the corpses. They fed off them, burrowing into the shallow graves and then into the cavities of bodies. Long a symbol of corruption, the hordes of rats left new soldiers revulsed, and even old hands never grew to like the rodents. Lieutenant W.B. Forster, a former bank clerk from Calgary, confessed in one letter that the uncountable rats, with their scurrying bodies and weird sounds, "frighten one more than bullets."[18] One of the nearly universal informal games of the trenches involved killing rats—with revolver shots, bayonet stabs, poisoned bait, elaborate traps, or trained terrier dogs—even though it never made much impact on the mass of little monsters. The rats carried diseases like infective jaundice as well as more deadly plagues, and a barrage of lectures and orders were given regarding the proper disposal of food using anti-rat measures, although No Man's Land supplied enough rotting flesh that the vermin never grew hungry.

Another unsanitary nightmare were the clouds of flies in the summer months that swarmed the air, food, and wounds. They were tolerated as part of the vile landscape, and were easier to bear than the lice that infected almost every soldier at the front no matter how zealous each was about his cleanliness. Surrounded by other lousy men and with few opportunities to wash, it was not long before everyone was crawling with lice. The struggle against the parasites was continued daily with much enthusiasm, and for some this battle was an apt metaphor for the war—constant action, much killing, but little overall success. Each louse could be picked from the body and satisfyingly crushed between thumb and finger, but with the lice laying eggs and living in the folds of clothing, as well as in warm sections of the armpits and groin, the little vampires fed off their hosts and multiplied at an astonishing rate. Lice contributed to ailments and rashes, and most men were already coping with other skin problems, ranging from fierce acne for young soldiers to scabies, which was dismissively labelled as the "seven-year-itch."[19]

As the weather turned colder in late fall 1915, Canadian medical officers were warned to combat the lice more systematically for fear of the transmission of disease.[20] One of the bedevilling illnesses along the Western Front was an undiagnosed "trench fever." The virulent flu caused fever, headache, and body pain, and its origin was a mystery. After a few days of feeling poorly, men were beset by a weariness so deep that they could barely stand. A sharp pain in the shins stood out from the full-body ache. The medical officers in the field studied the disease, as did medical scientists further to the rear, because most affected soldiers had to be sent out of the line for an extended rest and it was a drain on the fighting power of units. Sometimes the symptoms were misdiagnosed as typhoid. The fever tended to pass after a few days and the men regained their strength, but then the fever and aches returned, often in several cycles, which drew comparisons to malaria.[21] Doctors hypothesized that it was a type of plague spread by rats, although it remained known as PUO—pyrexia of unknown origin. It was not until 1918 that Allied medical authorities, aided by Captain Allan Coats Rankin, a prewar professor of pathology at the University of Alberta, discovered that lice were responsible for the fever and that the causative agent was a new type of bacteria, *Rickettsia*.[22] While this was a significant medical breakthrough, it was impossible to kill all the lice. To combat the disease, the supply of mobile baths was increased on the Western Front to reduce infestations, although it was a losing battle and no cure for trench fever was ever found during the war. Over 20,000 CEF soldiers were diagnosed with PUO and trench fever, with the terms often used interchangeably, and many times that number would have been rendered horizontal by the sickness in civilian life, but they were forced to stagger on in service.[23]

"A man suffered continuous pain in his feet, yet was afraid to take off his boots, unwind his sodden puttees and look to confirm his fears that some of his toes were turning into soft, offensive-smelling mush, and about to drop off joint-by-joint."[24] So wrote Victor Wheeler of the 50th Battalion about the horrifying effects of a new ailment called "trench foot." Although the Canadians were lucky to miss the first winter in the trenches in 1914–1915, two divisions of Canadians suffered through the long, cold months as 1915 became 1916. Many of the trenches remained rudimentary, with poor drainage. Having no means to dry their feet in the slurry of mud and chilly water, soldiers developed a type of frostbite that affected the extremities.[25] Toes went numb; feet suffered from loss of circulation. Amid the shelling and sniping, and with everyone cold, the tough soldiers often did not complain. They had faced worse. But the pain could be striking, with bolts of agony shooting through the feet and legs until feet went numb. Deadened feet hidden in the boots suffered from cracked skin,

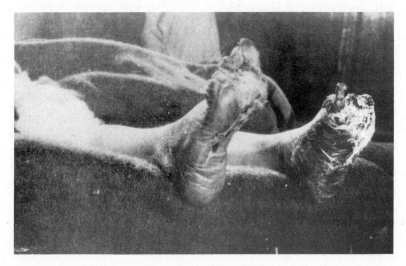

A severe case of trench foot.

oozing blood and pus. The contaminated soil sometimes got into the wounds, which led to more serious infections. In advanced cases, the skin began to turn dark, and gangrene set in.[26] If unchecked, toes had to be amputated, and in extreme cases feet were removed.

The casualties resulting from frostbite began to mount, and the high command became worried. They issued monumentally stupid orders, like "men should not remain wet more than 24 hours," which everyone already knew, but this could not be avoided because of the dreadful conditions.[27] A more successful approach was to place the burden of care on the regimental officers and their supporting doctor. A 1st Canadian Infantry Division order thundered, "The prevention of 'Trench feet' and loss of men from this cause is almost entirely a matter of discipline."[28] While the generals demanded stronger surveillance and punishment of offenders, the most important preventative act was the issuing of whale oil to be slathered on the feet. The gunk had the consistency of glutinous lard and was loathed by all. But the medical officer and his senior orderly had the unpleasant task of monitoring that it was applied daily, with everyone holding their noses as soldiers removed wet boots and soaked socks. Vats of whale oil were transported to the front, which were used up rapidly in the winter months, and even more so when soldiers learned the oil could be employed as a fuel. These new precautions, attention, and punishments greatly reduced the incidence of trench foot by 1916, although by the end of the war the Canadian forces recorded a total of 4,987 cases, resulting in dozens of amputations to the toes and feet, and two deaths.[29]

———

From battlefield surgery to the study of feces, with no small attention devoted to lice, rats, and rotting feet, the medical officers at the front had an unglamorous if essential role in an infantry battalion. But the doctors' driving force was their desire to ease the soldiers' suffering, even if this had to be balanced against ensuring that the regiment did not disintegrate as legitimately sick men were allowed to leave the unit for rest and care. The enforcing of discipline was a part of the doctor's duties. Many of the citizen-soldier-doctors did not want to be the army's mallet used to hammer soldiers who sought to escape the front because of exhaustion or illness, and the struggle was often discussed among medical officers. It even played out in their professional publication, the *Canadian Medical Association Journal*, which argued that "a man cannot serve two masters and so the military side should have ultimate precedence."[30] Doctors were frequently torn between their duty to their patients and their role within the military system.

The regimental medical officer had the power to relieve a man from his duties and to send him to the rear for a rest. But everyone at the front was exhausted, worn down, and on the verge of a mental breakdown; they could not all be sent from the firing line. Another problem was the malingerers and fakers: soldiers who were fed up with service and just wanted to escape the front. While some of these men had truly been pushed too far, others were trying to trick their way into securing an extended sick leave with a feigned illness. As a Canadian medical officer remarked of the regimental doctor, he "must be tender to the weak and harden his heart against the malingerer."[31]

It was during the daily sick parade that the medical officer began his assessment of those who claimed they were unable to continue in their duties. In the first few weeks at the front, many

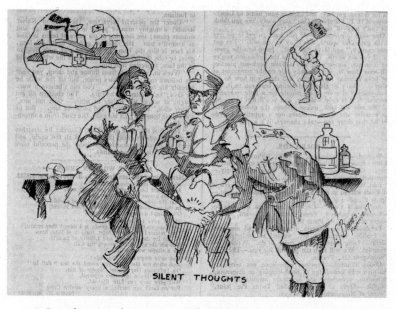

SILENT THOUGHTS

A Canadian trench newspaper, The Iodine Chronicle, captures the difference of opinions between a patient, who hopes to be sent back to England, and the medical officer, who feels the man is "swinging the lead."

of the medical officers were sympathetic in their "rounds," but they soon discovered a game was afoot. "Old soldiering," "swinging the lead," "shirking," "scrimshanking," and "working your ticket" were all soldiers' phrases for malingering. Whatever the label, it was the medical officer's job to separate the frauds from the legitimately unwell. While the ideal doctor–patient relationship is one based in trust, the exposure of malingers was about unmasking fakers and upholding discipline. The medical officer was thus often placed in an adversarial relationship with his patients.

Those malingerers who simply lied about ailments were usually found out quickly, as the doctor asked questions and queried claims that led patients to reveal some incriminating evidence. The more intelligent dodgers found ways to produce physical reactions that mimicked disease or illness. As infantryman George Bell explained, removing cordite from a rifle cartridge and chewing it "produced a pallor, quickened heart action and frothing at the mouth."[32] Cleaning solution could be ingested for a poisoning effect and an unpleasant internal smell; eyes were irritated with dirt or chemicals; skin was scratched to cultivate a wound; and some men deliberately ate rotten food to stimulate illnesses. Others jabbed themselves in the eye, deliberately twisted a finger out of its socket, or stabbed their gums to bloody them.[33] Some of this was quite dangerous and it was no mean feat to nurture botulism in canned meat and to know exactly when to seek medical care. But these men were out to succeed.

While only a minority of soldiers sought to escape the front by tricking an overly sympathetic medical officer, some of them framed the task as a game of wits and will, seeing it as the worker's right to dodge a hard job if not properly compensated. And nor was this practice—part dance, part duel—a secret. For example, an undercurrent of discussion emerged among soldiers looking to beat the system, and an informal soldiers' network shared the best means of simulating a malady or injuring oneself.[34] So common was this discourse that the soldiers' newspapers offered many stories, poems, and cartoons about the rank and file's jousting battle with the medical officers. *The Listening Post*, a popular Canadian soldiers' trench newspaper that was written and published by the soldiers for one another, not only brought malingering into the open but encouraged it, albeit with satire, jokes, and hyperbole. One story dedicated to "The Ancient Order of Lead Swingers" described a fictional society geared towards deceiving the doctors, offering the newspaper's more than 20,000 readers tips on deceiving those in power.[35] Another newspaper for No. 1 Canadian Field

Ambulance, *The Iodine Chronicle*, which was more friendly to doctors, offered a printed joke under the title of "Something Wrong." The patient before a medical officer remarks—"'I feel quite fit now, Sir, and I want to go back to duty.' M.O. replies— 'Take this man's temperature, there must be something wrong with him.'"[36] No one, the joke implied, ever wanted to go back to the front, with those that did obviously having a mental illness that should have paradoxically kept them from the firing line.

The high command was increasingly worried that their army was degenerating into a band of cowards as news of this complex social ritual played out. Increased pressure was exerted on the medical officers to keep soldiers in the line, with high rates of sickness—like trench foot or trench fever—interpreted as a sign of poor discipline. Moreover, the regimental officers, with whom most doctors felt an affinity due to the shared responsibility of their commission, needed soldiers for all the manual labour and duties required, from digging and sandbag-filling to sentry duty and raiding. Most medical officers were also concerned about acquiring a reputation as being too lax and therefore becoming easy targets for the rank and file, which was interpreted as an indictment of their commitment to winning. All in all, the medical officer felt enormous pressure to declare that the soldiers were not sick, or at least not sick enough to be excused from the fatigues or the firing line. "There's no point in going to our medical officer," raged one unhappy Canadian soldier, "unless the blood's running out of you."[37]

All of this led to medical officers frequently being overly harsh in their treatment of those who came before them in the sick parade. Major George S. Strathy from Barrie, Ontario, who served as a regimental medical officer, recorded in his diary that because

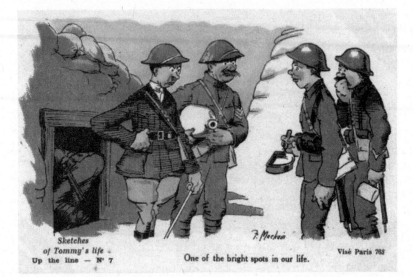

*A popular postcard series, Sketches of a Tommy's Life, depicts
the importance of rum: "One of the bright spots in our life."*

of soldiers' unsympathetic reception during the daily ritual of
inspecting the ill, "a large percentage of the men carry on too long
when they are sick, rather than go in the sick parade, for they look
on it almost as a disgrace to go sick."[38] But both the legitimately
unwell and the malingerer often found that the battalion doctor
did not have much medicine to treat a man in any case. Rum was
an important tool for both maintaining morale and fending off
illness, and it was, as one Canadian medical officer wrote, one of
the few "cheery" things for men who were pushed "almost beyond
human endurance."[39]

The regimental medical officer had a store of rum in his aid
post to be given to men on parade if he deemed it necessary. While
rum had restorative power, most doctors avoided doling it out
because once the rankers learned that he gave rum to sick men,

the line outside his dugout would stretch down the trench. Instead, the medical officer issued castor oil or the No. 9 pill—a laxative. One British journal observed that the medical officer was engaged in preventative care—"endeavouring to tackle small evils early"—but doctors didn't have much medicine to offer and the No. 9 pill was all but useless.[40] Over time, the No. 9 became a symbol of the medical officer's supposed callous nature, for when it was combined with the army diet of an overabundance of canned meat and lack of fresh fruit and vegetables, the pill could have an explosive effect on the body's digestive tract. The No. 9 was so ubiquitous that a running joke held that if the medical officer did not have a No. 9, you instead got a No. 4 and a No. 5, adding to nine, as all pills were believed to be useless.[41] In a letter to his mother in

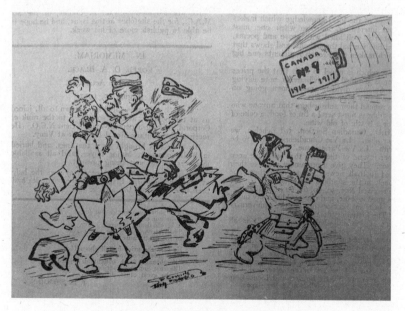

A cartoon depicting the fanciful effects of the
No. 9 pill on terrified Germans.

December 1915, Gunner James Fargey, who did not survive the war, shared his unhappiness about his unit's doctor, noting, "No matter what is wrong with you he gives you the same pills."[42]

———

While regimental medical officers were recognized for their important work and bravery during the course of the war, they remained ambiguous figures for front-line combatants. Soldiers often had an antagonistic relationship with their doctor, both admiring and resenting him for keeping them in the line. The medical officer was respected for the forward care he provided in the face of dangers similar to those of the officers and privates, encountering the same shellfire, sniper bullets, and chemical agents as those under his care. During the course of the war, some thirty medical officers were killed, thirty-one died of disease, and ninety-nine were wounded.[43] And yet the doctors in uniform were also viewed warily by the rank and file. *The Listening Post* offered this taunt to the medical officers: "When a doctor leaves the civilian life for the military, he becomes a different person altogether. Just like Dr. Jekyll and Mr. Hyde."[44] In the eyes of the soldiers, the good and the evil doctor resided in the same man.

Balancing the care of the soldiers with the demands of the army, the medical officer sought to offer treatment and compassion to his physically wounded charges, and by most accounts he succeeded, although the medical officer also served in the military hierarchy, which led to a tension between being a healer and an enforcer. In the eyes of the high command, the medical officer's primary goal was to keep soldiers in the line, fit for fighting. The privates were forced to negotiate their interaction with the medical officer, with some dismayed when their doctor turned on them, Jekyll to Hyde, denying them their own illness, offering panaceas as medicine, and leaving them to suffer at the front. None other than Sigmund Freud captured the medical officer's dilemma: "The physicians had to play a role somewhat like that of a machine gun behind the front line, that of driving back those who fled."[45]

And yet the relationship was not always a combative one. Many of the medical officers had deep sympathy for the soldiers in the line, even as they realized that the strength of a unit could not be allowed to drain away through the funnel of the sick parade. However, long-service men were often treated more sympathetically than a man new to a unit. Captain Robert Manion interacted with many soldiers during his time as a regimental medical officer, and he offered thoughts on how to walk the fine line: "If he is an old soldier and knows the game well, he may get away with it, sometimes with the tacit consent of a sympathetic medical officer."[46] But it was the medical officer who was always the gatekeeper in deciding who would escape the trenches and who would continue to face the storm.

CHAPTER 4

VICE AND THE MEDICAL CORPS

The Western Front was bloody awful. Day in and day out, the infantry sweated in the summer and froze in the winter. The 1,000-strong infantry battalion, which was usually at a strength of around 800 due to soldiers' casualties, sickness, and periodic leave, was spread over hundreds of metres of front-line trench that also connected to units on its flanks. It also extended back to the rearward areas in a series of secondary trenches to a depth of hundreds of metres, although this changed from sector to sector depending on geographical terrain and enemy strength. This was a lot of ground for 800 men to cover, and they were dispersed in sections of ten or platoons of fifty. "We are all mud from head to foot, everything we own and wear is wet, and our dugouts are caving in from the rain," wrote Private Douglas George Buckley of the 19th Battalion to his sister in Toronto soon after arriving at the Western Front in late 1915.[1] He would survive but would be medically invalided out of the army by late 1917 from a virus, picked up in the trenches, which rendered his left wrist immobile and his fingers curled into a claw.

Every trench was different, but a common element was the sandbag. Stacking the jute bags was an endless task because the sandbags became flaccid over time, leaking mud like grey blood and losing their consistency because of rain or annihilation by shellfire. Soldiers were continually filling and restacking the bags. Corrugated iron, wood, twine, and wire were all meshed together to reinforce trench walls to prevent wholesale collapse in these makeshift underground homes.

Mud was under fingers and in most body crevices. The assault on the olfactory sense was even worse, and the stench of gathered men could make one's eyes water as soldiers went weeks without bathing, lived in wet wool uniforms, and engaged in hard labour without the benefit of deodorant. And yet soldiers freely huddled together for warmth, comfort, and company despite the malodorous stench. Songs of all sorts, from the nostalgic to the smutty to folk and hymns, could be heard at night as groups of men came together in the trenches or in deep dugouts twenty to thirty feet in the earth that offered protection from all but a direct hit by a high explosive shell.

Other soldiers were skulking in No Man's Land, crawling amid the craters, using their heightened senses to avoid the putrefying dead, although occasionally employing a corpse hanging on the barbed wire as a rotting signpost. In No Man's Land, the uncanny feeling of being exposed was never shaken, even by the most experienced of the patrol sergeants. A full moon could bathe the apocalyptic front in dangerous luminosity, and soldiers preferred to creep about in the gloom. Most nights multiple working parties toiled in front of the forward trench system. Packs of men, their boots wrapped in sandbags for warmth and to deaden sound, dug new trenches or unspooled barbed wire that acted as a

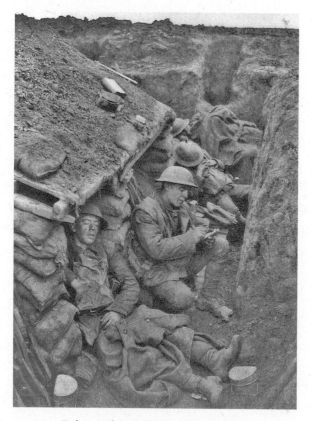

Exhausted Canadians in the trenches.

forward defence against raiders or channelled attackers into kill zones. The defenders on both sides periodically fired flares into the night that temporarily cast the front in a ghostly white glow, whereupon experienced soldiers whispered to the new men to stand still, for any movement might draw the attention of snipers who sought their human prey. Far from civilization and up close with brutality, the soldiers in this strange twilight world lived by their wits, by skill, and by chance.

The infantrymen in the front lines dreamed of being released from the death and destruction. Soldiers did not—and could not—spend the entire war in the trenches. They would break under the burden. In fact, the length of service in the forward trench was usually four to six days, and even this was a strain for all the officers and men who were hyper alert for the possibility of enemy raids, forced to carry out patrols in No Man's Land, and always prepared to dive for cover from incoming shells and mortar bombs. No more than a few hours of sleep were snatched at night. After the tour, the battalion moved to a rear area for rest and restoration for about the same time period as they were in the front lines, and the units in reserve shuffled forward. The cycle continued, week after week, sometimes with longer stays in the open countryside away from the barking guns.

————

When exiting the forward trenches, the survivors walked single-file under the cover of darkness, below ground and back along the winding communication trenches, staggering like the undead, eyes red-tinged with exhaustion. They usually had between five to ten kilometres of marching to reach a village. Barns were a common billet, but not always an appreciated one since they were often shared with animals. Sleep was crucial to restoring the soldiers, and most hardened young men had an amazing resilience. The next day, as the sun rose on a landscape where soldiers did not have to walk bent over to avoid a sniper's bullet through a sagging sandbag, the company cooks laid out a feast of stew, fresh bread, and whatever eggs or vegetables might be purchased from the locals.

The battalion's medical officer was in attendance to examine bodies, and often men had minor injuries like boils, skin irritations,

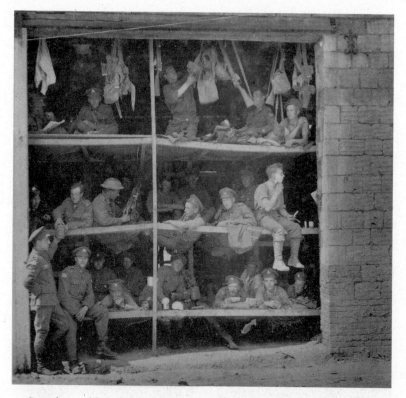

Canadian soldiers billeted behind the lines in a barn adapted for them.

and infections that needed to be treated. An important aspect of returning to normalcy were the showers arranged for the lice-infested homeless men, which were often established in converted breweries and followed by sporting matches. Soccer, football, and baseball were the most popular leisure activities. After one bout of vigorous sports in the summer of 1917, Major D.J. Corrigall of the 20th Battalion believed that "for the time being everyone forgot about the war."[2]

The soldiers soon lined up before the paymaster to draw upon their bank accounts that had swelled with their $1.10 a day in pay for privates and more for higher ranks. There were about five francs to the Canadian dollar, and so the soldiers were flush for a period of time. But it went fast, first to gambling, and then to secure food and drink. The Canadians were paid almost five times as much as British troops, who growled at the cheeky colonials who drove up prices among the locals. "We are fortunate in being billeted quite close to a fair-sized town where we can buy nearly all the necessaries of life if we feel so inclined," expressed Lieutenant G.E. Scroggie in late 1916.[3] Postcards, battlefield souvenirs, and silk scarves were popular with soldiers, who sent them home to loved ones.

Vice was also a part of soldiers' lives. After the hard living at the front, soldiers looked for pleasure where they could find it. With 80 percent of the Canadian Corps consisting of single men, it is no surprise that they sought women's company behind the lines.[4] The female bartenders in the informal French estaminets

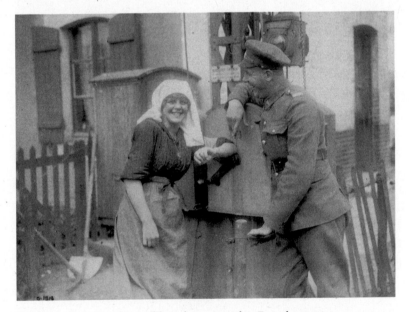

A Canadian soldier chatting with a French woman.

that served food and beer were pursued with desperation, charm, and not a little bit of vigour. Manual labour or gifts were thought to woo women on farms, although with the thousands of soldiers passing through the area, female civilians developed well-honed means of turning back amorous advances.

Most soldiers—whether old or young, serving at the front or in bomb-proof jobs in the rear—had opportunities to seek out prostitutes if they wished. Tens of thousands of what we now call sex workers were housed behind the lines, many of them refugees as the warring armies destroyed or occupied their communities.[5] They were forced to sell their bodies for survival, and soldiers were eager clients. Some men in uniform craved human emotional connection, while others looked for pleasure or a temporary escape from the drudgery of war. Young soldiers spoke of not wanting to die as virgins and felt that intercourse might be another way to grasp hold of life that could be extinguished during the next tour to the front lines.

Along with sex came the scourge of venereal diseases, which had become a significant problem over the winter of 1914 on Salisbury Plain. There were 1,249 cases among the 31,000 Canadians, a situation that had left the authorities worried and turning to the medical officers to sort out the randy mess of men.[6] While the figure was high, somehow over the decades it has become garbled, and an often reported statistic is that the First Contingent had a venereal disease rate of over 29 percent.[7] It is unclear where that erroneous figure came from, but it is significantly inflated at about ten times the actual rate of infection. That said, many soldiers had entered the ranks already infected with the "leprosy of lust," as one prewar morality tract described sexual diseases.[8] And those who went on leave to the big cities of London and Paris

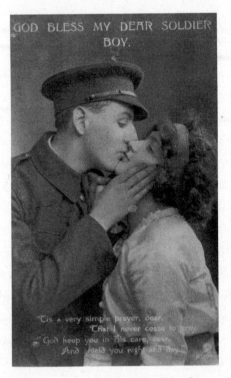

*Postcards were available for sale behind the front lines to send to loved
ones. Many of the postcards made reference to missing those at home.*

faced much temptation, with some areas of England, such as the
Strand, described as "a veritable Devil's Playground" infested with
prostitutes.[9]

The medical officers warned that there was no easy solution to
the threat of these diseases, and that measures for curbing this
blight would need to extend far beyond medical care and into the
realm of social control. Nonetheless, it fell to the doctors in uniform to address the issue. They faced two primary enemies. The
more common disease was the bacterial infection of gonorrhea, or
"the clap" as it was known for centuries, which led to pain in the
genitals, a pus-like discharge, fatigue, and exacerbated effects of

other diseases. Far deadlier was syphilis, caused by threadlike spirochete bacteria in the blood that attacked the body, including the brain, with the acute form of the "pox," eventually leading to madness and death. Chillingly, syphilis could be passed on to children through an infected mother, causing blindness and deformities.

The high command viewed these diseases as a moral and a disciplinary problem, although the loss of diseased men—usually for fifty to sixty days of treatment—was also a significant drain on manpower.[10] Restraint was preached to the soldiers, with the hope that army discipline might curtail action, but men in uniform exerted their own agency. By the mid-point of the war, with the numbers of Canadian soldiers reaching 100,000 in the Canadian Corps, as well as another 150,000 in England as part of the system of training camps, hospitals, forestry units, or working in administration, the issue of venereal disease had to be addressed.

———

Senior staff officers and commanders were anxious about the growing loss of soldiers to sexual diseases, but this was also viewed as a barometer of morale in a unit, much like occurrences of trench foot. High rates of sexually transmitted diseases were interpreted by the Canadian and British senior officers as a sign of low morale. While the infected soldiers were usually evacuated to England in the first half of the war, the policy changed in 1916, when more patients began to be treated in hospitals in France to avoid congestion along the lines of communication and to dissuade any hope among soldiers that venereal diseases might lead to an escape from the front.

There was also a moral dimension to the issue, with the army not wishing to be accused of recruiting young men to serve and then exposing them carelessly to the sexually diseased harpies—as concerned moralists in Canada depicted prostitutes—who were preying on the helpless soldiers. The soldiers were, of course, not that helpless, although many in that repressed age were surprisingly naive about sex and transmissible diseases. While a diseased army can still fight, with painful urination not stopping a rifleman for some time and syphilis not destroying the brain for years, the high command felt a moral obligation to care for all wounded soldiers. The social contract between the civilian soldier and the armed forces, according to which the soldier rightly expected to be restored to health for all manner of injury, extended to these more shameful wounds. However, sexual wounds were met with moral outrage. This plague, some claimed, would lead to race suicide.

To stem the rising tide of sex-based diseases, the army ordered the medical services to end the problem. Regimental officers lacked both the expertise and the interest necessary for giving lectures or examining their soldiers' genitals, and so these tasks fell to the medical officers. They were also the only ones who had the knowledge, professionalism, and expertise to combat these diseases. And so it was the doctors in uniform, one article in *CMAJ* noted, who were charged with preserving "the health of the troops," and this extended to sexual wounds.[11]

As with other forms of medical treatment, it took time to create a coherent medical policy to combat the diseases, and the Canadians relied heavily on the British for guidance.[12] But the venereal disease outbreak in the First Contingent in 1914 had attuned the Dominion's military and medical services to the disease's wasting effects. Almost from the start of the war, medical officers educated the soldiers in the evils of intercourse with "lewd women" and the diseases that might follow, often lecturing hundreds of men at a time.[13] The medical officers were joined by the chaplains, who would approach the issue with even more zeal, warning of everlasting shame and of souls lost to damnation through immoral acts. Soldiers wrote about the lectures, impressed by their shock and awe, but men on leave temporarily exiting the horror of the front, with pockets filled with francs and usually deep into the drink, were often guided by other urges.[14] Sergeant Frank Maheux, a South African War veteran and logger from near Maniwaki, Quebec, wrote to his wife that after listening to his chaplain, he believed that the English women were "snakes from hell with fire in their mouth all over."[15] No doubt the sermon was a memorable one, although Maheux's personnel file indicates he contracted a sexual disease during the war.

—

Education about venereal diseases was a war-long process. If chaplains, medical officers, and others in positions of authority told the soldiers over and over again about the importance of abstinence, then perhaps this would have an effect, thought the high command, much like the relentless marching or drill with arms. Pamphlets were also issued to the men as part of the barrage of education on self-restraint. The YMCA contributed considerable resources to these printed documents, with one of them, *Facts for Fighters*, stating that "all loose women are dirty, in spite of their attractive, alluring attire."[16] A British silent film, the thirty-eight-minute *Whatsoever a Man Soweth*, was shown to hundreds of thousands of the Empire's warriors—a stark morality tale of a soldier who chooses sex with a prostitute and then heads down the pockmarked road to ruin, while another man stays pure, avoids temptation, and is saved to enjoy a happy life after the war.[17]

Despite the enormous resources and energy expended in the form of lectures, pamphlets, and films, the spread of sexual disease was not curtailed, and, in desperation, the high command redoubled efforts and demanded that the regimental medical officers use their authority to identify soldiers with the disease by monitoring their bodies. Because of the stigma associated with these diseases, most soldiers did not willingly reveal their affliction, and so, employing one of the most hated aspects of soldiering, the medical officers conducted a weekly review, known as the "short arm inspection" or "dangle parade." Soldiers were ordered to

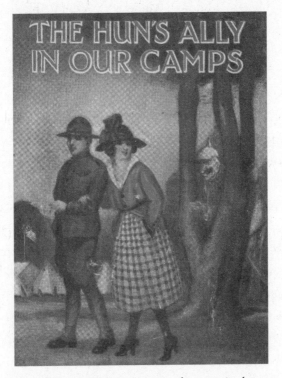

"The Hun's Ally in our Camps" warns of weaponized women who are part of a German plot to poison soldiers with venereal disease.

diseases. Continued appeals to honour and abstinence went hand in hand with punishments, such as reducing pay by half for the duration of a man's recovery in hospital, but soldiers' sexual behaviour seemed little diminished.[22] While an early-war policy had the military contact wives of soldiers to explain why their pay was temporarily reduced, after a few suicides among humiliated husbands the cruel policy was revoked.[23] To ratchet up the pressure, group punishments were also used, such as withholding leave for an entire battalion to pressure individual soldiers into conformity. That did not work either, and only led to strife in a unit.

The military high command relentlessly attacked the problem for many reasons, with some senior officers particularly in a lather over the fear that venereal disease was no more than a self-inflicted wound that allowed soldiers to escape from the front. Venereal disease was indeed a ticket to a hospital, even if the treatment was painful and long. Becoming intentionally infected was no easy thing to accomplish, as prostitutes were often under medical examination in French towns, though the rumour mill among soldiers promised it could be done. Perhaps it was true. "Men on leave discovered a further form of ingenuity, and deliberately consorted with promising women," believed a Canadian medical officer. "This practice was hard to check, as venereal disease is the least difficult of all self-inflicted wounds to inflict."[24] Soldiers also learned other means to make it appear like they were diseased. The least painful act was the delicate work of souring milk, injecting it into the urethra, and holding it until an inspection, with the white discharge tricking the medical officer into thinking that a disease was present.[25] A more painful means of escape was to damage the penis: striking it, smashing it, even burning it to create lesions. It took a brave man to carry through with these harmful deceptions, and it was also a sign of the despair of some soldiers.

The epidemic of sexual diseases required a special Canadian hospital of 1,060 beds to be created at Etchinghill, near Folkestone on the southeast coast, with a second hospital established at Witley in 1917 providing another 600 beds. Officers, granted the privilege of not being treated with the ranks, had a smaller hospital in Hastings, while a CAMC-run centre was established at Le Havre in France. Isolated and humiliated in these special hospitals, patients were treated harshly and housed in shabby quarters devoid of books and magazines save for moralizing tracts that shamed and preached a horrible fate if abstinence was ignored. One Canadian doctor observed that the patients were sneeringly accused of "rendering themselves unfit for service," while another wartime report revealed that the unsympathetic medical staff at these facilities viewed their patients as "moral lepers."[26] Furthermore, nurses were not allowed in the special hospitals for fear of their being exposed to these "depraved characters," as one doctor recounted with disapproval.[27] It is not surprising that these were not complacent patients, and some of the men felt that the punishment did not fit the crime. Of able body, they sometimes escaped the confines of their hospital wards, roaming the local town in search of drink and other pleasures.

Some of these patients were also running away from their medicine. An arsenic, salvarsan, had been discovered in 1910 as an effective means to combat syphilis. The arsenic was injected directly into the urethra and it caused considerable pain. This "magic bullet," as some believed it to be—despite documented cases of patients suffering organ damage or death—was injected several times a day, usually for a full month. It left the weary warriors with cramps, vomiting, bloody urine, and rotting teeth.[28]

Salvarsan had more success than the previous mercury-based applications, but it was most effective in reducing the potency of syphilis in its early stages. The treatment of these diseases came with much indignity, and the injury was viewed as being different from almost every other wound that was associated with an honourable release from the front. Furthermore, the long method of curing the infected soldiers was dreadful, and at least eleven Canadians died from the treatment.[29] Investigations and autopsies revealed the usual cause of the death to be arsenic poisoning or jaundice brought on by the "medicine," although the chemotherapy regime was not modified even after these findings.

———

The Canadians had the highest rates of venereal disease infection in the British forces, at slightly over 15 percent during the course of the war—about five times that of British soldiers, although only somewhat higher than the Australians'.[30] Prime Minister Sir Robert Borden was horrified by these revelations, and he was also under considerable pressure from forces at home —morality crusaders, religious organizations, and temperance groups—to rectify the situation. Soldiers' wives were also apprehensive about the crisis, with fears of infidelity added to the long list of worries caused by extended separation.[31] Heroic soldiers fighting overseas keeping the Hunnish beast at bay made for good propaganda posters, but real life, with all its loneliness and the sorrow of separation, led to mental anguish between wives and husbands that could never be fully addressed in letters and postcards.

The venereal disease issue was exacerbated by the moral fervour of a renewed social purity movement animated by the patriotic war effort, with the two often twinned in battling societal evils—the Germans and the germs. Venereal disease in the CEF also revealed difficult truths about sexual desire, tension, and the transformative effects of war on people. While Prime Minister Borden was not a shrinking violet, he was like many Canadians of the time in agonizing over sexual morality. To make his point, Borden railed in April 1917 at the Imperial War Conference, "If I should be Prime Minister of Canada on the outbreak of another war, I would not send one man overseas if the condition were such that prevailed during the progress of this war. . . . I am absolutely astonished that no steps of any reasonable adequate character have been taken here to prevent these women swarming around our camps all over this kingdom."[32] That diseased women were portrayed as a greater enemy than the Germans or the machine gun reveals the propensity of the issue to cause fear and warp perceptions.

Lieutenant-Colonel George Adami, a McGill professor of pathology and a champion of better understanding diseases and their social dimensions, starkly observed at the time that the "position regarding the venereal diseases" was "terribly costly, with unnecessary failure."[33] The medical services were aware that no victory would be achieved via the relentless calls for abstinence, and so the CAMC advocated to move the discussion from stigma, guilt, and punishment to identification, treatment, and legitimizing the wound.[34] Despite the high command's fear of moral decay, the best weapon against sexual diseases was the issuing of prophylactics. However, when condoms could be found, they were not popular with the soldiers, and the "French letters" were not formally distributed by the military. If the military did make the decision to dispense them to soldiers, some worried they would be condoning the men's actions and, thereby, as one CMAJ editorial noted, "encouraging vice."[35] The French had already disregarded such notions and had established official army brothels where doctors inspected the prostitutes, and these sites were often available to the Canadians.[36] Identified with red lamps, the brothels followed the hierarchy of the army, with different houses for officers and enlisted men. A long-service soldier wrote in his diary about a "whorehouse" where the "girls were inspected (medical) once a week. The soldiers were marched over to the whorehouse and lined up to await their turn with the girls."[37] Another Canadian soldier remarked that lining up for the prostitutes was not for the bashful: "Each Sunday afternoon, a long queue is formed in front of a certain house. . . . One by one these soldiers are admitted, inflamed by the jibes and jests shouted out by the men behind them in the line, and each one is given ten minutes for the whole business."[38]

The CAMC worked with other national medical services to create treatment centres to combat potential infections, which were illuminated in many cities behind the lines with a blue light (in contrast to red lights that hung over the entrance to a brothel). After intercourse, soldiers were told to visit these clinics, where early cleaning and disinfection of the penis proved successful in reducing the infection caused by venereal disease. Those who willingly crossed the blue-light threshold were given soap, potassium permanganate, and calomel ointment. After lathering up the penis, a mercury-based solution was injected directly into the urethra, to be held there for ten minutes. The pain likely dissuaded many men from ever again visiting the centres, and others heard about the burning sensation from their comrades who were treated, or via the rumour mill. The shame was likely an even greater deterrent.

———

The CEF had 66,346 individually recorded cases of venereal diseases, although some men were infected multiple times.[39] Medical study also revealed that a venereal disease was only likely to be transmitted from one partner to the other 3 percent of the time through unprotected sex, meaning there was no shortage of action behind the lines.[40] While around one in eight Canadians sent overseas was infected, that figure needs to be put into perspective, as it is not very different from the 10 to 15 percent infection rate among civilian Canadian males in major cities during that time period. The CAMC often raised the contextualizing figure with military authorities, but it did little to dampen the military's ardour for stamping out this plague, and the generals were no doubt motivated by the unending pressure coming from the home front.[41] Another official report by civilian and Canadian medical officers studying the problem observed that venereal disease stimulated "greater public interest . . . than all the other questions combined."[42] There was no medical victory in this field of soldiers' health prevention, though no one could assess how many soldiers curbed their behaviour because of medical teachings and interventions. Colonel Kenneth Cameron, commander of No. 1 Canadian General Hospital, argued that the "record reflects credit upon the restraint and morals of the men under tremendous temptation," but the medical services could not work miracles.[43] As these diseases were subject to complex social and cultural pressures that far outstripped the approach of strict care and prophylactic protection, the Canadian medical corps was ultimately defeated in this unwinnable war against the pox and the clap.

CHAPTER 5

CLEARING THE WOUNDED, 1916

The Battle of the Somme—a series of campaigns from July 1 to mid-November 1916—involved several million German, British, dominion, and French soldiers. The carnage was unimaginable. The Canadians were lucky to miss going over the top on the first day of battle, a titanic disaster for the British forces in which 120,000 set off into the German guns and almost half of them were killed or wounded as they were caught on the barbed wire, torn apart by shells, and cut down by sweeping fire. But Canadian medical units supported the offensive, and at No. 2 Canadian General Hospital 235 injured men arrived on July 2, 1916, with the matron nurse writing in her diary that they were "mostly stretcher cases and all very badly wounded."[1] It only got worse as hundreds of gravely ill soldiers arrived in a crush of humanity in the coming days and every operating room was in use, both day and night.

Following the Battle of Mount Sorrel in June 1916, where the Canadians suffered close to 9,000 casualties from the 2nd to 13th of June, their turn at the Somme came in late August, when they

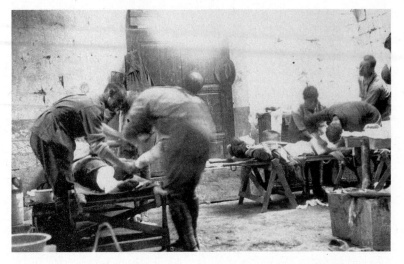

An Australian aid post where the wounded are being treated (July 1916).

marched southwards from the Ypres salient. The rising crescendo of the guns sent shivers down the spine. This was an altogether new type of warfare. For as far as the eye could see, there were armies of soldiers, gunners, and engineers milling behind the lines, working, and digging amid the ruins of an eviscerated landscape. "There is every kind of infernal machine at work here," observed one Canadian serving in a British machine-gun company of the Somme. "Gas, liquid fire, whiz-bangs, aerial torpedoes, high (very high) explosives, mines, bombs, and a multitude of minor 'diversions.'"[2] The French, British, Australians, New Zealanders, and other Empire troops had fought valiantly in August 1916 to advance the line, with little success and no little horror. They were cycled out to allow fresh troops to continue the fight, and units of the 1st Canadian Division took their first turn in the forward trenches from August 31. Almost immediately the casualties ramped up. The shellfire claimed dozens of lives, with soldiers doing little other than crouching in the trenches for safety, where, as one Canadian believed, the only course was to "sit tight, hold your breath, and pray to God it won't hit you."[3] Despite this holocaust of sight, sound, and smell, Charles Edward Clarke, a lieutenant in the 2nd Battalion, recounted his excitement at having a chance to strike at the enemy. After the "punishment" in the Ypres salient, he said in a postwar memoir, "we just itched to get a good lick at the enemy."[4]

Behind the front lines, in the shattered city of Albert, the Canadians set up a medical dressing station in a school that was on low ground and had therefore escaped much of the German shelling. Medical units often jostled over limited structures, competing for space with headquarters or other logistical formations. The field ambulances usually had priority, but not always, and on the Somme these units had to be out of range of most artillery fire but close enough to the forward battalions to take in the walking wounded. With the dressing station about 7 kilometres from the first-line of trenches, it was further from the battle lines than ideal, but its large brick building and open courtyard could accommodate hundreds of injured soldiers. With so many armies crammed into the battle space, the Canadians could fit only a single field ambulance unit near the front, although the CAMC senior officers pooled resources, drawing together the most experienced staff from three field ambulance units (each of which usually had about 190 ranks and 10 medical officers). As in previous battles, the doctrine underlying the evacuation of the wounded meant a funnelling from the battlefield and forward regimental aid posts back to the field ambulance—which had advanced dressing stations closer to the front and the main one in Albert—from where patients would be driven by motor or horse-drawn ambulance to surgical care at the casualty clearing stations out of range of shellfire.

Method of evacuation of wounded from front line to base.

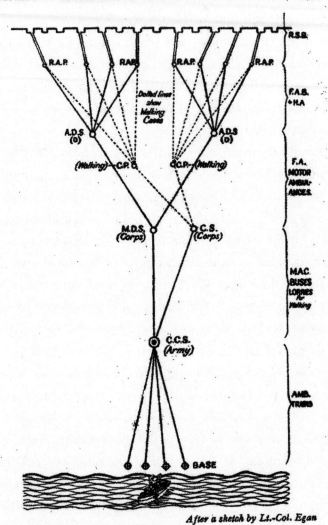

After a sketch by Lt.-Col. Egan

Echeloned medical services funnel the wounded from the front to units
behind the lines. The system moves from R.S.B. (stretcher-bearers) to
R.A.P. (regimental aid posts) to A.D.S. (advanced dressing stations as part
of field ambulances) to M.D.S. (main dressing station as part of the field
ambulance) to the C.C.S. (casualty clearing station) and base (hospitals).

With three infantry divisions in the Canadian Corps, and a fourth to arrive in October, the medical services were also expanding. At this midpoint in the war, the regimental medical officer remained attached to the battalion, aided by sixteen stretcher-bearers. It was hard living in the field, and as medical officer Charles Willoughby observed, "it is a young man's job."[5] At the sharp end of the medical battle, these doctors closest to the front were supported by the field ambulance, which kept them supplied with dressings, iodine, and splints.[6]

"We see some cruel sights," said CAMC stretcher-bearer James Ford.[7] At Albert, the pool of medical officers was close to thirty, although, because of the relatively unsanitary conditions, surgery at a field ambulance was discouraged except in the case of soldiers who arrived close to death, exsanguinated, and in shock. A lesson learned from the British and dominion forces' fighting over the previous two months was that survival rates increased when the wounded from the field ambulance could be rapidly "cleared" to the casualty clearing station so that surgeons could begin operating as soon as possible. The clearing station had at least 150 beds, several operating rooms, and even X-ray machines for locating metal shards in bodies. The system of clearance and care shifted slightly from battle to battle, but the medical chain of evacuation remained relatively constant from the Somme onwards.

———

The shocking violence and wastage to shellfire in the trenches were dwarfed only by the unfettered slaughter as soldiers advanced into No Man's Land. In the trenches, soldiers were relatively protected; outside these underground shelters was where steel met flesh.

Shells were the great killer in the war, but on the Somme machine guns had already mowed down tens of thousands of infantrymen. While the Germans had suffered heavily in the fighting to date, their defences remained situated around hardened positions behind rows of barbed wire, all of which was difficult to destroy with shells because of faulty fuses that often did not allow for detonation on contact. For Field Marshal Douglas Haig's British forces, the battles in July and August had been a series of disasters or brutally costly advances for limited gains. In the hope of breaking the enemy lines, a new British weapon, the tank, was added to the arsenal of artillery, mortars, machine guns, rifle fire, and hand grenades. Tanks would be a part of a new major offensive to be launched on September 15, an assault that would be the first significant operation for the Canadians on the Somme.[8] Although these metal beasts—rhomboid-shaped, 8 metres long, and weighing 28 tonnes—would aid the infantry by flattening barbed wire and overcoming German resistance, only seven were assigned to the two Canadian divisions that prepared to assault. The tanks were not a game changer.

A far more important innovation was the creeping barrage, whereby gunners carried out the difficult task of firing a moving curtain of shells in front of the advancing infantry, which would rake through the enemy lines at a slow, measured, and methodical pace of usually 100 metres every four minutes. Behind these shells, infantrymen were to march slowly to hug the wall of fire, allowing them to cross No Man's Land with fewer casualties as the Germans took cover in their dugouts to escape the bombardment. But even with the new tactic—which was difficult to achieve and often included Allied shells falling short and landing on the Canadian troops—the clash in the enemy trench was fierce. Former teacher

Lance-Corporal Charles Savage wrote about how, despite the planning involving tens of thousands of men, success in battle came down to a "tired mud-stained man in a trench, waiting for the Zero Hour to arrive when he will rush across a few hundred yards of shell-churned soil and try to kill another tired mud-stained man in another trench."[9]

When the 298 field guns and heavier howitzers opened fire along the Canadian front at 6:20 A.M. on September 15, the sound was a sonic blow through the gut. High explosive shells sent up slime and slain soldiers in the enemy trenches, while the cacophony of noise meant that it was almost impossible to hear officers' orders. The acrid smell of cordite and the copper-like scent of rum and blood wafted over the battlefield. And into the furnace went the 2nd and 3rd Canadian Divisions, attacking with seven battalions of some 3,600 infantrymen in the first surge as they climbed up ladders from their trenches and scrambled over the trench bags.

The battlefield seemed to boil as thousands of shells rained down every minute, hurling up clods of earth and creating steaming craters that varied in size, some housing a man while others could swallow a truck, and all the while whirling metal sailed over the battlefield. Along the front, the advance was not uniform. Some platoons and companies encountered little resistance, snatching enemy positions from dazed Germans lying among their dismembered comrades. Other Canadian platoons were annihilated by shellfire or a single machine gun that survived the bombardment.

Canadian infantryman James Kirk was wounded on the 15th, and from a hospital he wrote of the battlefield, "In some places it is beyond a man's imagination and can't be believed until it is seen by your own eyes. They speak of a place called Hell. If they can

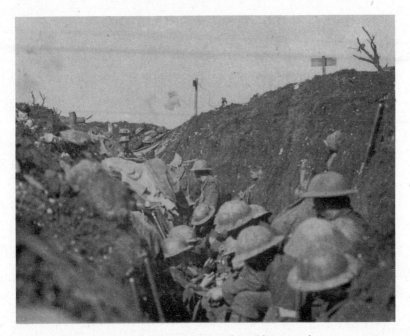

A forward trench with infantry burrowed
deep into the shattered landscape.

beat this they will have to show me."[10] The exploding shells cast a flicker of weird lights within the clouds of dust, like a rippling electric storm. Many soldiers in No Man's Land found they had to avert their eyes from the otherworldly exploding shellfire, as one avoids the retina-scorching effects of a lunar eclipse. Countless unseen bullets zipped through the air, while others kicked up dirt and sparked on the barbed wire, but some found flesh. Louis Keene, a prewar artist who survived the war, noted grimly, "A bullet hitting a man in the head will smash it as effectively as a sledge-hammer."[11] The thud of bullets in bodies was lost amid the banshee shrieks and wails of weaponry, but the sight of a man's head exploding was never forgotten.

In the face of this horror, many soldiers pulled down their steel helmets that had been issued earlier in the year as they began to march, their Lee-Enfield rifle with its 17-inch bayonet pointed at the enemy, chins tucked in as if in a fierce gale. Weighted down as they were with up to fifty pounds of equipment, every step required considerable physical strength and unknowable internal courage. All across No Man's Land, the blast from detonating shells knocked soldiers down. Training took over as they patted themselves down in the frantic search for an injury, returned to their feet, and set off again, moving forward and around the barbed wire that was torn up by the shellfire and sometimes looked like giant shards of tumbleweeds. When bullets ripped past them or a shell exploded nearby, they dove for cover in shell craters. There, they caught their breath, shook their heads to clear the ringing noise, and waited for the next lift of the barrage to signal the new drive forward into the blizzard of steel.

As the Canadians advanced in the open, it was the enemy artillery shells, fired by gunners hidden several kilometres to the rear, that initially did the most damage. Shrapnel shells detonated to scatter hundreds of iron balls the size of marbles. High explosive shells were even deadlier, with Lieutenant-Colonel E.J. Williams of the CAMC observing that "shrapnel wounds do not manifest such a destructive nature as those from the high explosive shells, where we often find a whole limb or the head completely separated from the body, or where the whole body is blown to pieces."[12] There were all manner of ghastly sights as steel and iron tore through human flesh. Amid the shells, German machine guns firing hundreds of bullets a minute also cut through the ranks. Bullet wounds to the extremities, such as arms and legs, and even necks and heads, could initially produce surprisingly little blood. But a severing of one of the key arteries or veins in the body—the jugular in the neck or the femoral in the thigh—led to spurting blood. The victim turned into a crimson fountain.

The advancing infantry were ordered not to stop for their wounded comrades, even though they knew that every minute counted in saving a mate, which could be done with the swift application of a shell dressing bandage to slow bleeding. The officers instructed them to keep moving. If every infantryman halted to help a wounded man, the operation would rapidly degenerate into a mob scene. Though some infantrymen refused to leave their best chums, often checking to see if they were alive and dragging them into a shell crater, most kept going, fuelled with a new vengeance to make the enemy pay. But before they set off, they often stabbed the victim's bayonetted-rifle into the ground to act as a marker for the follow-on stretcher-bearers who were to administer medical aid.

———

The stretcher-bearers went into battle wearing their steel helmets but without rifles. Instead, they were armed with first-aid kits, multiple field dressings for wounds (often carried in a sandbag), morphine and rum for the pain, and a huge dose of courage. They wore a white brassard armlet emblazoned with a red cross on their left arm to alert all to their non-combatant status, although bullets and shells made no such distinctions. One of the bearers, Private Ralph Watson, who enlisted in Ottawa, reflected on his role as a battlefield medic, noting, "It's a rotten job, of course, and nobody wants it, but I rather think I would be more use binding up wounds than I would be just carrying a gun in the ordinary way."[13] The "rotten" aspect to the job was that bearers were expected to aid their comrades no matter the danger, exposing themselves to enemy fire in order to save soldiers caught in the kill zone. Another bearer, Private Peter A. Hughes, remarked, "I intend to do my duty as far as in my power. I shall experience many trials and I shall be where death lurks, but our duties are duties that perhaps are not appreciated as much as they should be, because we not only run the risk of the ordinary soldier, but do our best to save lives that otherwise would be lost."[14]

Unlike at the Battle of Second Ypres in April 1915, on the Somme the regimental medical officers were ordered to remain in their aid post to wait for the wounded. They were too precious to lose to the shot and shell of the open battlefield, and too many British, Australian, and New Zealand doctors had already died on the Somme. Aware of the mass of wounded in the large-scale campaigns, battalions increased the number of stretcher-bearers to thirty-two in preparation for an assault. Further carriers came forward from the field ambulance, and most were issued armlets with the letters "SB" to denote "stretcher-bearer," but without the red cross because they were infantrymen.

On the morning of the battle on September 15, the medical officer's sixteen core stretcher-bearers, whom he had trained in first aid and emergency care, went over the top behind the assaulting forces and almost immediately encountered the wounded men, those lying still and those writhing in pain. Some of the injured soldiers close to the jumping-off trenches were already limping back, using rifles as crutches or crawling through the chalky dust. The bearers passed them as they set off towards the enemy lines, looking for other wounded men, "with machine gun bullets whistling by their ears," one recounted, "and shells bursting all about them."[15]

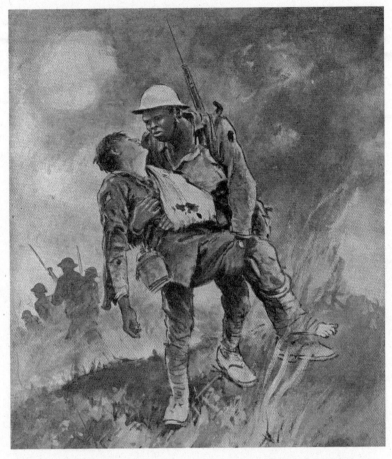

This remarkable wartime drawing was published in Canada in Khaki, *an official Canadian magazine. The image shows a Black Canadian infantryman carrying a wounded man to medical care, with the caption "A White Man." The term "white," at the time a racialized term applied to something good and outstanding, is used here to describe this brave Black soldier, although it is firmly rooted in racist discourse that raises the soldier to white status. Despite facing racial barriers at the start of the war, at least 1,300 Black Canadians served in uniform, in all service arms. Many soldiers received gallantry awards and were seen, as this cartoon suggests, as comrades equal in status through shared hardship.*

The stretcher-bearers ran to the wounded. Soldiers lying face down were turned over, their pulse examined, and their bodies studied for the location of the wound with its telltale spreading crimson. The first step was to apply a bandage to control the bleeding. Tourniquets were sometimes used, but they were not officially issued to stretcher-bearers because it was found that soldiers who had tourniquets applied for many hours suffered further damage due to the slowing of blood, with a majority of patients being subject to amputation of their limbs after a tourniquet had been left on for longer than three hours.[16] These were, again, lessons learned from painful experience. Instead, iodine was splashed over the wound to clean it—bathing the skin in a weird orange tint—and then a bandage was wrapped into place with the dressing. The bearers had been trained by the medical officer on how to wrap a head, arm, leg, foot, or hand, although some wounds were harder to cover than others, especially those to the torso. The bearer first used the soldiers' field dressing, which was sewn into the right front of their tunic and was usually wisely loosened by soldiers before a battle to ensure easy access. Containing a cotton wool pad wrapped in gauze and stitched to a bandage four inches wide and almost a metre long, the field dressing was the most important medical tool of the war, saving countless lives. For long or deep gashes, the bearer double-wrapped a wound with one of his own dressings, or an even larger "shell dressing." As the cut-down soldier took in the sight of his own lifeblood, torn flesh, and broken bones, stretcher-bearers observed that almost all were calmed as the medical man worked on them. "A clean white dressing . . . seems to reassure a wounded man strangely," felt one British medical orderly at the front. "It makes him feel that he is being taken care of, gives him a kind of status, and stimulates his sense of personal responsibility."[17]

Most soldiers lost their helmets when they were hit, but a bearer made sure that a gas mask was at hand in case the enemy let off the chemicals. The medic was also armed with an important tool—the cigarette. With most soldiers addicted to their tobacco, the nicotine brought instant relief and a small kick of energy. Conscious men were also usually terribly thirsty, and the medical man gave them liquid from one of his canteens, some filled with water, others with rum. Only those with stomach wounds were denied drink as it hastened death. In those cases, and with other "bad" wounds, some bearers were entrusted with tablets of morphine that were put under the soldiers' tongue to dissolve, reducing the suffering. Absent from historical records are these many lethal doses of morphine given in quiet acts of mercy to screaming men who had no chance of survival.

———

The sound of war is often lost in histories. But the noise of the Somme battlefield was an unholy terror. The weird shriek of shells was described by soldiers who tried to make sense of the disharmony as akin to a drumbeat of smashing sounds or to the passage of invisible trains above them. The dropping of mortar bombs created a deep crunch followed by a bang, while bullets passing close were likened to bees or hornets seeking their prey. The sound of the wounded men had its own quality. There were those who screamed in uncontrollable agony, out of their mind with pain, although they seemed to be in the minority. More often men only groaned and whimpered, clamping down their jaws to stifle their tortured sounds. It was easier to sit or lie still when movement brought white-hot hurt, and many prayed that relief was coming from the hands of a stretcher-bearer.

And yet to remain immobile in No Man's Land was to invite death. The only hope of survival lay in rising up through the slurry of misery and setting off for care. Every minute counted, and the long voyage to receive aid was easier with a mate. Sometimes a blinded man carried out a friend with a broken leg; sometimes a soldier with a shattered arm used his good one to keep his comrade's intestines in his torso, each leaning on the other as they grew faint from traumatic shock. Men with wounds that should have left them stretcher cases drove onwards. What propelled them forward we can never know. Some thought of their mothers, wives, and children; others focused on a future that might never be; others displayed a bloody-mindedness of simply refusing to join the legion of corpses that already polluted the battlefield. Through drive and a toughness that only a select unlucky few will ever know, the bleeding and battered set off across the fire-swept No Man's Land, down trenches, stumbling, falling, rising, and setting off again.

Some did not make it. The pain was too great or the trial too difficult, and they found refuge in a shell crater and prayed for help. Others were cut down by the arcing fire of machine guns or the non-stop shelling. Private Henry Ruddock of the 28th Battalion, a twenty-one-year-old farmer who enlisted in Regina, Saskatchewan, was wounded in the arm by shrapnel early in the assault and sent back in the direction of a dressing station with a comrade. "Neither were seen again," noted one report, "and it is believed that they were caught in a barrage laid down by the enemy and blown to pieces."[18] Ruddock's body was never found and his name is inscribed on Canada's National War Memorial at Vimy Ridge.

Many of the walking wounded threaded the shells and sniper bullets, making their way to the regimental aid posts, where medical officers were waiting to offer treatment. "From the inferno they come, battered wrecks of humanity," observed a Canadian private at a dressing station. "Limping along, they are supported by others, some with heads swathed with bloody bandages, others blinded, led by those who can see. Legless men, barely alive, are borne by stretcher bearers. Some do not survive the trip."[19] The doctor's orderlies offered warm tea, saturated with sugar for some energy. Sometimes it was fortified with overproof rum, which was usually enough to bring a smile even to a dying man. Wounds were

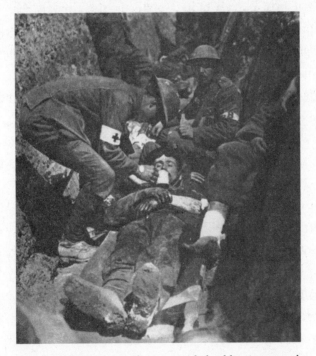

A stretcher-bearer cares for a wounded soldier in a trench.

examined and rebound with fresh dressings, and soon the floor of the aid post or dugout was littered with crusty bandages and occasionally puttees that had been unwound from the ankle to better secure a bandage.

The medical officer rarely carried out emergency surgery in the front lines. While this practice had been more common during the Battle of Second Ypres a year earlier, it was not sustainable in the larger operations of 1916, where it was better to get the mass of wounded rapidly to the rear hospitals where surgery could be conducted in antiseptic conditions. But if a soldier was slipping into shock, to be followed by death, or was suffering from a traumatic wound to the brain or gut that had to be addressed immediately, sometimes the medical officer went to work on site with his scalpel.

Each battalion had only one doctor, however; and there were so many in need of assistance. This necessitated triage, the appraisal and selection among wounded men to determine who would be treated first and which soldiers—often those with the most awful wounds—would have to be pushed aside. "Those nearly dead were put to bed and given morphine if necessary, and left to die," recounted one Canadian medical officer who, though sympathetic to the men's suffering, nonetheless understood the brutal choices that had to be made between those who could be saved and those who were too far gone and who would consume precious time on the surgical table.[20] The life-giving front-line medical officers thus sometimes had to decide who would die. Few caregivers could emerge from such an environment unaffected by the awful ethical choices that were thrust upon them.

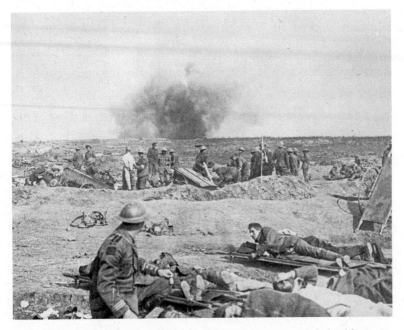

A stunning photograph of a shell detonating near wounded soldiers.

Captain Norman Guiou, a recent graduate of McGill's medical school and serving at the front in the later part of the war, wrote that he did not like the term "killed in action." Instead, he observed, "Men died of wounds, some faster than others. It was our job to get them before they died."[21] While some soldiers died almost instantly in combat, the key to the survival of the wounded was to clear them from No Man's Land and the enemy trenches as rapidly as possible and get them into surgery. However, with the stretcher-bearers and regimental medical officers overwhelmed almost from the start of battle, the soldiers at the front took matters into their own hands. The Canadians pressed the German prisoners of war into service to carry the wounded.

While this had occurred in other battles, it was a key feature of the Somme, where hundreds of German prisoners were captured in each engagement. Fraught with danger, the surrender process was a grey area in combat, a situation where it was up to the attacker and captor to accept the surrender or not.[22] With adrenaline pumping, and with justifiable fear of large groups of prisoners overwhelming small bodies of attackers, it was often safer to slay the enemy even as he came forward with hands raised and pleading for his life. Canadians who fell into German hands also often suffered the same fate. In such circumstances, it is not surprising that the prisoners from the Kaiser's armies often volunteered to carry wounded Canadians back to their lines. It was a factor in currying favour with their captors, and it also made it less likely that some follow-on Canadian would plug the German as he stumbled over the broken battlefield to the rear. To kill one of the two or four Germans carrying a stretcher would be to leave a bleeding comrade stranded in No Man's Land. The converting of prisoners to stretcher carriers saved lives—those of both the wounded man and the German prisoner.

The Canadian stretcher-bearers, having offered first aid over several hours while they traversed the craters looking for their wounded comrades, followed that exhausting action by turning to carrying in those too badly injured to walk. A foldable six-foot canvas stretcher with two wooden poles was equipped with a shoulder strap to allow for the torso and back to bear some of the crippling weight.[23] "Mud and blood are congealed together all over a man," said one Canadian medical man.[24] Entrails, gore, fecal matter, and all manner of filth mixed with the chalky mud that slathered the wounded, adding to the burden of the two or four stretcher-bearers, walking or shuffling as they carried the deadload. Most soldiers weighed between 150 and 175 pounds, but sweat, water, and mud could add considerable weight. Even bearers who had done the job for months, with hands calloused like sandpaper from hardening drills, found that the long carry left oozing blisters and weeping sores. Within a few hundred metres of carrying these great bleeding weights over the cratered ground, shoulders were on fire and backs were in agony; but still the bearers continued the journey to the field ambulance. To this physical strain was added the emotional load of confronting the mass of dead and dying men in a race against time. Years after the war, Sergeant Frederick Noyes of the 5th Canadian Field Ambulance remembered, "What man who carried wounded . . . could ever forget the terrible groaning, cursing and pleading of the poor fellow, half rolling off a shoulder-high stretcher? Who could ever forget the dark brown and purplish stain that seeped through the stretcher canvas and all too often dripped down our backs and arms?"[25]

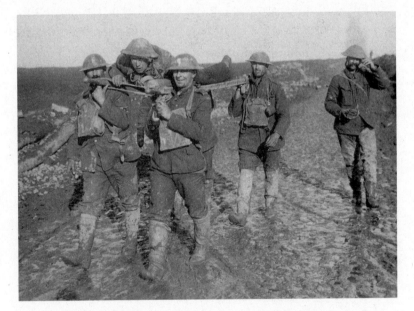

Four stretcher-bearers carry in a wounded comrade through mud. He likely has a wound to his posterior.

In preparation for the two-division assault on September 15, the CAMC had laid out a series of staggered aid posts in advance of the main dressing station in Albert. Most soldiers had been wounded hours before they finally arrived at the field ambulance in the school. A senior orderly or a medical officer surveyed each man and a tag was attached to the patient, providing scribbled notes about the wound. These cards became important, as stretcher-bearers and doctors, and later nurses and surgeons, looked to them for information.

The wounded were triaged at the ambulance unit to allow for streamlined care, and all were jabbed with an anti-tetanus serum through a few increasingly dulled needles used over and over again as the patients rolled in.[26] The medical officers worked on the wounded throughout the day, examining and irrigating wounds with saline solution to clear away some of the debris, applying new bandages, and perhaps sewing up a gaping wound to slow blood loss. The war diary of the No. 4 Canadian Field Ambulance reported on the 15th that, despite recording 1,544 cases treated, including German prisoners, "at no time was the dressing station unduly crowded."[27] This seems an optimistic assessment as most of the doctors worked two days straight, with almost no breaks. One surgeon with Herculean stamina pressed on for a full seventy-two hours before he eventually sank to the ground and was moved to a stretcher. He slept so deeply that his pulse was occasionally checked to ensure he was still alive.

"The duty of the advanced dressing station staff was to stop bleeding and to patch up the wounded so that, if possible, they wouldn't die while being taken to some place farther back," wrote

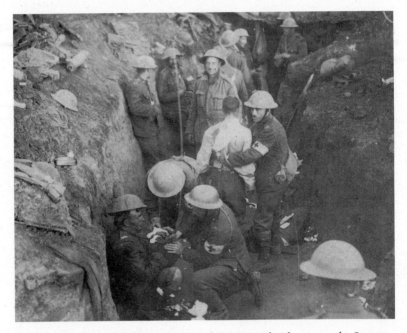

Stretcher-bearers offer medical care at a regimental aid post on the Somme.

a Canadian infantryman wounded during the attack and destined to survive.[28] With the pooled medical resources in this first battle, the Canadians had at their disposal some eighty-four motor ambulances and thirty-six horse-drawn ambulances to transport the injured to centres of care further to the rear.[29] Behind the lines, the terrain was chewed up by old shellfire or reduced to paste by the tramping boots of tens of thousands of infantrymen. It was no mean feat for the motorized vehicles to transport the wounded to the clearing station, and so the horse-drawn ambulances played a key role. The Canadians used the Mk VI ambulance, which was drawn by two or four horses and had fittings for four stretchers. With their "cargoes of suffering," as described by Private George Bell of the 1st Battalion, these ambulances ferried the "wreckage of war."[30] Painted on the side of the ambulance was a large red cross,

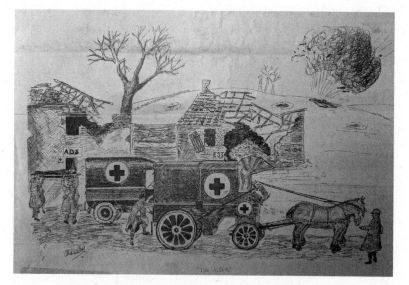

A sketch published in the Canadian soldiers'
newspaper NYD, *depicting the loading of a horse-drawn*
ambulance at an advanced dressing station.

and in the rear carrying space there was a lamp to offer some light, but it was rarely used for fear of attracting enemy fire and perhaps due to a reluctance to reveal the broken men who agonized there.

With the roads in better shape further away from the combat zone, the motor ambulances waited at a remove for the relayed package of patients from the horse-drawn ambulances. From there the motors took them to the designated casualty clearing station, although the roads remained in rough shape from overuse. As one Canadian with shrapnel in his leg said of the motor ambulance ride over rough ground, "Every jerk goes through my leg like a knife."[31] Another infantryman, Charles Brown of the 4th Battalion, had an arm shattered in battle that would later be amputated. He reflected back on the ambulance ride over the shell-pitted road as "the most God-awful part of the war."[32]

The wounded arrived at the clearing stations covered in mud and blood, filthy with dirt and crawling lice, bearing breaks that were set with makeshift splints, wounds compressed and covered with blood-soaked dressings. The struggle for survival was not over, and it was at the clearing stations and other forward hospitals, as we shall see in the next chapter, that surgery was conducted to save the lives of soldiers with horrendous wounds.

———

While the Canadian offensive on the 15th was a celebrated victory, the Battle of the Somme did not end there. Two more months of combat followed, in which hundreds of thousands of Germans and Allied soldiers were killed and maimed. Losses eventually topped one million casualties. In the seesaw combat over blasted trenches, most of the Canadian casualties fell on the infantry, which suffered 93 percent of the total losses until the fighting stopped in mid-November.[33] "I have escaped unharmed so far but cannot go through much more like that without getting hit because it is simply a miracle one gets through," felt Private Walter H. Dyment, a prewar merchant from Winnipeg who enlisted at age twenty-six, writing to his sister as he recovered from exhaustion after the long campaign. "All my best chums have been killed with shells or buried alive, others wounded."[34] Dyment would not survive the war, being listed as missing in action in August 1917.

Major Georges Vanier of the 22nd Battalion, destined to survive the war and later become governor general of Canada, reflected on two stretcher-bearers in his company who were awarded the Distinguished Conduct Medal—second only to the Victoria Cross—for carrying out a severely wounded soldier with a head injury, in daylight, over trenches and through barbed wire, with the Germans firing at them: "It is extraordinary that they were not killed."[35] They survived, but many soldiers of medicine did not, including Lieutenant-Colonel Roland Campbell of the No. 6 Canadian Field Ambulance, whose life was ended by a piece of shrapnel that tore through his upper chest. He was one of the most senior medical officers killed during the war. The losses of the CAMC were added to the butcher's bill for a total of 24,029 killed and wounded Canadians. The ratio of dead to missing, which was usually about one to four, was much higher on the Somme, with 8,096 Canadians killed, 296 taken prisoner, and 15,637 wounded—or 1 killed to every 1.93 wounded.[36]

In battle after battle, the dead lay splayed over the killing ground, sometimes almost in the evenly spaced lines that marked their advance as a machine gun caught them in the open. So many

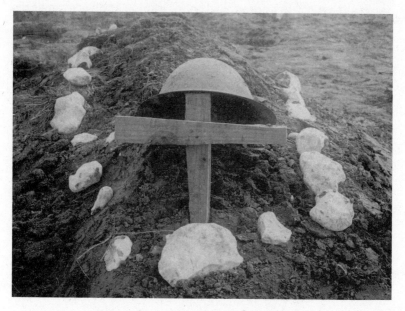

A Canadian soldier's grave on the Somme.

corpses lay in No Man's Land that the Germans and Allied forces occasionally engaged in brief truces to collect them. Arranged by a complicated series of white flags, shouts across No Man's Land, and brave soldiers emerging from trenches with their hands up, the gathering of the dead marked a pause of a few hours amid the long mass killing.[37] Sometimes wounded men were found too, days after an attack, having survived by gathering water or food from the dead, fending off the rats that sought to make a meal of them. Too often though, the bodies of soldiers were located in shell craters, having died alone and whispering for their mothers. They could not always be carried in due to the sheer number of slain, but always their identification tags (known in later wars as dog tags) were separated, with one left on the body for future identification and one gathered up as evidence of a soldier's fate. And spread across the battlefield was the haunting sight of rifles stabbed bayonet-first into the ground, leaning at diverse angles, a sea of weapons turned grave markers that revealed the many who could not be saved.

CHAPTER 6

SAVING LIVES THROUGH SURGERY

T he human body can be remarkably fragile. Small pieces of steel passing through it often lead to death. But the body can also be shockingly resistant, withstanding horrendous injuries that leave brains exposed, limbs ripped from bodies, and all manner of sickening wounds. In this war of industrial might, death was delivered most commonly by the blast of a high explosive shell, with bodies mangled or internal organs ruptured by the force. High explosives reduced men to scraps of flesh, shards of bone, and messy viscera that could be shovelled into a sandbag for a burial of sorts. There were, however, many ways to die at the front, and sometimes even deep scratches could become infected, eventually leading to an agonizing and drawn-out contagion that slowly consumed the afflicted alive. It fell to the surgeons behind the lines, at the casualty clearing stations and the hospitals further to the rear, to bar death's door and bring these soldiers back into life's embrace.

Bullets, shrapnel, and shell splinters were the three primary conventional weapons that wounded soldiers. Burns were infrequent save for those sustained by troopers in tanks and airmen coming down in their flaming planes, while caring for soldiers suffering from poison gas came with its own massive challenges, which will be addressed later in the book. This chapter will examine the peculiar characteristics of injuries sustained as steel, lead, and iron tore through human flesh, shattered bone, and punctured organs. The putrid wounds on the Western Front also frequently led to potential life-ending infections, and with no antibiotics available surgeons were forced to develop new techniques and tactics to defeat this bacteriological enemy. The location where these weapons struck the body—the head, torso, or extremities, for instance—also had an impact on the surgical approach used and on a soldier's ability to survive. Throughout the war surgeons underwent a learning process on how better to save lives, leading to evolutions and even revolutions in treatment. The treatment applied was often brutal but effective, and sometimes amputating a limb was the only way to save a patient. Colonel J.M. Elder of No. 3 Canadian General Hospital noted that he and other surgeons struggled to strike a "just balance between the saving of a limb and the saving of a life."[1]

The hospitals in France varied in size, but they were always large organizations. Established along the lines of communication, as the military called the rear area that supported units at the front, the base hospitals were generally the component of the medical system in Europe that was furthest from the Western Front, and many were located along the French coast in permanent structures such as schools, prisons, or convents. Each Canadian division was served by two general hospitals, usually of at least 1,200 beds each, as well as smaller stationary hospitals of about 500 beds, although because they were semi-permanent they served all Allied wounded and sick soldiers. Closer to the front, the casualty clearing stations were initially a halfway clearing unit between the field ambulance and the hospitals further to the rear, but they took on greater responsibility by mid-1915, especially as the importance of forward surgery for saving lives was recognized. The four Canadian clearing stations were equipped with sophisticated medical equipment, had multiple operating theatres with twelve or more tables, and emerged as crucial sites for emergency surgery. These were rarely quiet places. Respected Canadian surgeon Colonel George Armstrong of Montreal, who was sixty-two years old when he enlisted in 1916, wrote of surgeons working under "great physical and mental strain" and operating for up to forty-eight hours without a break.[2]

———

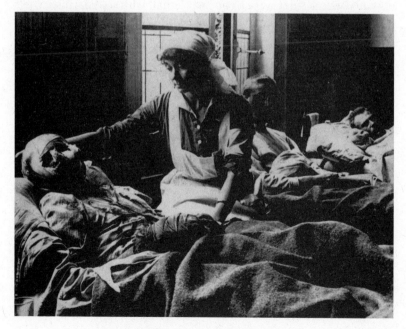

A gravely ill patient cared for by a nurse.

Among the welter of wounds to bodies, surgeons commented on the curious absence of identifiable bayonet gashes on their patients. Many historians have mistakenly concluded that the bayonet was never used, and that it was better suited to opening tin cans. However, while hand-to-hand fighting was rare in this war of shell and bullet, the bayonet remained a frightening weapon. Any study of unit war diaries or operational reports, or even of letters and memoirs, makes it abundantly clear that the bayonet was often wielded in battle. The British and Canadian 17-inch steel blade, attached to the Lee-Enfield before every major attack, was used to stab the enemy, to herd prisoners, and to offer some psychological protection as men advanced into the fire. Even though bullets and shells caused the vast majority of bodily wounds, bayonets were still plunged into flesh. Surgeons often did not see the bayonet wounds because they were frequently lethal, with soldiers instructed to aim for the centre mass of the body—the chest and abdomen— which were among the most fatal places for injuries.[3] Furthermore, the extraction of the blade was done by twisting it out of the body, causing an awful, corkscrew tear to major organs and to flesh. Major H.E. Munroe, a prewar surgeon at Saskatoon City Hospital who was serving with various medical units, wrote during the war, "The majority of bayonet wounds are abdominal, causing death on the field."[4]

Bullet wounds in the British and Canadian forces were thought to account for over a third of the total injuries at the front. While it was never easy to tabulate wounds on bodies, and soldiers who were killed in combat and left where they fell were not included in these statistics, one large study of soldiers passing through medical units determined that artillery caused about 58.5 percent of Allied wounds, with bullets accounting for 38 percent.[5] However, these figures would shift in the course of the war, with more Canadians suffering bullet wounds in the last year of the war, when the British and Canadian artillery batteries gained dominance over the Germans through weight of shell and improved counterbattery work that targeted, harassed, or destroyed enemy guns. In the fateful year of 1918, the Germans were forced to rely more heavily on machine guns than artillery, and the wounds to Canadians reflected that battlefield reality.

A high-velocity round fired from a rifle at several hundred metres caused terrible mutilation to muscle and bone. But not always. Bullets sometimes passed through the arm, the leg, even the neck, shoulder, or torso without inflicting too much trauma. A small entry wound with a blueish tinge to the skin and a small exit wound was a "through and through." That was good. While there was copious blood and excruciating pain, rapid medical treatment with minimal contamination sometimes allowed soldiers to return to their unit within eight weeks. This type of wound was seen as a Blighty—the soldiers' slang word for England—as it offered a welcomed rest from the trenches, in an English hospital, in a bed with fresh sheets, and under the care of a nurse. Many tired men embraced receiving such a non-fatal wound, considering the alternative in the trenches.

Other bullet strikes caused ghastly injuries, as when the small head of the bullet, about the size of an adult fingernail, penetrated the body, deforming on impact, ricocheting and fragmenting, shattering bones and gouging internal organs. In many cases, the ferocious burrowing power of a bullet meant it exited the body in a burst of gore. Soldiers who witnessed the horrendous wounds sometimes believed that the Germans were using special explosive bullets, but there is no evidence of that—it was just that stunned soldiers could not square the dreadful wounds with the small bullets.[6]

Major Edward Archibald, who was chief of surgery at the Royal Victoria Hospital in Montreal when he enlisted at age forty-two to serve at No. 3 McGill Hospital, conducted hundreds of operations during the war. He wrote up his findings in scholarly papers for other doctors, often published in the *Canadian Medical Association Journal*. In one such piece, Archibald noted, "The damage done, first of all, varies enormously from patient to patient according to the size of the shell fragment or the velocity of the bullet, and of course also according to the location and direction of the missile, and finally according to the presence or absence of other severe lesions of the body. There are good cases and bad cases."[7] Good and bad, indeed, and everything in between. Bullets struck bodies with such force that sometimes the skin was liquified, to the point where, as Archibald explained, "the explosive force of the missile radiated laterally by the passage of a high velocity bullet not only devitalizes the tissues (so that often one can wipe off muscle tissue with a swab) but also separates them, as one might fluff out a feather duster by blowing into it."[8] These were nearly incomprehensible sights.

In addition to bullets, shrapnel shells were a deadly antipersonnel weapon. Smaller calibre shells—the 18-pounder for the British or 7.5cm for the Germans—were usually packed with several hundred iron ball bearings, each about the size of a marble. The gunners gauged the distance to the target several kilometres away and set the shell fuse to detonate at about 20 metres above the ground so that the shotgun-like blast exploded downward, hurling the hundreds of balls over a wide area. While the vast majority sank into the former farmers' fields with no effect, when flesh was hit the impact caused devastating harm. As one Canadian surgeon wrote in November 1915, "If a vital part of the body is severely injured by shrapnel the patient usually succumbs on the battlefield."[9] The introduction of the British steel helmet in early 1916, with its wide brim for protection, was a direct response to shrapnel, shell case splinters, and bullets—although this helmet still left the neck and brain stem exposed.

Shell splinters were even more lethal than shrapnel. Sometimes mistakenly called shrapnel, the splinters were metal casings from a high explosive or shrapnel shell that upon detonation became weapons in themselves. "Even tiny splinters could do great damage," wrote one Canadian. "A small splinter hit one of our gunners . . . penetrating his shrapnel helmet in front, passing completely through his skull and out through the tin hat behind."[10] These were jagged pieces of steel, warped into weird shapes by the force of the blast, and when they passed into a soldier, they created the worst wounds. Lieutenant-Colonel E.J. Williams, who commanded No. 1 Canadian Stationary Hospital, wrote of the fragments, "The missiles being of many different sizes and shapes and travelling at low velocity when coming in contact with the body, produce wounds of different appearances. A sharp piece of steel may cut its way right through the tissues, while on the other hand a large, rough, jagged piece will cause extensive laceration and contusion—besides carrying with it into the deeper parts, pieces of clothing, dirt, etc., and so causing infection, which is a constant condition in all wounds of this class."[11]

Doctors also faced the challenge of dealing with patients with multiple wounds. Machine guns fired hundreds of bullets a minute. In these bursts of fire, soldiers were often struck by many bullets. Shrapnel blasts and shell splinters also were clustered as they rained down destruction. Captain F.R. Hutson recounted his experience in battle: "I was hit while lying down, when the bullet entered the centre of my tin hat and then instead of going into my head, took a side-slip, came out at one side, exploded and entered my left shoulder and neck, taking with it some pieces of my helmet. Altogether, I had about twenty-five bits of metal in me."[12] The medical staff often encountered patients with so many wounds that it looked like someone had stabbed and slashed their bodies with a knife over and over again.

———

The Western Front was filthy, and almost every injury caused by shell splinters and shrapnel balls was infected, as were many of the bullet wounds. The soil in Flanders and France had been enriched with fecal matter for centuries, and so when a bullet or piece of shell splinter struck a soldier, passing through his dirty uniform, his dirty skin, and into his body, it often carried bits of bacteria-ridden soil, cloth, wool, and waste into the wound. A soldier who lay untreated for a long period, wrote Captain Donald Hingston of the CAMC, almost always arrived with an infection that "rapidly becomes more foul and more virulent."[13] There were even cases in which high explosive shells, dismembering soldiers, transformed bone shards and teeth into projectiles that were embedded within other soldiers.[14]

It is said that generals of a current war prepare by training to refight the last one; the same might be said of military surgeons, who begin by planning for surgical procedures in the new conflict that mirror those of the last one. In the British army, the injuries in the South African War had been caused largely by rifle bullets.

Surgical experience on the veldt from 1899 to 1902 had found that the bullet wounds were often remarkably small, healed without major surgical intervention, and rarely infected.[15] A decade and a half later, on the Western Front, Lieutenant-Colonel John Alexander Gunn, a prewar militia officer and surgeon at the Winnipeg General Hospital, wrote that "in the early days of the war, when not only the medical service but the entire military organization was more or less handicapped by the delusion that the experiences gained in South Africa should form the basis of all wars in the future, conditions were such that this application of these ordinary surgical principles, which sounds most simple and easy, was, on the contrary, a most difficult undertaking."[16] Another surgeon observed more succinctly, "All the lessons of the South African War had to be unlearnt."[17]

Behind the Western Front, surgeons were confronted by infection almost every time they opened up the body. Although physicians' understanding of the germ theory had made vast improvements since the nineteenth century, this new plague of infected wounds was frustrating for doctors who had never encountered such horrors in civilian life. From the start of the war, tetanus killed many soldiers, with the victims suffering intense muscle spams. Soon the British and Canadian medical services were giving high doses of anti-tetanus serum to all patients to prevent lockjaw, with vaccination also assisting soldiers in fighting off the tetanus bacilli.[18]

While the war against tetanus was a great medical victory, the bacterial infection *Clostridium perfringens*, known as gas gangrene, was an insidious killer. Wounds became infected with a bacillus that broke down human tissue, releasing gas bubbles that swelled surrounding flesh to a grotesque size and produced a

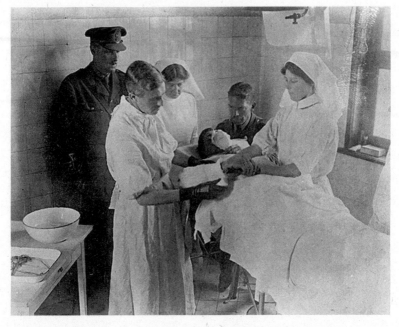

This Canadian surgical team of two nurses, a surgeon, and an anesthetist
work on a wounded solder from the Battle of the Somme.

gagging stench and staggering amounts of pus. With shell fragments lodged far within the body, along with the soil and dirty
bits of uniform dragged into the gaping hole, the septic infection
went deep. "The progress of the infection naturally varied a good
deal, but it generally worked with a frightful rapidity," said one
medical officer.[19] Another surgeon wrote about gas gangrene with
its "raging and often rancid suppuration," noting that once it took
hold it was almost impossible to save the patient.[20] A postwar
medical history concluded that when the infection was "deep-
seated," the infected limb became "hard, glistening white, and
cold as marble, and death always followed."[21]

Surgery was conducted in antiseptic theatres where patients
were mercifully rendered unconscious by chloroform or ether,

and, later in the war, by gas and oxygen anaesthesia. Nurses were trained in this difficult art; administering too much could lead to death, and Canadian women in uniform were among the leaders in the field.[22] While attentive care was given to the cleaning of wounds with saline solutions, this proved largely ineffective in preventing infections because the bacteria were driven too deep into the body. As a frustrated Canadian surgeon wrote early in the war, regarding the failure to stop the infections, "We are thus hurled back to the pre-Listerian era; to the era of unsutured wounds, early amputations, spreading cellulitis, and gangrene."[23] After skillfully wielding their bone saws and scalpels, surgeons watched in dismay as soldier after soldier died from infection, the nauseating stink of their rotting bodies filling the ward.

The medical services in all armies were forced to adapt. In early 1915 some success was achieved by radically cutting away the flesh around a wound. Through a process known as debridement, surgeons removed necrotic flesh and tissue to stop infection from spreading and to allow oxygen to kill the bacteria. A deep hole was gouged into the body, diseased flesh scooped out, and the pit continually flushed with saline. If injuries to arms and legs began to go black, with the discolouration indicating the infection coursing through the area, amputations were performed in the hope of lopping off the afflicted area. Men lost feet or hands, and if that did not stop the infection, the lower leg or arm was taken. A high thigh amputation was nearly impossible, but usually at that point a man was so weak from the previous interventions that he could not survive in any case.

British medical orderly Frederick Pottle described one operation to remove a shell fragment from a soldier's leg: "The surgeon goes after it with scalpel and scissors, excising all the damaged tissue with what looks like reckless abandon. As he cuts into muscle the blood spurts up like juice. . . . The surgeon probes with his finger between the muscle bundles for the shrapnel, and finally dislodges it, a jagged chunk of metal an inch square each way, with a great wad of cloth from the man's breeches clinging to it. He goes on, painstakingly removing every particle of clotted blood and tissue that has been damaged by the missile or the resulting infection."[24] The surgeon's assistant would raise and lower the leg, shining a light into the gaping wound, which grew with each scalpel cut. By the end of the operation the initial small entry wound was six inches long and four inches deep. While many surgeons acknowledged that this radical cutting away of flesh would deform bodies and make for a long recovery, in the age before antibiotics it was this or a gangrene death of horror beyond imagination.

———

"The head injuries were the most frightful," wrote Lieutenant-Colonel William Boyd, a trauma surgeon for part of the war, "for in some cases the greater part of the face was smashed in by shrapnel, while in others the nose, eye, and greater part of the cheek had been torn away, leaving a great red, bleeding cavity."[25] Patients arrived at the casualty clearing station or the hospital with appalling wounds to the head and brain, and these were usually only the men who had a chance at survival. Major Archibald, a recognized expert in brain surgery, wrote, "A man suffering from a direct hit going through and through the head rarely lived to get to the base."[26]

During the first two years of the war, no consensus emerged on how to deal with brain wounds. Most were fatal, especially as the trauma broke the skull and pushed parts of the swollen brain

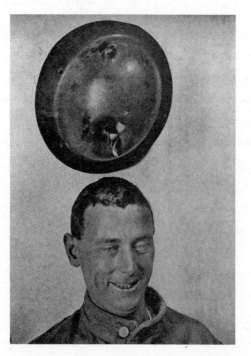

This lucky Canadian soldier shows his helmet that reduced the worst effects of a shell splinter.

through the hole, like toothpaste squeezed through a narrow opening. Irreparable damage was often done. But, surprisingly, not all died or suffered permanent brain damage. Through experimentation, surgeons found the chance of survival improved when the brain was left exposed for several days or even weeks and irrigated with saline.[27] The insertion into the brain of an aluminium tube, which was then left to drain, was found to be useful, especially since, as one surgeon wrote, "there is frequently present a lot of destroyed mushy brain tissue which sometimes in the course of a few days becomes mixed with a small amount of pus."[28] However, the course of treatment changed by 1917 through more study and practice, and it was felt that patients had a better chance of recovery if brain wounds were closed, with the hope that infection would be fended off by the body's immune system. Other types of head injuries were prevalent as well, although beginning in early 1916 steel helmets saved many soldiers. But the loss of an eye was distressingly common. Offering one of the many understatements of the medical war, surgeon Percy Bell of the CAMC remarked, "The pulping damage done to the eye by a rifle bullet is of course great."[29]

In the first half of the war, most soldiers shot in the chest or abdomen died before reaching surgical care. Early in 1915, Major Thomas Archibald Malloch of the CAMC, who enlisted at age twenty-eight and served at the front and in England, wrote that wounds to the abdomen almost always resulted in death, either from the trauma or from the perforated bowels emptying waste into the body, leading to sepsis. Of one sampling of wounded men, Malloch wrote early in the war that "all have been operated on and all have died."[30] Moreover, the pain was so terrible for these men with gut wounds that they were often not moved by stretcherbearers, who could not bear their screams of agony. Corporal Alfred Andrews, a prewar lawyer from Winnipeg, recounted the death of one friend: "The Hun shelled the mine head and Sonny got a piece in the stomach. Poor chap! He died hard. We gave him morphine but couldn't deaden the pain. I never saw any one in such pain as he was."[31] Even with many soldiers left at the front to die, Major Edward Archibald observed in 1916 that only about a third of patients with these wounds arriving at the clearing station lived: "The causes of death are shock, haemorrhage, peritonitis, intestinal obstruction of the paralytic type, gas gangrene of the wound, and pneumonia. It is a fearful gauntlet to run."[32]

In response to autopsies, lectures, official reports, and published articles, a consensus was built by mid-1916 that the only hope of saving more of these patients with abdominal wounds was to move surgery closer to the front, with the casualty clearing station increasingly becoming the surgical epicentre. Operating rapidly to remove fragments and foreign matter, clean the wound, and sew up the torn torso—abdomen or chest—led to survival rates rising dramatically.[33] Other surgical procedures were positively affected by this forward treatment, with the amputation rate for gunshot wounds to limbs, for instance, dropping from 25 percent in 1916 to 7 percent in 1917.[34] Often these soldiers were left to heal for a week and then moved on to a hospital further to the rear, where they were opened up again to ensure that infection had not set in. Even with this evolution in care, gut wounds were among the worst in the war, in terms of both pain and mortality rate. Nonetheless, doctors traversed a grim learning curve throughout the war, and as Major Archibald wrote of these wounds, "experience taught us gradually what to do and what not to do."[35]

Chest wounds also included injuries to the heart, and these were rarely mentioned in the literature, no doubt because almost all but the freakishly lucky did not survive. Wounds to the chest, torso, and thorax had been major killers early in the war, with as many as half of victims dying in hospitals and many more never making it to the surgeon.[36] As the war progressed, however, those struggling to breathe through blood-filled or collapsed lungs were given oxygen, which raised the odds of survival, although oxygen was in limited supply in most clearing stations or hospitals, with awful choices forced on doctors in deciding which patients should receive the limited stock.[37]

Lieutenant James Walter Skidmore, a prewar accountant from Cobourg, Ontario, was wounded in battle with a bullet through the upper thigh. It was a small entry wound, he wrote to his mother, but "it turned sideways and ripped quite a chunk of flesh, leaving a hole at the back nearly two inches in diameter." Though he had applied a tourniquet, he was still bleeding to death as he was transported to a casualty clearing station. Viewing the mass of soldiers on stretchers, he observed, "Many die before their turn comes, some though living can only be comforted."[38] He watched anxiously as doctors studied wounds and then sent some soldiers to the operating room while directing others to an area where they were left to perish, their injuries too grave or complex to be treated in the limited time available to deal with the crush of the wounded. Skidmore was one of the lucky ones and he survived the war. In these times of *Sturm und Drang*, the triage system was always in effect, and as one surgeon noted, "one abdomen, one laparotomy, means a whole hour devoted to an altogether uncertain result; it means, at most, half a chance of saving one man. An hour given to three other severe wounds means you will save three at least."[39] These were the grim odds of war, and ones that surgeons were forced to weigh during the mad rush of battle. It was often at the casualty clearing station that lives were saved and lost, with records revealing that 55 percent of deaths from wounds occurred in the clearing station or the field ambulance.[40] Later, in the quiet moments, the decisions over the soldiers' fate played out in nurses' and doctors' nightmares.

———

Shell explosions caused other almost unbelievable wounds. Sometimes the dead were found to have their bones nearly liquified and their bodies stretched far beyond their normal height. Corporal Archie MacKinnon of the 58th Battalion wrote to his sister after being knocked out on the Somme when a number of shells arrived in rapid succession to wipe out his entire machine-gun section. "I thought I was done for," MacKinnon confessed. "My leg was twisted around my neck and the blood was dripping down my arm. . . . My leg was not hit with the shell. It was the concussion that broke it. The skin isn't broke and will most likely be O.K. again as it is getting on fine and my arm only had 3 holes in it. That ain't much. I was lucky."[41]

One of the deadliest wounds was that of a fractured femur, and it was even more lethal if bone protruded from the skin. Early in the war, these injuries were almost always fatal because of the trauma to the body, the likelihood of infection or blood poisoning, and the difficulty of healing. "A bullet hitting the femur splinters the bone, as it does a glass bottle," wrote a Canadian radiologist who made a study of X-rays that captured bone damage. "At the same time the bullet breaks into pieces, and its fragments and those of the femur are scattered through the limb, or blown out through the skin as if an explosion had taken place."[42]

The frequency of leg wound cases gave surgeons new and intense experience in honing treatment, and revolutionary techniques were tested in special wards where the femur-wounded were grouped. In the first eighteen months of the war, surviving patients were usually sent to England for intensive care following attempts in France to set the bones and control infection. But the number of shattered femur cases rose with the increase in wounded

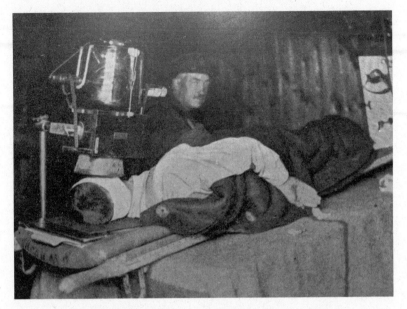

*A rare photograph of a patient with a head wound in
an X-ray machine at No. 3 General (McGill) Hospital.*

soldiers in the battles of 1916, and the high mortality rate meant that hospitals experimented with keeping patients in France to avoid the long and often lethal travel to Blighty. Gradual improvements in treatment were achieved and more patients survived, especially with the new techniques of cutting away flesh and the constant irrigation of wounds. A significant lifesaver was a new splint that allowed for the setting of bones more effectively. The Thomas splint, which was first used by the Canadians at Vimy Ridge in April 1917, provided a revolution in treatment. The splint encircled a damaged leg, allowing for fixation to a frame in an ambulance that decreased jostling of the patient. This revolutionary device was credited with reducing fatalities in femoral factures from 80 percent early in the war to 15.5 percent by 1918.[43]

The removal of foreign metal, clothing, and bits of uniform

was important for preventing infection. While X-rays were discovered in the late nineteenth century, the war saw the first mass employment of radiologists and their machines to provide a view into bodies that were often peppered with metal. "Two stretchers do nothing all day but carry cases to the X-Ray room to locate the exact position of the pieces of shell or bullet," wrote one Canadian orderly.[44] One of the most accomplished radiologists was Major Alexander Howard Pirie of Toronto, who enlisted at age thirty-nine and served with No. 3 Canadian General Hospital. His findings were published in medical journals during the war, including an important September 1917 article based on some 10,000 X-ray plates that he had taken of patients.[45] Pirie noted that, of that large number, "pieces of casing of shells, bombs, grenades, etc., . . . were shown on 3,846 plates." Highlighted by the X-rays, this metal could then be removed by surgeons.[46] Also found were foreign matter like belt buckles, the backsight of a rifle, chalk, and pewter (likely blown into the wound from a shattered drinking mug). In the latter part of the war, surgeons had success using X-ray plates and magnets to extract slivers of metal from internal organs.

If surgery failed or infection took hold, at some point only amputation would be left as an option. The surgical theatres often had pools of blood beneath the operating tables, with buckets filled with soiled bandages and occasionally an amputated limb. Official records tabulated the number of Canadian amputations performed by medical staff throughout the war. There were 2,780 cases of amputations, with 141 losing a hand, 667 losing an arm, 6 losing both arms, 11 losing both feet, 242 losing one foot, 1,675 losing one leg, 47 losing both legs, and 1 losing both arms and both legs.[47] These figures include only those who survived the operation, and they also exclude those who had limbs blown off

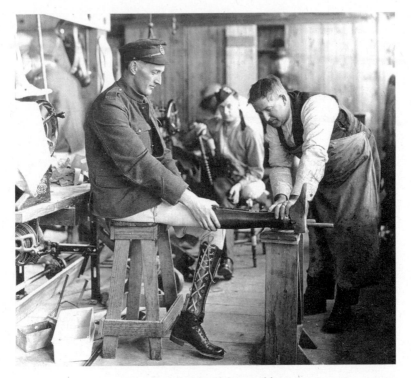

Prosthetic leg fitted for a soldier.

in battle by high explosive shells and those who received multiple bullet wounds, which could tear extremities from bodies.

———

The revolution in surgery was a staggering accomplishment that saved thousands of Canadian soldiers who would have died in earlier wars. By 1918 major advances in medical care had been achieved, so that wounds to the brain, gut, and femur that likely would have killed a soldier in 1914 or 1915 were now routinely survived. Of the 149,732 cases of wounded soldiers who arrived at a Canadian medical unit, all but 17,182 were saved.[48] This survival rate of over 90 percent was a triumph of care in such unthinkable circumstances. A soldier's odds were vastly in favour of living if he made it to surgical care, although more so at the end of the war than at the start. And British statistics show that about 82 percent of the wounded and 93 percent of the sick and injured were able to return to some form of duty.[49] Medical interventions that saved lives and returned soldiers to the front were a significant contribution to the ongoing manpower shortages, even if statistics must always be interpreted, interrogated, and contextualized. For instance, the statistics do not include the countless Canadians and others who were left to die on the battlefield, who expired at the regimental aid post, or who did not survive the journey to the field ambulance.

"The war demanded a constant evolution in care, treatment, procedures," wrote CAMC surgeon John Alexander Gunn.[50] Medical staff underwent an intense learning process, and most doctors wrote openly about their struggle to adapt in the middle of the storm, lecturing and publishing about their successes and failures and drawing widely upon French, British, and other medical advances. New surgical techniques pioneered in the charnel house of the Western Front led to many victories in innumerable battles against wounds and infections. And yet few surgeons would have disagreed with Colonel George Armstrong of the CAMC, who remarked, "Medicine has advanced—but at what a cost."[51]

CHAPTER 7

COLLECTING SOLDIERS' BODY PARTS

When George Gibson enlisted in July 1915, he was twenty-six years old and living in Winnipeg with his wife, Ethel May Gibson. He gave his trade as a farmer and an electrician, stood five foot six, had blue eyes and fair hair, and weighed 130 pounds. He served overseas as a private with the 78th Battalion and was shot in the spine near Vimy Ridge, on April 7, 1917, two days before the titanic battle. Gibson survived the initial wound and was rushed to medical care. Following emergency surgery at a casualty clearing station, a doctor assessed his condition and noted "immediate loss of power in both legs."[1] Paralyzed from the waist down, his wounds were dressed daily, but the damage to the spine left him "with no sphincter control and with complete loss of motion and sensation in his limbs." On April 22—more than two weeks after the terrible injury—he was still listed as "seriously ill." Four months later, in August, his doctors expressed optimism when he was able to wiggle the small toes on his left foot. But he would soldier no more and his personnel file notes he was discharged on August 22, 1917, by a medical board at the Ontario

Military Hospital in Orpington, Kent, from where he was to be invalided to Canada. He did not make it. At Orpington on September 29, nurses found the first signs of an infection, and his weakened body was unable to fight it off. After weeks of intermittent fever and seeming recovery, Gibson died on October 23, 1917, at age twenty-eight. He was buried at Orpington (All Saints) Churchyard, with his headstone reading, "HE LIVES WITH US IN MEMORY AND WILL FOR EVERMORE BY HIS LOVING WIFE."

"In the event of my decease," Gibson's last will and testament read, "I hereby bequeath all my property and effects to my wife Ethel May Gibson." The widow received her husband's personal goods—and, after the war, his medals. Like so many widows and loved ones, Ethel knew that her husband was buried overseas, and her selected epitaph provides a brief glimpse into her pain and her desire to remember George. What Ethel May Gibson did not know was that her husband's entire body was not buried in the graveyard. George's spine had been extracted from his body and sent first to London, England, and, later, to Montreal, Quebec, as a pathological sample for a future museum.[2] While it is unlikely that Ethel ever visited her husband's grave, as international travel was very rare in the 1920s, curious medical students at McGill probably studied her husband's shattered spine.

This harvesting of body parts was done without the consent of slain soldiers and their loved ones, none of whom were alerted to these actions. While enlistment in the Canadian Expeditionary Force gave the army control over a soldier's body, the military's snatching of body parts for medical study is a shocking revelation. This was not grave robbing in the deep of night, but an open act of forcing dead soldiers to once again serve their country: having fallen in combat they were now to contribute to victories in future medical battles. This story is told here in full for the first time, drawing upon long-buried archival records to provide a better understanding of the medical war that raged in the name not only of saving lives but also of advancing knowledge through the snatching of soldiers' bodies. It is troubling in many ways, as the reader shall see.

———

The dead held many secrets to life. There was a long tradition in medicine of studying bodies ravaged by disease or traumatized by injuries, in the interest of advancing knowledge. In civilian hospitals, post-mortem autopsies were so common as to be almost obligatory when patients died from injuries or illness that was difficult to determine, with pathologists ordered to open up bodies to ascertain causes of death. As part of this process, which was deeply embedded in physicians' education, museums of pathology and medicine had been established across the world since the 1800s.[3] These museums displayed specimens of tissue and bone for study and schooling.[4]

McGill was Canada's leading medical university in the early twentieth century, having made its reputation under the internationally renowned Canadian-born doctor William Osler, the foremost physician and medical scholar of his time. Osler taught at McGill from 1874 to 1884 before moving to Johns Hopkins Medical School, where he became a celebrity. He taught extensively from the cold autopsy room, cutting open cadavers and explaining to his students how diseases presented in the body, how they might be diagnosed, and how they might be better treated.[5]

Medical schools in Canada and around the world relied on corpses stolen from freshly dug graves or on shady deals involving the bodies of the poor and indigent. These remains were sold by "resurrection men," body snatchers, and other grave robbers, although this was a great outrage to many Canadians who saw this as a desecration of the body and an affront to societal and religious norms.[6]

At McGill, professor of pathology John George Adami instructed countless students turned doctors after he began teaching there in 1892 at age thirty. As a recognized leader in the field of medicine throughout the British Empire, Adami created a cutting-edge department, and in 1899 he hired Maude Abbott as assistant curator of the McGill Medical Museum, which had been

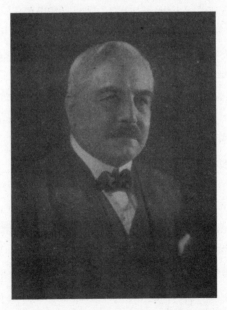

Dr. John George Adami, who served as a colonel in the CAMC and was responsible for coordinating the collection of Canadian soldiers' body parts during the war.

created around a core of Osler's teaching specimens.[7] Professor Abbott would become a leading expert on congenital cardiac disease, and Adami and Abbott would be involved in the curation, study, and display of Canadian soldiers' body parts.[8] With the act of collecting pathological samples for study and display long established in the medical profession, neither Adami nor Abbott gave any thought to the ethical ramifications of harvesting these citizen-soldiers who had already given their all in the crusade for victory.

The Canadian program of collecting body parts overseas was led by Adami, who had acquired some fame at a young age for being exposed to rabies and publishing an account of the disease as it coursed through his body. Much admired in the medical profession, he researched widely and published in many journals.[9] His *Textbook of Pathology* (1912), co-written with John McCrae, who would go on to worldwide fame with his wartime poem "In Flanders Fields," was much consulted, and one doctor commented at the time that it was "easily one of the best and most widely known" texts on pathology.[10] Adami was a fellow of Britain's Royal Society and the Royal Society of Canada, and he enlisted in Montreal on March 5, 1915. The burly five-foot-five-inch-tall professor was fifty-three years old and in no shape to serve in France, but his influence ensured a spot in the CEF.[11]

Lieutenant-Colonel Adami had many duties as a staff officer in England, although primarily he served as assistant director of medical services in charge of records at the CAMC headquarters in London. In that capacity, he worked closely with the British medical services, with which the CAMC was intricately entwined through the sharing of knowledge and the interchange of patients and medical practitioners both along the battle front and in England. The Royal Army Medical Corps (RAMC) had established the British Medical History Committee in November 1914, and it was mandated to gather information for a forthcoming series of histories to document the medical legacy of the war. In fact, Adami had written to his friend William Osler, who from 1905 was Regius chair of medicine at Oxford University, to urge the British to write a multi-volume history of the medical war for future generations of students.[12] With an eye on an unwritten historical series, documents were to be archived, along with medical information, especially statistics on aspects of wounding and healing.[13] Grounded in empirical data, the medical struggle to save lives also involved the study and processing of information.[14] As part of this creation and codification of knowledge for wartime use and postwar lessons, the Imperial committee agreed that it would also encourage the gathering of pathological samples—its traditional teaching tools—to illustrate case studies in the histories.[15] From the first months of the war, the senior British medical generals put plans into place to use the great clash as a teaching experience and to select body parts from those soldiers killed in battle to not only inform the history but to be put on display in a future medical museum.

On April 19, 1915, the Committee on the Medical History of the War issued its first circular to the Empire's medical services, advising doctors in uniform of the comprehensive history to be written. It also asked that "pathological specimens from Medical or Surgical cases illustrating points of Military interest" be sent to the Royal Army Medical College in London.[16] The history committee was especially interested in "specimens of entrance and exit wounds to the skin," "wounds of nerves," and "wounds of jaws." Lieutenant-Colonel Adami was included in these discussions as the Canadian representative on the committee. Upon his arrival in

1915, and were directed especially to the casualty clearing stations and hospitals, as these were the units where surgery was conducted most frequently and many already had a pathological section. But what authority did the military have to collect slain soldiers' body parts? The truth was that the signing of the attestation paper by every member of the CEF gave the military control over the soldier's body. Few if any soldiers seem to have given any thought to the implications of this permission-granting, as the act of signing is almost entirely absent from descriptions in enlisted men's letters, diaries, and memoirs, but they came to understand the consequences of accepting army discipline as they were ordered about, forced to accept vaccinations, and even subjected to punishment outside of civilian law. In fact, military discipline and punishment allowed for penalties as harsh as death by firing squad for military crimes like striking an officer or deserting one's post. Very different rules indeed governed the lives of those in uniform, and one articulate Australian officer, Frederic Manning, was not wrong in observing that soldiers no longer had control over "their own bodies, which had become mere implements of warfare."[21]

Amid the avalanche of wounded soldiers, the headquarters' demands for body parts were not initially a high priority for most medical units.[22] However, thousands of soldiers were killed or injured every day along the Western Front, even in the quiet periods between the large campaigns, and the Canadians' share of that daily total was usually several dozen casualties. A number of Canadian specimens began to arrive at the Royal College of Surgeons by late summer of 1915, among the first noteworthy organs being corrupted lungs that revealed the novel and devastating effects of chlorine gas.[23] As a gifted orator and writer, not to

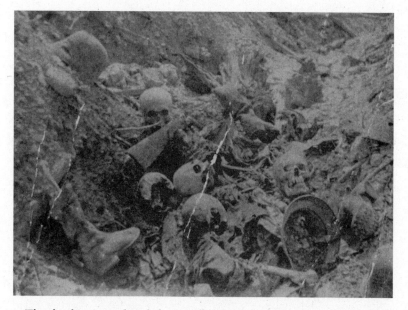

*The shocking casualties led to a callous attitude towards the dead, with
their remains often left unburied on battlefields or interred in mass graves.*

mention a leader in the field of medicine in Canada and Britain,
the influential Adami was not satisfied with the slow trickle of
body parts to London, and he continued to push his fellow
Canadians to gather pathological samples. Moreover, Adami was
energized after seeing the first battlefield specimens at the Royal
College in late October, and the professor believed that Canadian
universities, especially McGill, should receive their fair share of
these pathological samples for educational purposes. He pressed
Keith, the Royal College's curator of the new collection, for control of the Canadian body parts and he succeeded, noting in his
diary on October 23, 1915, "The agreement is that men may now
collect specimens in the different Hospitals for their own museums, these to be recognized as national property."[24]

With this new verbal agreement among Canadian doctors to gather Canadian body parts to keep for their universities or hospitals, further orders went out to the CAMC officers, instructing them to redouble their efforts to select organs and bones. These pieces of young Canadian soldiers were viewed as teaching tools that would offer lessons for future generations and that could even be used in this wasteful war to save lives through the application of better surgical techniques. For safe-keeping, the samples would first go to the Royal College, where they would be treated, preserved, and put on display for all the Empire's medical officers.[25] Canadian doctors sometimes dropped into the college to read from its medical library and to view the specimens, but Adami had concerns over the fate of these pathological samples once they passed into Imperial hands. As these medical samples were priceless, he feared the Imperials would never part with them. Adami was increasingly adamant that they had to be transferred to Canada—perhaps, as he argued from late 1915, to form the basis for a new national medical museum. Adami revealed his thinking when he wrote on November 23, 1915, to Major John James Ower of No. 1 Canadian General Hospital that the pathologist should guard the specimens for a future Canadian war museum. To increase their value, medical officers were also to record the names of the slain soldiers "to whom the specimen belonged in life." Adami finished the letter with an admonition to remain vigilant: "Wherefore hang on to your specimens by all the excuses you can make until this letter comes out. And keep a good heart!"[26] By that, he meant to encourage Ower, although Adami was particularly interested in the collection of hearts for future study, especially those with the bedevilling ailment known as "soldiers' heart"—a weakening of the cardiac muscle, caused by the strain of long service, that seemed both a physical illness and a psycho-somatic one as it was sometimes linked with mental injuries.[27]

Throughout 1916, memoranda instructed Canadian medical officers on how better to engage in the work of dissecting, stabiliz-ing, labelling, and transferring the soldiers' organs. As a promi-nent McGillite, Adami leaned heavily on his former students and colleagues, and he often wrote personally to them in a mixture of praise, pleading, and scolding. They responded with promises to collect more pathological samples, and the surviving archival doc-umentation has yielded no evidence of objections or concerns raised about the morality of such actions. That is not surprising since all of Adami's medical colleagues had been trained to under-stand both the importance of the post-mortem in revealing the trauma inflicted on bodies and how this knowledge could be used to save more lives. While these medical officers often responded to Adami's letters with an affirmation that they were carrying out the work and that they had specimens preserved at their medical units, many had not figured out how to transfer them to London. There were cases like that of Captain F.M. Auld, who was serving with a British medical unit and who had discovered an interesting case of tuberculosis of the lungs.[28] The captain had carefully extracted the lungs and was anxious to show Adami the fascinating disease-induced deformities, but the organ had to remain with him until a courier could get the preserved lungs safely out of France. Auld's letter reveals that some pathological samples were selected not because they exposed war wounds but instead because the cadaver had been opened and the doctor had encountered something worth preserving to explain some other medical mystery.

To rally support and stimulate the collection of good pieces of killed soldiers, Adami toured the front in the early summer of

1916, visiting hospitals and medical units. He met one group of medical officers in June 1916, in the aftermath of the Battle of Mount Sorrel, where some 8,000 Canadians had been killed or wounded in a two-week-long battle. He told them brightly that, to date, "quite a good collection has been brought together, containing some valuable specimens."[29] Adami continued to emphasize the importance of the doctors' including the clinical history of the soldier, information on the autopsy (how long, for instance, did the pathologists wait to harvest the organs after death?), and information on the surgeon performing the work.[30] At the same time, Adami encouraged the officers at the front to use the body parts in the emerging teaching symposiums that were occurring in units. For some young doctors, this was a continuation of their studies, as senior physicians offered lectures and demonstrations, and often the speakers presented the pathological samples as part of their learned talks with the goal of improving treatment.[31] For instance, at No. 1 Canadian General Hospital on November 1, 1916, several cases were presented—including a set of preserved lungs showing a bullet's trajectory. Major John James Ower, with whom Adami communicated frequently, spoke to a group of medical men about the wound path of bullets burrowing through the lungs, which were halved to reveal the interior. He spoke about other wounds drawn from human specimens, including an autopsied brain that showed an unusually "large ulcerating tract in the front lobe," as the brain had been savagely pulped by a shell splinter.[32] Major Ower was one of the most enthusiastic supporters of the program, and in 1917 alone he conducted 260 autopsies, many of which led to the removal of pathological samples for the future Canadian museum.[33]

The Canadians and the British were not alone in this scientific pursuit of gathering pathological samples, with the French having

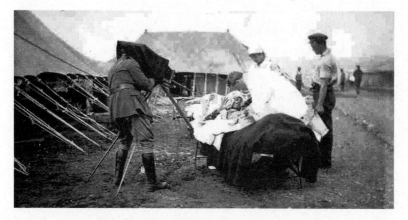

A wounded patient being photographed, possibly for
propaganda, documentation, or as part of a medical study.

their own program that collected over 10,000 specimens from
their own soldiers by war's end.[34] American medical authorities
also engaged in the practice after arriving on the Western Front in
late 1917, with doctors first visiting Adami, among others, for
guidance on best practices. The Germans, too, were carrying out
these autopsies through their own medical networks, eventually
collecting some 6,000 specimens.[35] Little of this was known to
soldiers at the front, but a virulent and malicious rumour was
planted by the British to be used against the Kaiser's armies, which
said that the slain German soldiers were being ground up and
melted down into fats for the war effort.[36] It was a macabre story
that spread rapidly and that was only revealed to be a hoax after
the war, although, as indicated in the multinational body-part
collecting programs, what was described was not far beyond the
known reality of how some soldiers' bodies were treated on the
Western Front.

Throughout early 1917, more samples moved from the British
and dominion medical units to the Royal College of Surgeons in

London, with the collection growing to 1,500 objects by mid-year.[37] "As the specimens arrived," curator Arthur Keith explained, "they were numbered, registered, and suitably stored, every effort being made to obtain and keep a full history of each specimen." The collection revealed all manner of injuries, and Keith was most pleased with the 688 wet samples—organ, tissue, and flesh—that revealed damage wrought by projectiles, shrapnel, and shell fragments. Another 467 items were reconstructions of shattered bones.[38] Keith shared his vision for these teaching resources, noting that "such specimens are original documents; they constitute an original and reliable source of knowledge for all time and they supply the most valuable basis possible for present and future medical and surgical treatment of the diseases and injuries of war,

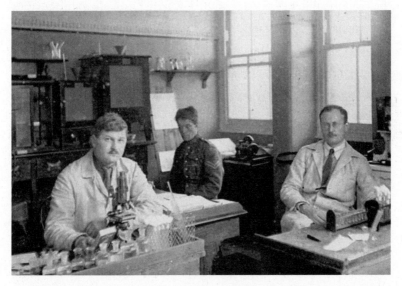

All of the Canadian hospitals had a pathological section where medical officers engaged in scientific study of bacteria, infections, and other medical mysteries. This photograph captures researchers in the pathology laboratory at the Ramsgate hospital in England.

and are, therefore, to be recognized as the basis of its medical history."[39] Few medical men would have disagreed with his assessment, though the general public would likely have been less enthusiastic about the harvesting of body parts from citizen-soldiers fighting in the defence of Crown and country and using them as medical samples to be displayed in jars.

Within the CAMC were a number of doctors who took to the work with zeal. Pathologist Major Laurence Joseph Rhea served at No. 3 General Hospital, which had been raised at McGill and had close ties to Adami. Major Rhea selected samples with much enthusiasm, applying his professional focus on the delicate process of arranging bone specimens. After a bone was removed from a soldier's body, the flesh was cleaned from it and the sample was then mounted for observation. The process was akin to making models of human bones, and the doctor was skilled at reconstructing broken bones to illustrate how steel and lead had cracked and shattered them.[40] Throughout the war, Major Rhea gave lectures to other doctors using pathological samples extracted from the corpses of soldiers, and he wrote an important report on brain injuries and the need for steel helmets after studying fifteen autopsied soldiers' brains, some of which were later sent to the Royal College.[41] He thought the work so important that for a while he refused to send his collection of bones and brains to the Imperials, instead hatching a plan with another surgeon to take it out of the country in their luggage. Adami had to lightly scold him and insist that the British could be trusted to send the samples to Canada after the war, although in private he expressed his worries too.[43] As a testament to the value of Rhea's work, Sir Andrew Macphail, a wartime medical officer, professor at McGill, and man of letters, described his pathological samples as "unique in the history of

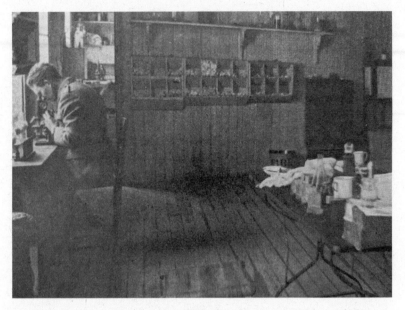

Major Laurence Rhea looking through a microscope in the pathology department at No. 3 Canadian General Hospital. Rhea was one of the champions of collecting soldiers' body parts for a future museum.

war, and a brilliant example of the triumph of personal skill and intelligent collaboration over serious difficulties."[43]

———

The unprecedented mass death caused by industrial weapons was creating unique learning opportunities, and these lessons would be codified in both a multi-volume history and the pathological collection. "The amount of material promises to be of extraordinary extent and value," wrote Lieutenant-Colonel Adami of the many pathological samples from slain soldiers.[44] Adami occasionally referenced the importance of the American Civil War collection of human specimens at the Army Medical Museum in

Washington, which he had visited before the war, as well as its display of war-related objects, artifacts, photographs, and material.[45] Beginning in late 1915, Adami wrote repeatedly to senior military medical officers in Ottawa about the need for a suitable medical museum in Ottawa.[46] The headquarters staff officers in Canada's capital were at first little interested in a museum, as they were scrambling to raise and equip new units, but Adami kept up a steady barrage of progress reports on the pathological collection and its enduring worth to the medical profession. Persuaded by Adami's leadership in the field, his considerable wartime influence, and evidence of the success of the Royal College collection, authorities in Ottawa agreed in January 1916 to a future museum that would memorialize the actions of the thousands serving in the medical services.[47] The heart of the museum would be the pathological samples, which would remain as unique teaching tools.

Adami was inspired by the work of the multi-millionaire expatriate Sir Max Aitken (Lord Beaverbrook from early 1917), who had been appointed the Canadian official "eye-witness" at the front, a designation that he expanded to include record keeper, archivist, and publicist of the Dominion forces.[48] Aitken was a mischievous kingmaker who was a newspaper baron and a friend to the leading Canadian and British Conservatives. Seeking to raise the profile of the Canadian forces, Minister of Militia Sam Hughes made him an honorary colonel and Aitken travelled the front in early 1915, writing newspaper accounts of the Canadians, especially their heroic and costly actions at the Battle of Second Ypres in the face of the enemy gas attack.[49] These accounts were popular among English-language readers, with Aitken turning them into a best-selling book, *Canada in Flanders* (1916), which sold over 250,000 copies.

In early 1916, Aitken began to grapple with the British high command because of its stringent desire to control the message around the fighting through censorship. The little Canadian millionaire wanted to have official painters, cinematographers, photographers and historians, all in uniform, who would go to the front to publicize and document the war effort. Aitken defeated the generals, and in the summer of 1916 he sent his band of artists and historians to the front to, as he later wrote, lay "down the bedrock of history."[50] Seeing Aitken's success, Adami tried to follow suit by creating a medical officer position whose full-time role would have been to gather body parts. But even though Ottawa had signalled its commitment to establishing a museum,

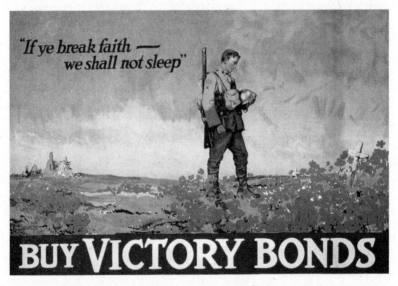

"If ye break faith — we shall not sleep"

BUY VICTORY BONDS

A Victory Bond poster that draws on John McCrae's poem "In Flanders Fields" in urging Canadians to support the war effort. In this image, a Canadian soldier pays his respects at a comrade's grave, surrounded by poppies. Few Canadians could imagine that fallen Canadian soldiers were being dissected, their organs removed and used in medical study.

they evidently did not see the value in a body-snatching officer, and the request was denied. Adami took the setback in stride and agreed that Canadian pathological samples would continue to go to the Royal College, to be cared for, catalogued, and stored, and then sent back to Canada at the end of the war.[51]

———

"You can hardly move anywhere without stepping into a pile of bones or some other sign of our dearly beloved departed, very few of them English though, all German and French, we can always tell by the clothing and equipment they have on." A former medical student at the University of Toronto, Claude Williams wrote to his mother in Edmonton, Alberta, revealing his "morbid" fascination with corpses. "I used to go searching about everywhere for good specimens of bone for my collection, I now have nearly a whole skeleton rigged under my bed, the worst of it is he is a composite of a French and Hun." This was not a normal activity, even if soldiers became calloused to the unburied dead who jutted from trench walls, hanging respirators off a femur bone or striking a match off the leathered scalp of a corpse. Williams, with his medical training and perhaps other urges, tried to justify his actions, noting, "It is funny how hardened and accustomed you do become to these things though, the sight is so familiar that you never think twice about it, but I must stop."[52] While he understood that his bone collection was likely an indecent act among his fellow soldiers, perhaps he was using it to better understand the human body for his eventual return to medical school. Lieutenant-Colonel Adami also had no such shame, with his bone and organ collection drawn from Canadian soldiers harvested in the name of advancing medicine. Given the circumstances of the mass death in the war and the need to further knowledge, he gave little thought to consent or to the sanctity of the body. Despite the setback of being denied a body-snatching officer to assist in his work, Adami would continue to pressure Canadian doctors to harvest corpses throughout the war in the name of progressing scientific medicine and drawing tangible medical lessons from the killing fields of the Western Front. Canadian soldiers would not likely have been so supportive of the possibility that, should they be wounded in action and brought to a lifesaver, and should the doctor fail to save them, their bodies would be ripe for scientific scavenging.

CHAPTER 8

THE MANY BATTLES OF THE MIND

"Real shell shock is a horrible thing," wrote Sergeant Lawrence Rogers to his wife in August 1916. "If you ever saw a man suffering from it, I don't think you would ever forget it."[1] Rogers was a senior orderly to a regimental medical officer, and he often joined his officer in assessing the wounded during the daily sick parade. In that capacity, he observed soldiers who had broken down from debilitating wounds to the mind. The prolonged stress of trench warfare eroded men's ability to endure, a problem exacerbated by the lack of sleep, the harsh conditions of living outside all year round, the dirt and deprivation, and, most importantly, the constant fear of death and maiming. The mental collapse was labelled "shell shock" early in the war, a term that emerged in the language of soldiers and physicians who grappled with this mystifying wound that laid low combat soldiers and gallant leaders. Once healthy and vibrant soldiers became increasing gaunt, red-eyed with fatigue, slow of speech, and plagued with strange facial tics and twitches. A dazed stare, increased stammering, frequent trembling, and wild mood swings followed. And then it got worse.

One British medical officer noted that, in the early part of the war, "We did not bother about men's minds," and the generals initially put little stock in doctors who specialized in explaining away the breakdown of the fighting man through psychoanalysis.[2] Through training and discipline, the military system pushed soldiers physically and mentally, and the ethos of the army demanded that soldiers tough it out no matter the strain.[3] It was therefore perplexing to see men succumb to this unseen injury. To explain the mental collapse, soldiers and doctors at first diagnosed shell shock as a physical wound to the brain caused by a high explosive shell blast—the "shock" of a "shell." In some

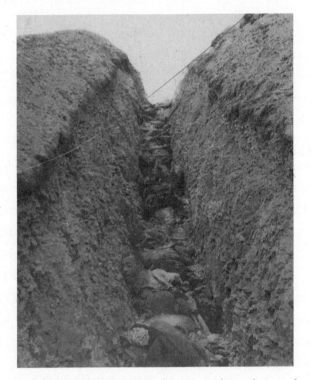

The relentless brutality at the front wore down the morale and fighting efficiency of even the most resolute of soldiers.

soldiers that was in fact the case, and there was ample evidence of the concussing blast of shells rendering men insensible. In the aftermath of bombardments, survivors were sometimes unable to walk, had trouble concentrating, and presented other physical ailments. These were tangible wounds and thus an acceptable reason for the victims to exit the front for recuperation. However, shell shock also manifested itself in soldiers who were not blown up by a shell and who were instead steadily worn down by the combat experience.

A complex and contested wound, shell shock could be both physical and mental, and it also seemed to affect soldiers differently, making it even more difficult to understand, diagnose, and treat. Some civilians and soldiers believed that the shell shocked were simply faking their symptoms to get out of the line, while others saw links to prewar discussions around hysteria—often ascribed to women—or other mental imbalances. Viewed through this lens, the individual, not the war, was to blame. At the same time, other experts believed it was the frightening and lethal environment that was scarring men's minds. Captain Colin Russel, a professor of clinical neurology at McGill University and a specialist responsible for shell-shocked patients at Granville hospital, believed it was "exposure to, or the expectancy of being exposed to grave danger, danger clothed in such terrifying forms as a human nature has seldom been called upon to face previous."[4] In the absence of a clear diagnosis or treatment, shell shock remained a puzzling injury. The generals turned to the medical officers to make sense of these wounds, but then turned on the doctors, viewing them as part of the problem because of their perceived leniency.

———

The generals had little sympathy for soldiers who suffered from mental collapse, often blaming the men for having failed to live up to the ideals of the warrior. These masculine concepts infused all aspects of the army—from recruitment to training to sticking it out in the trenches. In the eyes of many senior commanders, breaking down in response to the ordeal must be the fault of the individual and not the environment. And some military medical officers agreed, looking for defects in the victims: a lack of character, education, or breeding; prewar signs of mental illness or venereal disease; a propensity for drinking; or a lack of "the right nerve," however that was defined. Sometimes these features were present; more often, the doctors could not find the flaw and began to suspect other factors were at play.

Soldiers were also unsure about these wounds, although all witnessed the shattering effects of shellfire and the slow drumbeat of comrades felled by snipers, poison gas, or furious combat. Victor Wheeler, a rifleman and signals operator in the 50th Battalion, recounted one near-death experience when a mortar bomb landed in his trench. The explosion sent shock waves in all directions, hurling him into the mud. When he came to and looked for survivors, he stumbled upon his friend Tom, who was sitting upright in the trench, but, in Wheeler's words, had "lost his mind." Tom was carried out of the trenches to a dressing station. "He was in a pitiful state of shock," observed Wheeler. Each time a shell landed nearby, "Tom dived to the ground and tried to crawl under the trench mats."[5] His fingernail-ripping digging frenzy and wild stare left all the men shaken. Indeed, a bad case of shell shock was, in the words of Ernest Black of the 41st Battery, Canadian Field Artillery, "an unnerving thing to see."[6] When a soldier's mind was torn, it was a stark reminder to other worn-down soldiers of their own unending battle against a mental breakdown. Lance-Corporal Charles Savage, a long-time survivor of the trenches, wrote that what he "feared more than anything else was his own nerves. Every time he saw one of his old companions crack and go to pieces under the strain, the terrifying question arose, 'Shall I be the next one?'" His main worry was not that he might be hit by a bullet or shell, but "that he wouldn't be able to hang on until he did get hit."[7]

The war provided enough raw horror to drive men to insanity, but after months of attritional trench warfare, most soldiers at the front also believed that they had, in a phrase of the day, "done their bit." Though the concept of a limited tour for a soldier is a relatively recent one, what of the other men in uniform behind the lines, in England, or in Canada, and the many more who had not enlisted? Why, the soldiers at the front might rightly have asked, were they meant to suffer without end? Some came to see a Blighty wound as an honourable escape. As one trench warrior said of these wounds, "I suppose a man is justified in saying he's got off lightly when what he expected was death."[8] Another Canadian, George Ormsby, who was shot through the arm and back on the Somme, shared his thoughts with his wife in a letter: "I consider that I have done my share, 1 ½ years in the trenches and fought four big battles in that time—a record which very few can show. . . . The Somme is a dreadful place, the man that gets a decent wound there is lucky as I certainly consider myself."[9] The hope for a Blighty was well known to all soldiers and medical officers, and was such a commonly expressed sentiment that the high command worried that some desperate soldiers courted such

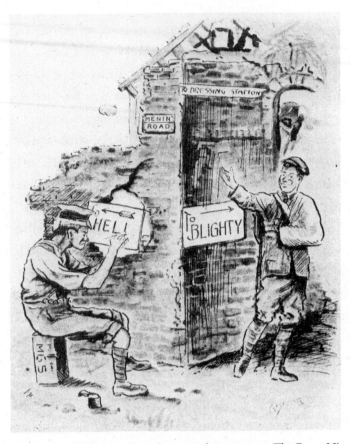

A wartime cartoon from a Canadian trench newspaper, The Forty-Niner, *captures the soldiers' dark humour. One arrow points to the front, "Hell," while the wounded soldier cheerfully wishes his mate goodbye as he heads to the rear with his Blighty wound.*

wounds to escape. As it took considerable courage to drink poison or deliberately injure oneself, faking shell shock was thought to be a less painful route to the rear.

Regimental medical officers held the role of gatekeeper in sending shell-shocked soldiers for medical help.[10] They were ordered to distinguish those who exaggerated symptoms from those with legitimate mental wounds, to be released from the line. Even though few medical officers had prewar exposure to injuries like this, many were sympathetic to the soldiers, especially to those who had been at the front for some time. A senior Canadian officer, John Taylor Fotheringham, who would command the medical services after the war, wrote about the doctor's challenge of assessing each man's "moral element"—from those whose "sensitiveness is due to faulty endowment and faulty training from his childhood up" to the deceitful malingerers—while balancing his desire to "avoid injustice to the deserving sufferer."[11] But even with their inclination to help the "old soldiers," as long-service men were sometimes known, the doctors worried, if all the soldiers of the front were allowed to go to the rear because they could not hack it, wouldn't the entire army eventually disintegrate?

From the start of the war, the medical officers worked with regimental officers in the domains of care, sanitation, and discipline. While it was a foolish commanding officer who did not follow his doctor's advice on those matters, a battalion's officers were more involved in dealing with the challenge of mental wounds. Writing on the subject, two Canadian medical officers noted that the unit's physician and the colonel could usually work out an arrangement on what to do with soldiers on the verge of breakdown, except "when the medical officer has a difficult commanding officer or where he himself is perverse or tactless."[12] The final comment here was meant to refer to medical officers who were not tough enough on the privates, letting too many slip through the sick parade to rest behind the lines. This softness implied that the medical officer was not committed to his task of protecting a battalion's strength. With such pressure, the medical officers were often forced to be rigid, although it should be noted that many of the commanding officers were also sympathetic to the soldiers in the battalion. And yet all of these leaders at the front were caught in the vice of war, where it was necessary to keep men in the firing line. One medical officer summed up the challenge: "To hold a middle course is difficult—between injustice to the man and injustice to the service."[13]

———

In 1915 the medical officers diagnosed and sent to hospital 642 Canadian soldiers for shell shock.[14] It was a significant number of the total non-fatal wounded, and many suffered from this injury in the aftermath of the Battle of Second Ypres with its many days of intense warfare. Medical officer George Nasmith observed that some of his friends in the infantry "were greatly changed in appearance, were very tired and could tell little of their experiences . . . one of my officer comrades had gone insane, and another had been so shell shocked that he was of no further use and had to be sent to England."[15] Even the tough and disciplined John McCrae was beset by deep exhaustion and a mental wound that smothered his prewar good humour and sunny outlook. Struggling with his dark thoughts, McCrae wrote, "One feels a kind of blind anger which one cannot vent upon anyone."[16] In 1915 and the first half of 1916, those men with invisible injuries were usually evacuated to England to be treated in special hospitals, although this meant that they were lost to their units for, at a minimum, months, and often for the entire war.

By early 1916, the problem of mental wounds was becoming more pressing. The April 1916 Battle of St. Eloi—a forlorn two-week struggle in soupy mud amid constant enemy shellfire—saw

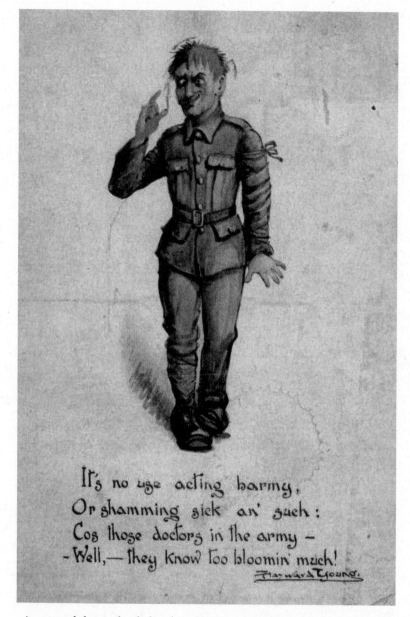

A postcard that makes light of a soldier malingering with a mental wound. It reads, "It's no use acting barmy, / or shamming sick an' such: / Cos those doctors in the army— / —Well,—they know too bloomin' much!"

heavy shell shock casualties, while the 3rd Canadian Infantry Division was thrashed in its first major engagement at Mount Sorrel, in the southern part of the Ypres salient, from June 2 to 13. The fighting cost some 8,000 casualties to the Canadian Corps, and Major-General Arthur Currie's battle-hardened 1st Canadian Division, which was thrown into the battle to stabilize the line and drive back the enemy, reported that 44.6 percent of its total losses—532 cases—were due to shell shock.[17] This was rightly viewed as a crisis by the high command, and other British and dominion forces reported much higher shell shock figures during the long and costly Battle of the Somme.

The generals, terrified that their army was collapsing, increasingly blamed the medical officers for being too lenient on the soldiers, and even some medical officers believed the diagnosis of shell shock to be overused. Captain Harold W. McGill, medical officer for the 31st Battalion and generally a friend to the privates, wrote that "a number of men [were] buried by shell explosions or otherwise put out of action without having sustained an open wound. . . . Of these there was [only] one to whom the much-abused term 'shell-shock' could properly be applied. Often the term was used to describe a condition that was nothing but terror."[18] Captain McGill's observation reveals the challenge of accurately identifying the wound but also the banality of terror at the front, where a massive shell explosion was simply part of the day-to-day experience and soldiers were meant to withstand such trauma no matter the physical or mental cost.

Private William Hemmings of the Canadian Machine Gun Corp wrote after the war about the difficult choices facing the soldiers at the front, remarking, "In the First World War you either went forward or got shot." There was no opting out, and in Hemmings's opinion, "some were just more mentally prepared than others. It was like a man who has led a scholarly life all of a sudden getting involved in a gang fight. It could be quite a scary experience."[19] It was indeed, and many medical officers came to this same conclusion. As the medical officers witnessed more and more cases, doctors believed that shell shock was often the result of a soldier's internal battle between his sense of duty in the face of awesome destruction and his need for self-preservation.[20] At the same time, while some of the contemporary literature and judgments were positively wrong in accusing these soldiers of cowardice, it should not surprise anyone that some soldiers were more able to stand the pressure than others. There was no easy solution to this vexing wound.

———

"I am witnessing terrible suffering," wrote Nursing Sister Sophie Hoerner of the shell-shocked men in her hospital. "Some of them go right to pieces. Their nerve has gone and they cry like babies."[21] These devastated soldiers with their nightmares, hallucinations, and more incapacitating effects were usually sent to specialists at hospitals in England in 1915 and 1916. Haunted by comrades slain, they cried out for friends. Patients would be found at night in the wards trying to dig a hole through the wooden floor to protect against artillery fire, or would beg nurses for a respirator that they could not locate as imagined gas seeped closer to their beds. They had left the battlefield, but it had not left them.

No accepted treatment for shell shock existed, and so as in other fields of wartime medicine, doctors had many opportunities to examine these wounded men and to test new practices. Captain

Edward Ryan of the CAMC, who treated and studied the shell shocked, believed that many patients suffered from physical faults that "lowered resistance," although the culminating effects of strain, including "nervous exhaustion due to mental stress, anxiety, insomnia, terrifying dreams, etc.," as well as "bodily exhaustion from heat, cold and hunger," also had to be factored into a diagnosis.[22] Other psychiatrists engaged in techniques of talking about the trauma with patients, who were frequently labelled with neurasthenia—exhausted nerves.[23] Though these doctors were products of their time and education, they often took a gentle approach to restoring a man's mental health. Moreover, a sustained break and distance from the fighting front helped in many cases.[24] Hydrotherapy through warm baths was a primary treatment at the Canadian hospitals at Buxton and Granville, both former seaside resorts. "My nerves have been giving me lots of trouble and sometimes they nearly drive me wild," wrote Lieutenant T. Stanley Jackson in June 1917, while recovering from physical wounds and exhaustion. "The doctors and nurses are exceptionally kind and attentive, so I am lucky to be in such a good place."[25]

With specialized treatment, greater success was achieved in dealing with men who often bore the stigma of cowardice, and Granville even had a room filled with crutches and sticks where soldiers with paralyzed limbs from extreme shell shock left their walking aids after successful treatment. For some, miracles seemed to be worked in the hospitals, although not all could be treated and some keenly felt the dishonour of having failed at soldiering and having let down their comrades who were still in the line. In a letter to his mother, Robert A. Horne, a stretcher-bearer in the CAMC who was diagnosed with shell shock, lamented, "I was one of the best 'dressers' in the unit and so got my full share of the

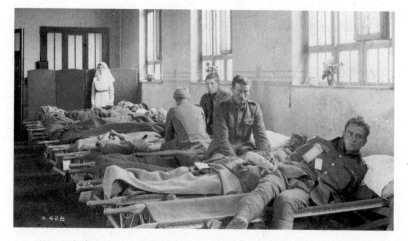

Wounded soldiers who have emerged from the cauldron of battle.

worst cases to do." Having dealt with the horribly mangled soldiers for over nineteen months, he testified, "My nerves gave out."
Confessing his guilt about breaking down, he declared, "I should
have preferred to have been wounded, even to have lost a limb
than to have suffered what I did."[26]

With tens of thousands of shell-shocked patients in the British
and dominion forces by 1916, two schools of thought emerged in
dealing with the injury, even though neither was rigidly defined.
The first looked for inherent failures in patients—in effect blaming
those who entered the army with pre-existing emotional problems
or a history of madness in the family. It was thought that these
"hysterical" men, innately unsuited to be soldiers, had similar
flaws to the many unfit men who were kept out of the army for
physical defects. They had slipped through the screening process
and the war had outed them. The most aggressive expression of
this view came from Canadian medical officer Captain Andrew
Macphail, who dismissed shell shock as "a manifestation of child-
ishness and femininity. Against such there is no remedy."[27] While

this conclusion has been much condemned over the decades, and it was an extreme view even during the war, there were certainly contemporary adherents who agreed with Macphail that some men were mentally unfit for the strain of service.[28]

The second approach to the subject held that these once healthy soldiers had suffered emotional trauma at the front, exacerbated by long service and usually triggered by a disturbing event. In many cases, it was felt that the mental wounds could be healed like physical wounds, to allow soldiers to return to the front. Major Henry Pulteney Wright of the CAMC, a prewar physician from Ottawa who enlisted at age twenty-six and served in almost every type of military unit, shared his thoughts with the profession about the challenge of classifying the mental wound. He wrote that "shell shock has been defined as the symptoms produced by exposure to the forces generated by the explosion of high explosives without visible injury. This is the only definition that I have ever heard given to shell shock, and while I have no quarrel with it as far as it goes my only concern is that it does not go far enough."[29] Through his mid-war study of soldiers, he found that many different types of patients suffered from shell shock, with all grouped under the same term. There was evidence of soldiers who collapsed because of nearby shell detonations, those men who were ground out through exhaustion, and others who broke down because of a single traumatic event. Wright was among a growing number of physicians who believed the injury could not be rigidly defined, even though this further frustrated some doctors and enraged the high command, who could not grasp the complex disorder.

As there was no accepted diagnosis—although by the mid-point in the war medical officers leaned towards accepting that an element of emotional attrition contributed to or triggered a mental collapse—doctors had an opportunity to try experimental treatment beyond the slower process of rest, hydrotherapy, and talking through trauma. With the British and Canadian medical forces so deeply entwined, lessons and treatment were shared freely. Major W.J. Adie of the Royal Army Medical Corps developed a reputation for taking on shell-shocked men who had lost the ability to speak. He lashed them to an operating table and put a constrictive gas mask on them, leaving them to agonize in isolation with their breathing rasping in their ears. Major Adie returned some time later and, in a soothing voice, promised to remove the mask when they said, "Take it away." For more stubborn cases, he injected ether through the mask to create a dreamy effect, and then, in his words, "pricked the skin over the larynx rather vigorously with a pin."[30] He sought to elicit a plea to stop or even a howl of pain. Another form of aggressive treatment came from Dr. Lewis Yealland, a Canadian neurologist who was not in uniform but who treated wounded soldiers with electric shock therapy to cure the "hysterical disorders of warfare."[31] He brutally electrocuted tongues, eyelids, and even genitals to draw a response and bring shell-shocked men out of their catatonic state. One doctor admitted in a chilling report that the pain of the electric shock delivered to patients strapped to a table was "as severe . . . as anything we know . . . the sting of a whip, no matter how vigorously employed . . . [is] almost nothing compared with the sudden severe shock."[32] While these treatments were ghastly by any standard, they had some success in forcing mute men to talk, albeit with their eyes wide with terror. In a war where the citizen's body was controlled by the state, doctors were pressured to send men of nerve, the Commander of the Division or other formation will decide whether the individual is to be tried by Court-Martial or not, care being taken that, except on grounds of urgent medical necessity, he is not evacuated out of the Army until a decision on this point has been arrived at."[34] In response to the high rates of shell shock on the Somme, which rose in the Canadian Corps to 8 percent of the total non-fatal casualties, the fighting officers were increasingly called upon to police the medical officers.[35] The high command felt that the rising number of mental injuries was because the doctors were too humane towards their patients.

To further take control of the worsening situation, British generals sought to rename shell shock to make it more difficult for medical officers to categorize it as a wound. The general public had become aware of this term that seemed to connote a battlefield so terrible that their fathers, uncles, sons, and brothers were being driven to madness. That was bad for morale in a total war. In early 1917, Sir Douglas Haig's headquarters issued an order announcing that "in no circumstances whatever will the expression 'shell shock' be made use of, verbally or in writing," except by specialists in rear hospitals.[36] "Only cases in which there is evidence of direct contact with the effects of explosion, although not producing visible wound (as, for example, cases which have been buried or blown up by explosion) shall be reported as Shell-shock, wound." In a battle to control language and more narrowly define the wound, patients exhibiting conditions of shell shock were now to be labelled "N.Y.D." for "Not Yet Diagnosed."[37]

Along with these changes in nomenclature came instructions to the medical officers in England to return soldiers to the front more quickly. But talk therapy was not effective if rushed, and

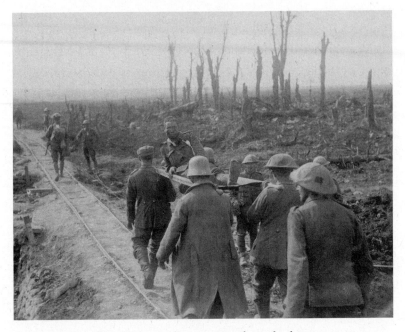

There was usually no escape from the front
unless one was carried or buried.

some experts refused to comply. While this sphere of medicine was a domain where the high command wielded little influence and was forced to rely on the medical experts, these authorities found that one method of getting soldiers back to the line more rapidly, and one over which they could exert some control, was not to let them leave France. At the site of a historic French fortress, No. 3 Canadian Stationary Hospital at Doullens became the centre of Canadian treatment for shell shock in Western Europe. It was headed by a British expert, Captain Frederick Dillon of the Royal Army Medical Corps, again providing evidence of the interchange of doctors between the RAMC and CAMC. Dillon ordered rest and hypnosis for soldiers, while also applying electric shock therapy, which allowed for the treatment of "larger numbers of patients."[38]

He claimed that 62.5 percent of the afflicted were returned to the front, even if he did not track how many later relapsed.

Sergeant Arthur Hickson recounted the story of Old Tom from his battalion, a friendly, balding man in his late thirties who was well liked by his companions. A shell detonated near him during one tour in the line, killing his two mates and leaving him shell shocked. He was evacuated from the front, but his comrades were surprised to see him back with the unit after only a short absence. "After a series of electric shock treatments at the base hospital he was returned to us though still very shaky," observed Hickson. "Lighting a cigarette for instance was very difficult for him. He told me that the patient would do or say anything to stop the treatment."[39] One wonders how many of the soldiers were like Old Tom, and how many more relapsed as they were rushed back into the maelstrom before they were even remotely ready

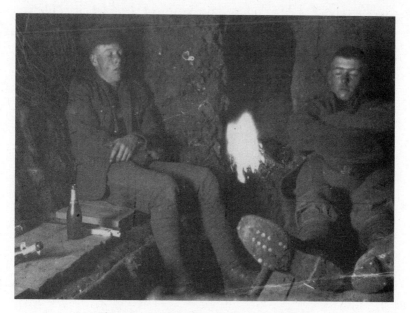

Sleep was essential for staving off collapse.

for combat. Captain Robert Manion, a medical officer who was awarded the Military Cross for bravery, wrote that a soldier with "a severe attack of this malady"—here purposely framing shell shock in medical terms rather than designating it as cowardice—is "rarely ever again fit to serve in the firing line."[40]

In addition to keeping most shell-shocked soldiers in France from 1917 onwards, field ambulances and casualty clearing stations created rest areas. The medical officers found that success in returning soldiers to units was more likely if they were treated behind the battle lines, and less severe cases of shell shock were often found to be deep fatigue that led to disorientation and hyper-anxiety. The institutionalizing of rest stations at medical units from late 1916 allowed mildly shell-shocked soldiers to be kept within the war zone while providing these exhausted men a place to sleep for twenty-four or thirty-six hours, often aided by pharmaceuticals. After a few days, many of the refreshed soldiers underwent light training and were then returned to their unit. There, if they had served at the front for any length of time or had a sympathetic medical officer, they could be assigned to a "bomb-proof job" at company or battalion headquarters and thus kept out of the firing line for a longer period in the hope of restoring their resiliency.

Those with more traumatic disorders not healed by sleep and a break from the forward trenches continued to be assessed at special shell shock hospitals, both in France and in England. Patients seared by the war experience were given various forms of treatment, although they were frequently also pressured to return to the front. Doctors were instructed to push them out of the hospital wards with assurances that they were fine. One expert in mental wounds, Thaddeus Hoyt Ames of the CAMC, believed that the medical officers' authority could be leveraged to convince the wounded soldiers that they had recovered, as soldiers were "trained to the habit of accepting without question the statements of those in authority."[41] While the physicians were torn between

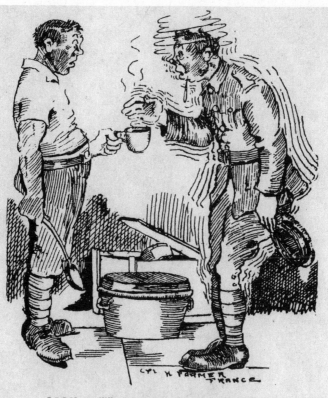

COOK: "What's wrong, chum, shell-shock?"
BILL: "No, back off leave."

A cartoon in The Listening Post, *a Canadian soldiers' newspaper, joking about shell shock. "What's wrong, chum, shell-shock?" asks the cook. Bill, the shaken soldier on the right, responds, "No, back off leave." The return to the battle zone was always jarring, but this cartoon is also revealing in that it openly references shell shock, which for the generals was increasingly seen as a taboo subject.*

their multiple senses of duty—to the army, to their profession, and to their patients—they exerted their own agency in deciding the fate of soldiers, and while some, like Ames, sought to send the patients back to the front as soon as possible, others refused to drive out the wounded until they were ready to return to the fight. Many never were.

———

Given the nebulous nature of this mental wound—and the fact that the high command actively sought to obscure it by renaming the injury and by making it more difficult for doctors to apply the label of "shell shock" in the last two years of the war—the recorded wartime figure of 8,514 Canadian cases of soldiers with "nervous disease" should be questioned.[42] More recent studies have determined that about 15,000 Canadians were treated in medical units for some form of mental war trauma.[43] We shall also never know how many more soldiers were killed because they were on the edge of collapse, or were taken down by a sniper because they were unduly reckless as a result of mental exhaustion. And even more soldiers would carry these invisible wounds back into civilian life, haunted by a war they could never leave behind. However, considering the constant horror of trench warfare, perhaps we should ask not why the number of mental wounds was so high but why it was so low. Why, we may well wonder, didn't all soldiers succumb to the emotional distress and mental ordeal of the trenches? Part of the credit for any success in this area must go to the medical officers along the front who supported the soldiers, worked with regimental officers, found safe spots for men teetering on a breakdown, and did their best to aid those who could not be pulled from the line. Wounds to the mind offered different challenges than those to the body, and they were the only type of wound that would pit the army high command against the medical practitioners.

CHAPTER 9

THE CANADIAN ARMY MEDICAL CORPS IN CRISIS

"The hospital work was so different from the hospitals in France," wrote Nursing Sister Katharine Wilson-Simmie of the Canadian Army Medical Corps while serving in the Mediterranean. "Here practically every man admitted was critically ill with fevers that left them eventually worn to skeletons."[1] Wilson grew up in rural Ontario and was an accomplished nurse from Ottawa when she enlisted in 1915, serving first in England and France and then sailing thousands of kilometres with No. 3 Canadian Stationary Hospital to the Dardanelles theatre of war. Stationed there along with 1,450 other Canadian medical service personnel, her experiences were unlike those of most Canadians who served in uniform.

With the Western Front stalemated in slaughter by early 1915, British politicians sought other fronts where they might knock Germany's ally, Turkey, out of the war. The champion for this was the brash adventurer, former war journalist, and audacious thinker Winston Churchill. As first lord of the admiralty, he advocated a daring naval operation to ram Royal Navy and French warships through the 65-kilometre Dardanelles Strait, which divides Turkey and connects the Mediterranean to the Black Sea and Asia.

The operation failed after Royal Navy warships were unable to take the narrow waterway in February 1915 due to sea mines and Turkish land batteries. Refusing to accept defeat, a force of 75,000 British, French, Australian, and New Zealand soldiers landed on April 25, 1915, at Gallipoli, hoping for a rapid inland expedition.[2] But firepower ruled that front too, and few further advances were achieved once the Allied soldiers drove off the beaches, climbing the rocky terrain that soon became their new trench positions. With incredibly long supply lines, the Gallipoli campaign was short of everything—from munitions and artillery pieces to water and medical supplies. While shot and shell would take its toll, the great killer was disease, a situation exacerbated by harsh climate and the static trench conditions. Unburied corpses and refuse created a breeding ground for the millions of flies that covered everything, which were described by Newfoundland infantryman Richard Cramm as "carrying disease and death in their trail."[3]

Although no Canadian fighting forces would serve on this forlorn front, the Newfoundland Regiment of over 1,000 men (coming from the separate dominion since Newfoundland would not join Canada until 1949) landed at Gallipoli in September 1915.[4] By that time, the campaign had degenerated into costly, attritional trench warfare with no hope of a breakthrough. In for a penny, in for a pound, the British also flooded new forces into Salonika, where French and British soldiers tried to protect Serbia and entice Greece into the war on the side of the Allies. Stalemate

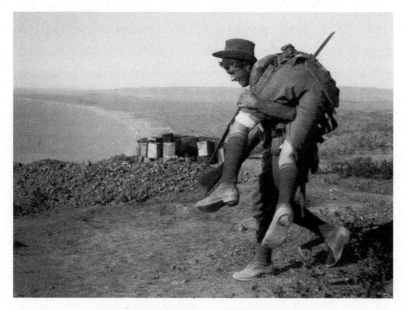

An Australian soldier in Gallipoli carrying
an injured comrade towards medical care.

soon ruled that battlefield too, and a growing Allied army was rendered useless after Austria defeated Serbia in October 1915. The Allied forces earned the title "gardeners of Salonika," largely for planting themselves in the ground where diseases like malaria and dysentery buried thousands.[5] The Germans were only too happy to draw enormous numbers of Allied troops to this region— ultimately some 300,000 soldiers who could have been used more effectively on the Western Front—letting them rot away in what they called "the greatest internment camp in the world."[6]

The Gallipoli operation had been badly planned in almost every way, but especially in terms of medical support. With initially only a handful of British hospitals available to treat the wounded and sick, these units were soon overrun. A catastrophe was in the making and one senior Australian officer later condemned the British high command's bungling, which resulted in medical services "so inadequate that they amounted to criminal negligence."[7] Desperate to avoid a humanitarian disaster that would shake public faith in the military that was demanding so much of every man, woman, and child in the Empire, in the summer of 1915 the British senior medical officer, Surgeon-General Sir Alfred Keogh, pleaded in writing to Surgeon-General Guy Carleton Jones, commander of the CAMC, for any medical units that could be spared. Jones understood the deepening crisis and he ordered three hospitals to the Mediterranean: No. 1 Canadian Stationary Hospital, which had served in France; No. 3 Stationary from London, Ontario; and a general hospital that had been raised from the professors and students from Queen's University. These hospitals arrived in sequence, and two more would follow. All were anxious to serve and to save lives, although few Canadians were prepared for the nightmare that greeted them in this fly-swept wasteland of armies.

No. 1 and No. 3 Stationary Hospitals arrived at the Greek island of Lemnos in late August 1915, while the Queen's University formation (later renamed No. 7 Canadian General Hospital) went to Egypt. For the Canadian medical personnel, both sites were hot, dusty, and utterly foreign. The Queen's students encountered the fleshpots of Cairo, and many men and women from the Presbyterian university were shocked at the debauchery for sale. But soon the wounded flooded in from Gallipoli, with injuries and diseases varying from gunshot and shrapnel wounds to infections and dysentery. There was even the occasional camel bite.

In Lemnos, a preindustrial island in the Aegean Sea about 115 kilometres from Gallipoli, the two Canadian hospitals set up camp near each other on the sandy plain at West Mudros. Not much was there, save for flies and sand mites. Mounds of rotting feces were also piled throughout this area where Egyptian labourers had been quartered with little supervision over matters of hygiene and camp sanitation. When the wind was blowing in the right direction, the Canadians burned the refuse and waste, and the hospital tents were erected by the last week of August, just as the first patients were flooding in. Many had travelled great distances and arrived in soiled uniforms, covered in lice and with suppurating wounds.

While the sanitation was deplorable, the water situation was lethal. Brackish water had to be trucked in on special carts, which were also filthy from overuse and lack of maintenance. The hospital's hygiene staff set to work and improvements were made rapidly, but dysentery and other water-borne diseases were soon to plague everyone. In such conditions, water was rationed, with baths non-existent and only a few basins of reused water available for hand washing. The patients suffered horribly, and what little water the Canadian doctors, nurses, and orderlies had they often gave to the patients with their sun-burnt lips, parched throats, and feverish eyes.

"The hospital received a convoy of dysentery cases," wrote Nursing Sister Constance Bruce of No. 1 Canadian Stationary Hospital. "One hesitated, to gather courage, before passing down the long rows of tightly packed beds, where sunken eyes were focused on every one who went by, or parched tongues held out in silent entreaty."[8] Within a week, some 500 beds were filled with these contagious patients. The infectious watery excrement produced by these suffering men required new safety protocols and isolation wards. In such rancid conditions it was not long before nurses, orderlies, and medical officers were infected.

Almost every Canadian medical practitioner was felled at some point by stomach ailments and more serious diseases. The low point for No. 3 Stationary Hospital was the death of Matron Jessie Brown Jaggard, who was born in Kings, Nova Scotia, and had worked as a nurse in Philadelphia. As the commander of the nurses, she inspired her staff and brought much expertise to the work of the hospital, walking the wards every night before bed to check on the patients. She contracted dysentery and died serving her country on September 25, 1915, at age forty-two, leaving behind a war widower and her grieving cousin, Prime Minister Sir Robert Borden. Many of the other Canadians were gravely ill, and it was felt prudent at one point to dig a number of graves in anticipation of more deaths. A sign was put up: "For Sisters Only."[9] It was not comforting for the sick nurses who passed the cemetery day after day as they continued to tend to even sicker soldiers.

"We surely saw active service at its worst," wrote Nursing Sister Laura Gamble in her private diary.[10] The medical teams never had enough bandages, disinfectant, or medical stores, although more water was available by late September after a pipe was laid between the camp and a far-off reservoir. At the same time, the Canadians set to trading what they had for essentials, and some of the hard-bitten sergeants of the CAMC went out to borrow, trade, or steal. All the while the Canadian medical staff worked long hours to care for the patients during intolerably hot days and shivery nights, cleaning and changing bandages, watching for fevers and infections, and offering kind words and encouraging smiles. "There is no doubt in my mind now that the person who does the most good in a hospital like ours," wrote a Canadian doctor in Salonika, "is the Nursing Sister."[11] These women were constantly caring for the patients amid the swarms of flies and the cries of the wretchedly ill. With bloodied and pus-soaked bandages needing to be changed frequently, every nurse required an orderly to shoo away the clouds of flies lest they become stuck in an open wound. Nursing Sister Mabel Clint wrote that it was "difficult to eat or drink without swallowing flies."[12]

In November, the blazing heat was replaced almost overnight by cold and rain, and on November 26, 1915, a freak storm struck Gallipoli. The temperature plummeted as a freezing torrential rain saturated the trenches, with soldiers swept away in a flash flood, after which a blizzard descended on the battlefield. By the end of the inexplicable storm, more than 200 soldiers had drowned in dugouts that filled with the water, or had frozen to death, again showing the sometimes bizarre ways in which lives could end during war.[13] Another 5,000 soldiers were evacuated for cases of hypothermia and trench foot. The frostbite wounds left patients in agony, wrote Canadian Nursing Sister Katharine Wilson-Simmie, who observed that "many of the cases became gangrenous, and many feet had to be amputated."[14]

After the evacuation of the Gallipoli front in January 1916, both Canadian hospitals left Lemnos, having treated many thousands of patients, with No. 1 moving in March 1916 to Salonika, where two other Canadian hospitals had served—No. 4, raised in Toronto, and No. 5, from British Columbia. At the Toronto hospital was a young medical orderly, Private Lester "Mike" Pearson. The son of a Methodist minister, Pearson had ached to enlist and did so at age eighteen on his birthday, although he rapidly became disillusioned with the horrors in the hospital wards: "We pitched our tents, spread our straw over the mud, and laid the casualties down on that, till there would be forty or fifty in a tent. Then the medical officer would come around with his lantern, the dead and dying would be moved to one side, the dangerous cases would be attended to at once and the less serious ones simply cheered up." It was service, in the words of the future prime minister, composed of "nightmare days when we all worked till we dropped."[15]

———

"Why has Jones sent so many Canadian doctors to Serbia?"[16] Sam Hughes got the destination wrong, but he wanted an answer from Surgeon-General Guy Carleton Jones, who had seemingly diluted medical support for the Canadian soldiers on the Western Front by ordering them on a disease-ridden misadventure in the Mediterranean. The unstable, angry, and often overwhelmed Sam Hughes thrived on chaos and was always at his best when looking for someone to fight. The minister of militia and defence had no shortage of opponents, and his sense of grievance was well honed against the Imperials, especially after receiving what he felt had been bad treatment in the South African War—where he had served bravely but had then revealed his true colours by arguing publicly that he deserved not one but two Victoria Crosses![17]

In the late summer of 1916, Hughes sent the respected University of Toronto professor of surgery Colonel Herbert A. Bruce overseas to investigate and write a report. Bruce was a skilled surgeon and an ambitious reformer who had founded his own private hospital in Toronto, the Wellesley. Surgeon-General Jones had little time for him and his secret mission for the minister. While the senior CAMC general no doubt viewed Bruce as an unwanted interloper, the surgeon-general was also busy as he headed the growing organization of the CAMC in London, with

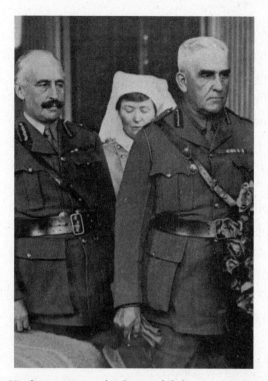

*Sam Hughes, minister of militia and defence (on right), with
Surgeon-General Guy Carleton Jones, commander of the CAMC,
as they inspect a hospital. Neither man liked the other.*

a staff of 28 officers and 158 other ranks, along with nurses who
were under the command of the matron-in-chief, Major Margaret
Macdonald. It was no bloated staff by any means, and it dealt
with matters of manpower, training, the movement of the
wounded, and logistics for all units, as well as providing support
to Colonel Gilbert L. Foster, the deputy director medical services
(DDMS), who was the senior medical officer attached to the
Canadian Corps.

In the field, the Canadian medical officers, orderlies, and
nurses treated all types of soldiers: British, French, Belgian,

Portuguese, dominion, Indian, German, and, of course, Canadian. Hospitals tended to be immobile, with the wounded from throughout the area coming to them by motorized ambulance or special train. In England, the ebb and flow of the patients who were recovering at different times meant that many of the Canadian hospitals and convalescent homes were full, although other Imperial or dominion hospitals had free beds. For the most part, Canadian soldiers did not seem to mind if they were cared for in British units, although some noted that the nurses there were more adamant about enforcing discipline and rules.

The CAMC, whose senior generals were almost all Canadian—unlike the four fighting divisions, which in 1916 still had many British staff officers—also worked closely with the Royal Army Medical Corps. The two medical services contributed to the recovery of British patients in Canadian hospitals, and the British were responsible for moving all the wounded by rail and water (save for the hospital ships that took the invalided back to Canada). Fruitful loans were also made, of Canadians to British units and of British to Canadian, with all sharing knowledge about the ever-evolving treatments at the front. Famed Canadian medical experts in uniform, such as George Armstrong, John Alexander Gunn, John McCrae, and John A. Amyot, travelled to other Imperial units to operate and lecture. William Boyd, a professor of pathology from the University of Manitoba, was pressed into service to head a British unit that specialized in infectious diseases, and he was one of 416 Canadian doctors who served with the RAMC.[18] Furthermore, two Canadian hospitals were in Paris, staffed with French-speaking Canadians, while two British general hospitals—Shorncliffe and Brighton's Kitchener Hospital—were situated near major Canadian training bases and treated the injured and sick who came to them. Wartime medical treatment was not to be confined by national boundaries.

———

Colonel Bruce came from the Hughes school of crashing down doors before asking to enter, and his report of September 20, 1916, excoriated Surgeon-General Jones. The Toronto surgeon noted many failures in the medical system in Britain, and some of his criticisms were legitimate, with the struggles he described being part of the trial of dealing with mass casualties. But others were unreasonable, such as his suggestion that recovering Canadian soldiers should only be treated in Canadian hospitals. All of it was written in incendiary language and garnished with cherry-picked outrageous examples.[19] He wrote, for instance, "There has been no medical inspection by the Canadian Medical Service of Canadian soldiers in Imperial hospitals, and there has been no efficient medical inspection of Canadian hospitals."[20] The statement was utterly untrue. He also condemned the surgical practices at the front, creating the impression that the Canadian doctors were amateurs. Bruce went so far as to accuse Jones of being derelict in his duty by allowing incompetents—"drug fiends or [those] addicted to alcoholism"—into the CAMC uniform, and he claimed that unqualified surgeons had honed their skills by carving up the bodies of Canadian soldiers. The British hospitals where Jones sent the wounded were, in Bruce's opinion, poorer than the Canadian ones, being little more than "marriage bureaus" for untrained VADS.[21] The Voluntary Aid Detachments, groups of dedicated women from Britain and Canada who provided important medical support, were not amused.

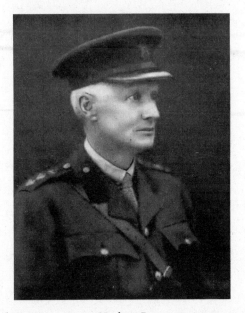

The respected Toronto surgeon Herbert Bruce went overseas and wrote a damning report of the CAMC medical system that caused a scandal.

Not all of Bruce's observations were incorrect, and he rightly noted that many of the drafts of soldiers coming to England since early 1916 had been made up of underage and overage soldiers, as well as many who were physically unfit for military service. He embarrassingly tracked down one seventy-two-year-old who could barely travel a few metres without wheezing, although he missed one of the oldest members of the CEF, seventy-nine-year-old William J. Clements, who, according to one report, was "very deaf" and "barely able to stand erect."[22] Thousands of these unfits, misfits, teenagers, and old-timers had enlisted out of patriotism or pressure, and were not suited for the hard life at the front.[23] These were in addition to the 100,000 or so men who were turned away in Canada, deemed too sickly or enfeebled to serve as soldiers.[24] However, as there was no master registry of those denied service, determined men went from unit to unit until they were accepted. One persistent thirty-three-year-old bushman, George Atkins, who suffered from curvature of the spine, claimed to have attempted to enlist almost 200 times before he was accepted by a tunnelling unit.[25]

Though the CAMC carried out more strident medical examinations on all drafts coming from Canada beginning in mid-1915, thousands of unfit soldiers still made it overseas by concealing an illness or slipping past the medical inspectors.[26] Some made good soldiers, while others were a drain on the system. Soldiers with tuberculosis were a particularly vexing problem, as they were potential spreaders of the killer disease and were unable to stand the hard living of the trenches.[27] These invalided men also became a postwar financial burden, and it was estimated that each of these veterans cost the state about $5,000 in treatment.[28]

The Canucks from the northern dominion had long forged an identity as warriors shaped by ice and snow—larger, more resilient, and stronger than the stunted men of Britain's inner cities. But the medical examinations of hundreds of thousands of young men put paid to this notion. Bruce's report shone a light on this crisis in masculinity, which terrified many Canadians who warned of "race degeneration" as the best and brightest were killed off in battle, leaving only the malformed and enfeebled to carry on. The increasingly visible number of soldiers turned away due to poor health, and the many thousands outed in Bruce's scathing report— along with the high venereal disease rates among soldiers—fired a new societal crusade in Canada that would extend into the postwar years and stimulate public health reforms.[29]

———

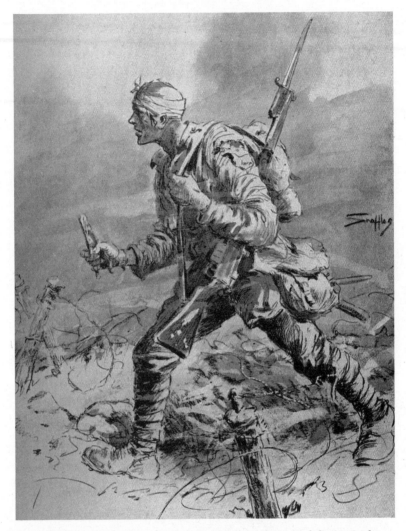

This wartime drawing depicts the tough, resilient, and determined "Canuck" soldier, who is advancing despite his wound. Fit and always ready for battle, Canadians were proud of their physical prowess. But Colonel Bruce's revelation that thousands of unfits and misfits were sent overseas, men too sick or malformed to serve on the Western Front, led to public debate and worry that Canadian manhood had been allowed to wither away through neglect of public health.

For a man used to wielding a scalpel, Bruce had turned freely to a hammer. The senior CAMC staff overseas were infuriated by his charges of incompetence, especially as they were struggling with the mangled bodies of thousands upon thousands of soldiers from the Battle of the Somme. Sam Hughes was not one to let a good scandal go to waste, and he blustered about protecting the vulnerable Canadian soldiers whom Bruce said were being poorly served by the doctors in uniform. To be sure, Hughes cared about "his boys," but he was also aware that the wolves were circling due to his mismanagement of the war effort. A public battle where he was the self-proclaimed protector of the wounded might raise his sinking reputation. In England, a Militia Council stacked with Hughes's cronies recommended that Surgeon-General Jones be removed from command and replaced by Colonel Bruce. This caused further shock waves among CAMC senior officers, who watched as Jones was removed in disgrace in early October. Matron Macdonald, commander of the nursing sisters, contemplated resigning over the "underhand intrigue" and "insupportable tyranny" in the surgeon-general's dismissal, but in the end felt it was her duty to stay on to support the Canadian women in uniform.[30] To many in the CAMC and RAMC, this looked like a political hit job.

Given to hurling outrageous comments, mounting unprovoked attacks, and wading into the fray with reckless abandon, Hughes gave an absurd and controversial talk at Toronto's Empire Club on November 9, 1916, in which he highlighted the "scandal," as he called it, using Bruce's report to allege that the medical services' failure had led to manpower shortages. "Canadian soldiers were allowed to go under the knife of first year medical men while the services of experienced surgeons in Canada were not utilized," Hughes railed.[31] In response to this war of words, the British medical services came to the aid of their Canadian comrades, emphasizing that the CAMC had helped the Empire in a time of great need in the Dardanelles and that the care offered in the Dominion hospitals was first-rate. Sadly, it was too little to save Jones, although the general was given a senior post in Canada.

After two years of Hughes's embarrassing scandals and outrageous attacks on friends and foe, Prime Minister Borden had been marshalling the case for months to depose the minister who had become a gross political liability. Hughes's attack on the medical services contributed to Borden's decision to demand his resignation. The fiery Hughes did not go gently to the backbenches, continuing to attack all his enemies both in and outside the party, but his removal from cabinet in November 1916 brought a more professional leadership to the country's war effort. Those around the cabinet table were relieved that the prime minister had finally acted, with Sir George Foster, a Conservative stalwart, summing up the feeling of many when he declared, "The nightmare is over."[32]

———

The removal of Hughes left Bruce swinging in the wind, especially when the CAMC formed its own committee to study his report. After the admired William Osler announced that he would steer clear of this mess—although he privately condemned the Bruce report, with his words carrying much weight in medical circles— Surgeon-General Sir William Babtie, a senior British medical officer who had served in India and who wore the Victoria Cross, led the investigation.[33] The committee hurriedly prepared a counter-report to bury Bruce's accusations, and its findings in early 1917 revealed that improvements could be made to the CAMC but that the matters were not as grave as the Toronto surgeon had depicted. Although the Babtie report, as it was known, attracted its own controversy as well as public attacks in Canada by some newspapers loyal to Hughes, the distraction was eased by the creation of the Overseas Ministry of Canadian Forces (OMFC) and the disbandment of Hughes's Militia Council. Borden's friend George Perley, then acting high commissioner, was appointed as the first overseas minister.[34] He began to clean up Hughes's overseas mess and the OMFC became an important administrative arm, which eventually, under its second minister, A.E. Kemp, led to the Dominion having greater control over its armed forces.[35]

Minister Perley immediately removed Bruce as acting commander of the CAMC. With no Canadian medical unit being willing to take Bruce on strength, he was banished to the Imperials as a roving surgeon, where he went back to doing what he was very good at: keeping men alive in the operating room. Bruce soon after met his future wife, Angela, and after being married overseas, he happily returned to Toronto to continue working at his private hospital, later becoming lieutenant governor general of Ontario and a lifelong champion of improving public health.

This internecine warfare led to change. The CAMC felt pressure to address some of its systemic problems, which it did, focusing on improving the examination of recruits coming from Canada, on reclaiming some of the convalescing Canadians in far-flung hospitals, and on beginning the process of pulling back the hospital units from the Gallipoli front to serve in England and France. Also, by late 1916, the CAMC slowed the transfer of trained Canadian medical personnel to British units, reflecting the increasingly desperate public complaints in Canada that a doctor famine

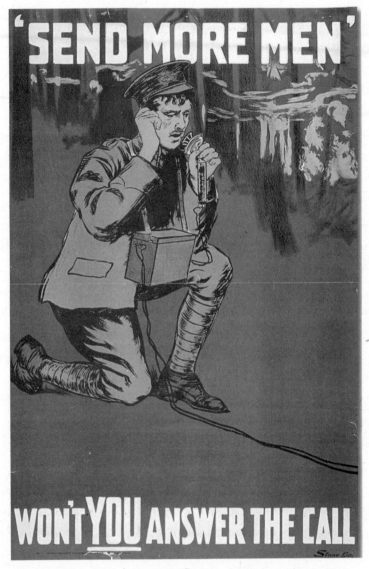

Wartime poster of an exhausted soldier calling for Canada to
"Send More Men." Some in Canada argued that there were already
too many men overseas, especially doctors, as this was creating a crisis
through a physician shortage at home.

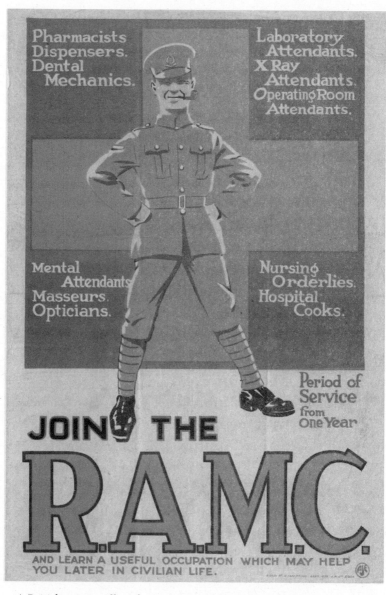

A British poster calling for recruits to enlist in the Royal Army Medical Corps. It advertises for many positions and promises that those who enlist will "learn a useful occupation which may help you later in civilian life."

was hurting rural communities.[36] About half of all doctors and about a third of all nurses would eventually serve in uniform, leaving many Canadians in want of medical care, a situation that was described in the pages of *CMAJ* as "intolerable."[37]

To sort out the administrative mess in England, Major-General Richard Turner was recalled from the front, and he successfully instigated new reforms to improve the overall training of soldiers. Turner would eventually become the chief of the general staff, bringing much order to the chaos in England, and he was guided by a council of OMFC civilian representative and generals, including new senior medical officer Major-General Gilbert L. Foster, who was transferred from France.[38] There was a growing sense among the senior generals in England of the important role of the medical services in caring for the wounded and, when possible, returning them to the front, which was crucial because of the manpower challenges that began in late 1916 as voluntary recruiting slowed in Canada.

Generals Turner and Foster also continued to authorize the establishment of new hospitals to meet the unending stream of wounded soldiers from the Battle of the Somme. For instance, No. 4 Canadian General was opened at Basingstoke, with an astonishing 2,500 beds, and several other hospitals were stood up at Kirkdale, Bramshott, and other locations in Britain.[39] Ontario taxpayers donated several hundred thousand dollars for the creation of Orpington Military Hospital in Kent, and it later expanded to specialize in tuberculosis victims and those with facial wounds. By 1918, Orpington had 2,182 beds, and by war's end, 32,294 patients had passed through its doors.[40] These hospitals took in the wounded from the Western Front, and each was larger than any hospital in Canada at the time.

In the aftermath of the Somme, the heavy casualties created shortages of trained infantrymen in the 100,000-strong Canadian
Corps. In early 1917, while Prime Minister Borden was in England
demanding greater influence over the Empire's war effort and putting in place agreements for Canadian autonomy after the war,
he visited more than fifty hospitals. Borden felt it was his duty to
meet the brave soldiers who pulled themselves to attention as he
passed through the wards or as he sat at the foot of their beds
to hear their stories. The prime minister was moved to tears and
anger that these Canadians, who had so clearly done their duty,
were being sent back into the line, sometimes with wounds not
fully healed or with mental scars that would never heal, while
more than a million men of military age were safe back at home.
His attitude hardened and he returned to Canada and announced
conscription in May 1917, with the law passed in late August of
the same year after fierce debate. Borden felt the "call from the
wounded, the men in the trenches and those who have fallen."[41]
The violence suffered by the wounded had a profound impact on
Canadians, and with conscription they would face one of the
greatest challenges in the country's history. Canada's total war
effort was shaped by an ongoing commitment to the fighting soldiers, the dead, and those who had been saved by medical services.

CHAPTER 10

FORCE PROTECTION AT VIMY RIDGE, 1917

The Canadian Corps dragged itself off the Somme like a great wounded beast. The final cost of the campaign was 24,000 Canadians killed and wounded, a grisly share of the more than one million Allied and German casualties in that swirling cauldron of ruin. Private David McLean, who enlisted in Toronto and served with the 15th Battalion, wrote about survival, fate, and chance on the Somme, confessing, "You never know the minute when you may get hit so I wish it was all over."[1] He would get his bullet on the Vimy front, killed on April 20, 1917.

The Canadians marched to the Vimy Ridge sector near Arras, some 40 kilometres to the north of the Somme. The dominating 7-kilometre ridge had been a cockpit of battle since the start of the war, a site where the French had several times hurled themselves against the dug-in Germans. Suffering some 300,000 casualties, including over 100,000 killed, the French had been unable to capture the ridge, but they had eaten into the deep enemy trenches so that the position of the *frontsoldaten* on the heights was now relatively narrow.[2] The Germans still had all the advantages as they stared down into the Allied lines, directing shell and mortar fire and even running off their dirty water to further flood the sodden trenches below.

The past campaigns at Vimy could be read in the countless shell craters that defaced the ridge. Amid rusty barbed wire that gave the appearance of weird, towering sculptures lay skeletons from the great 1914 and 1915 battles, as well as more recently putrefying corpses whose faces were distorted in death but still visible. The sickly sweet odour of decaying flesh was an assault on the senses. "There are all kinds of dead still lying round, every inch is torn up by shellfire," recounted Gunner William Ball of the 37th Battery, Canadian Field Artillery.[3] Sergeant W.L.M. Draycott of the Princess Patricia's Canadian Light Infantry observed how the living soldiers often "came across skeletons of Frenchmen who had so heroically defended the Ridge in former days and suffered enormously."[4] Only the dead held No Man's Land.

The Vimy front was known for its chalky soil, and while this substance made a glutinous mess of everything and everyone during the wet fall and winter months, it was easy to cut through to create caves and dugouts. When the Canadians took over the warren of subterranean French-made caverns, they expanded them to protect against enemy shellfire.[5] "The Canadian soldier looks today more like a drain digger than a soldier," penned Calgarian lieutenant C.B.J. Jones in a letter, "and those who are not on duty are busy with the shovels."[6]

The personnel of the medical services were excused from this hard labour as they waited for the patients to arrive. It was considerably quieter here than in the frenzy of the Somme, and many of the doctors used the time to write reports about how emergency medicine might be improved, such as by moving surgical treatment

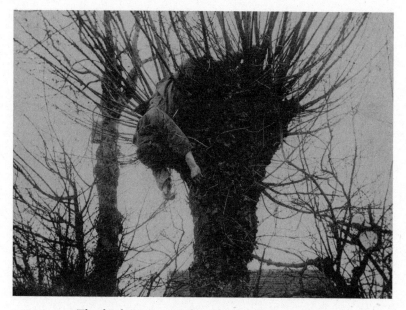

*The dead were everywhere: buried in the trenches,
lying in No Man's Land, or even, as in this case, blown into a tree.*

forward or hastening the removal of the wounded.[7] Symposiums were also held behind the lines. For instance, on January 5, 1917, at No. 1 Canadian Clearing Station, 130 medical officers came together to listen to lectures on evolving medical care and disease prevention.[8] Amid the raw destruction of violence and trauma, a systematic learning process about the art of healing and care occurred throughout the war.

Medical officers in the regiment and in the field ambulances also spent time instructing the stretcher-bearers in battlefield aid. Before the Somme, the bearers had been pestered by their comrades in the infantry, who accused them of shirking the fatigues and other back-breaking work projects that the bearers were excused from to save their strength. The low level of animosity was captured in barbs and bad chat, as well as in poetry and songs.[9] Frank Walker, a stretcher-bearer and poet, penned this poem, "Packing Out," which reflected some of the contradictions of service:

> We loaf around the Aid Post, on the sand bags in the sun,
> Taking the jeers and sneers of every passing son-of-a gun.
> We are the lousy stretcher-squads, the discards of the Pack,
> The idlers of the Army—til the Army's next attack! . . .
>
> Oh, then it's "Good Old Stretcher-Bearers: they're the boys for
>   trouble!"
> "Gangway for the Stretcher-Bearers coming on the double!"
> "Gangway for the Bearers!" goes trench to trench the cry,
> And everybody hops aside to let the "Bearer" by. . . .
>
> We go where men are falling in the awesome barrage-tract,
> We dig them out, and pick them up, and pack them safely back.
> Over the wire and through the mire and down the Line we go,
> And you can bet your old Tin Hat our pace is far from slow![10]

Walker's poem reflected the reality of service at the front, and when the shells had rained down on the Somme, the body snatchers had indeed raced forward into the fire. They had earned the respect of their comrades the hard way, and the criticisms were silenced. Stretcher-bearer Lawrence Rogers wrote home to his wife after the Somme, noting wryly, "It sure is great to hear someone speak well of the Stretcher Bearers for over here the majority have not much use for them until they get wounded[,] then they have an awful lot."[11]

Along the Vimy front, potable water was always in short supply, and the 100,000 soldiers and 20,000 horses in the Canadian Corps consumed 225,000 litres of it each day. The Corps' engineers laid new lines from spring-fed reservoirs far to the rear, with twenty-four pumping stations pushing water through 70 kilometres of pipelines that ran 2 metres beneath the earth to stations from which it was carried into the front lines.[12] While the risk of disease and infection was constant for static armies, proper water sanitation ensured that no significant outbreaks of illness occurred.

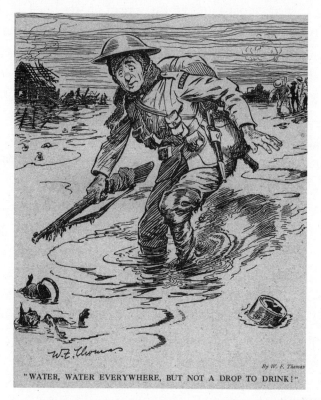

By W. F. Thomas

"WATER, WATER EVERYWHERE, BUT NOT A DROP TO DRINK!"

*A Canadian wartime cartoon lamenting the grim waterlogged
and polluted terrain and the irony, as the soldier laments,
of "water, water everywhere, but not a drop to drink!"*

Disease and pestilence had always been the great killer of armies, and the siege war of monumental proportions was the perfect environment to reap countless victims. But that did not happen in numbers high enough to wither the fighting forces. The outbreak of meningitis on Salisbury Plain had shocked Canadian officers into accepting the importance of preventative medicine and sanitation, with one of the medical officers later writing that the "epidemic was not an unmixed evil: it educated both combatant officers and men as to the necessity of observing the underlying principles necessary to prevent the spread of any contagious disease. It also showed them disease once out of hand could play greater havoc than a German attack."[13] Building on that teachable disaster, the regimental medical officers in the units had proven their worth by focusing on proper sanitation, an approach that enabled them to control everything from trench foot to new infections like trench fever. This message was also making its way back to Canada, and in the pages of the *Canadian Medical Association Journal* (*CMAJ*) the president of the Alberta Medical Association, Dr. T.H. Whitelaw of Edmonton, crowed about the doctors overseas and how the medical services had succeeded in limiting disease to the point where the war "has done much to raise the status of the medical profession to heights never reached in the world's history."[14] Even as Canada experienced a shortage of doctors because so many were in uniform overseas, there was a growing understanding among Canadians of the important work of saving lives and preventing disease.

Each division had a sanitary section consisting of an officer and twenty-seven other ranks, as well as roving sanitary units deployed to search for refuse, cesspools, and other potential breeding grounds for disease behind the front lines.[15] Canada's First Contingent had also included a mobile laboratory. Initially carrying the weighty name of the Canadian Army Hydrological Corps and Advisers on Sanitation, it was commanded by Toronto doctor George Nasmith, who had played a key role in the inoculation program at Valcartier. Lieutenant-Colonel Nasmith and several gifted scientists under his leadership, including University of Alberta professor of pathology Captain Allan Coats Rankin, who had for a time been adviser of epidemiology to the king of Siam, travelled the front with a mobile laboratory in a kitted-up van, conducting tests of water for pollutants. The group also studied lice and dissected rats in order to look for diseases like the bubonic plague or anthrax.[16] They periodically found these and other deadly diseases, especially among the Belgian and French population, and advised on the creation of quarantine zones. At the same time, the analysis of water kept the soldiers from the hospital or the grave, and the bacteriological organism that caused trench mouth—a disgusting disease that turned gums grey, made teeth fall out, and led to halitosis that would fell a horse—was discovered through scientific study, although the necrotizing ulcerative gingivitis was not easy to eliminate once it took hold in a man's mouth.

Poor diet, lack of sleep, and unsanitary conditions meant that everyone had digestive problems and many soldiers suffered from hemorrhoids. Watery feces forced soldiers to frequently run to the latrines. With no toilet paper, men sometimes used newspaper and magazines to wipe their arses, but more often they had little at hand. Underpants quickly became filthy and added to a man's revolting smell. The medical and sanitation officers faced the continual worry that dysentery would move from a few unlucky individuals to entire units, as it was passed through bowel movements and unsanitary practices. While the amoebic and bacillary forms of the disease plagued many armies in other theatres of war, it was not a significant issue on the Western Front because of close observation by the medical and sanitary officers. Another great killer of past armies, typhoid, was a constant source of fear among all senior medical officers. Having studied their history, they knew that Napoleon's soldiers had died in shocking numbers from this highly infectious and lethal disease in Russia in 1812, and that five times as many British soldiers had died of disease than weapons during the Crimean War in the 1850s.[17] The doctors of all armies were tasked with preventing such plagues from again decimating the fighting forces, although perhaps this was a factor that contributed to the extraordinary length and high cost of the war, as sick and wounded men were returned to battle over and over again. For the Canadians, preventative medicine, multiple wartime inoculations, and a keen attention to sanitation ensured that only 42 officers and 380 other ranks contracted typhoid during the course of the war, with only 16 related deaths.[18]

The periodic vaccination of Canadian soldiers against disease also shielded them. Lance-Corporal Charles Savage described the end of one tour of the trenches after which all the soldiers were lined up and jabbed with needles against typhoid and other killers.[19] "They must have been particularly potent for by noon of the day after taking them, most of us were feeling very bad indeed," Savage remembered.[20] Savage survived the slight fever and body aches, but never again did he mention typhoid in his postwar memoir. Vaccination was crucial in this war of attrition, and even the British increasingly restricted their soldiers' ability to refuse it despite some high-profile opposition in England to forced

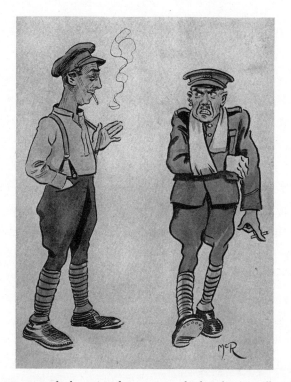

This cartoon spoofs the pain of vaccination by brushing it off with the worse pain of having to salute officers. It reads, "What's the matter, Bill—inoculation?" "No! Salutin' subalterns in London."

inoculation.[21] By November 1917, an order was passed in the Canadian forces that periodic vaccinations for typhoid, cholera, dysentery, and smallpox would be mandatory, and that any soldier refusing them would be punished under the Army Act.[22]

In that miserably cold and dark winter of early 1917, one of the great uplifters of morale for soldiers was a series of central and mobile baths. These were often huge showers in old breweries, where men were ordered to disrobe, enter a bathing area on mass, soap up, and be doused with water from an enormous overhead bucket. At best the water was tepid, but it was enough to lift the spirits of the great unwashed. "I bet you cannot realize how a bath feels after two or three months soldiering," wrote one Canuck to his mother.[23] As the refreshed soldiers exited, they were given underwear that had been steamed to kill the lice and their eggs. Here, too, innovations were achieved throughout the war. Colonel John A. Amyot, a professor of hygiene at the University of Toronto when he enlisted at age forty-seven, invented a modified and more effective disinfector that used heat and steam to kill the louse eggs. After the war, Amyot would become the first federal deputy minister in the Department of Health, applying lessons learned on the Western Front to save the lives of civilians.[24]

Wastage resulting from illness remained substantial, and good hygiene discipline could never eradicate all sickness in such hard-living circumstances, even though it limited losses. "Trench cough" became the informal term for a constellation of illnesses, flus, and colds, along with lack of sleep. Infantryman Claude Williams noted of the persistent cough that "the medical officer says there is very little harm in it. Their advice is to do without smoking for a while. Nobody does that, they had better take away our food rations first."[25] Private Gordon Robertson, a prewar student who enlisted at age eighteen, wrote home to his dad about spending all night in No Man's Land digging a trench and laying barbed wire beneath the shadow of the ominous ridge. He felt that although he was soaked through, frigid, and feverish, "You can't get sick in the army."[26] Robertson meant that mere illness did not relieve a soldier from his work, and almost all men toughed it out. He survived his illness and, later, a gunshot wound to the head.

There were always more losses to serious illness than to physical wounds. For example, in March, with relentless raiding against the enemy positions—known informally as "dash and destroy" operations—and constant shelling, some 1,435 Canadian soldiers were wounded, but 2,969 men were evacuated as sick from the cold and miserable conditions.[27] Microbes and viruses rather than snipers and chemical agents were the greatest threats to the Corps' fighting strength before the coming Vimy battle, and throughout the war a 1 to 1.32 ratio of battle to non-battle casualties was recorded for the rank-and-file soldiers.[28] But the situation would have been worse without the doctors in uniform, and a very low proportion of the sick died of their wounds. "The great, outstanding feature of the War," argued Colonel George Adami, "has been the triumph of preventive medicine."[29]

———

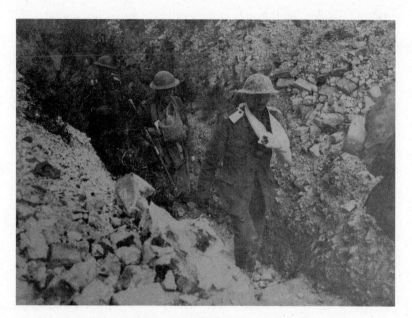

Wounded Canadians emerge from the trenches after a raid.
A stretcher-bearer has already provided aid.

Vimy would be a shell-driven battle. After systematically extinguishing strongpoints and barbed wire for over two months, the Canadian and British artillery commenced a more punishing and sustained bombardment on the German lines in the last week of March, and then ramped up the intensity in April, a week before the planned offensive. The introduction of the new 106 fuse, which enabled shells to explode on contact and thus vastly improved the process of clearing the barbed wire, was a major technological innovation in the war and likely more important to tactical success than the tank. The enemy fired back with less weight of shell but with the advantage of peering into the Canadian lines. Shells, mortar bombs, and snipers took their toll. Herbert Burrell, a prewar artist who had enlisted at the ancient age of forty-five from Winnipeg, served as a stretcher-bearer with the 1st Canadian Mounted Rifles, an infantry regiment that lost its horses early in the war. He kept a detailed diary and wrote on March 28, 1917, about an enemy shell exploding among his group as they moved to the front, "Wounding slightly the 3rd man from me and instantly killing his companion . . . blowing off the top of his head." Burrell noted, "We carried him as far as the dressing station. It was very heavy work owing to the awful condition of the road and the darkness of the night. We laid him amidst the ruins with a blanket over him, where he waits for burial like hundreds of others who have passed the same way."[30]

Like the infantry and artillery, the medical services prepared intensely for the coming battle. The doctors, stretcher-bearers, and nurses at every level understood that a full-scale operation that involved tens of thousands of soldiers would probably leave about a quarter of the attacking force wounded, with another 10 to 15 percent killed on the battlefield for a total casualty rate of around

35 to 40 percent. Only rapid clearing would save many of those cut down from the mass graves that had already been dug behind the lines in preparation for the expected losses. Under grey skies that frequently sent down snow and sleet in early April, the CAMC established advanced dressing stations, protected relay spots where stretcher-bearers could wait, and, closest to the front, regimental aid posts. Some of the caves that had been excavated in the chalk were outfitted with medical supplies and personnel ready to care for the flow of wounded soldiers. New maps were drawn to guide the infantrymen forward into the enemy lines, but also to aid the stretcher-bearers in finding their way back from the front through the labyrinthine passages while they carried their bleeding cargo to the Corps' thirteen field ambulances spread across the front.

A total of 983 British and Canadian artillery and mortars opened up at 5:30 A.M. on April 9 to crash down on the enemy's lines and rearward gun batteries, and to begin the creeping barrage that signalled the infantry to go "over the top." About 15,000 Canadians in 21 front-line battalions surged ahead, with another 20,000 behind them in the secondary and tertiary waves, and tens of thousands of gunners, engineers, machine-gunners, and soldiers in turn behind them. The infantry followed the creeping curtain of shells, plunging ahead over the torn-up ground. Most of the Germans were forced into their dugouts. While hundreds were killed in the initial barrage, defenders survived all across the front and, once the shells had passed over them, emerged from their protective spaces to fire into the advancing Canadians.

In the lead wave of assaulters was stretcher-bearer Private Herbert Burrell, who later wrote in his diary about running low through No Man's Land with enemy machine-gun bullets kicking up the mud and sometimes sparking off the barbed wire. "There

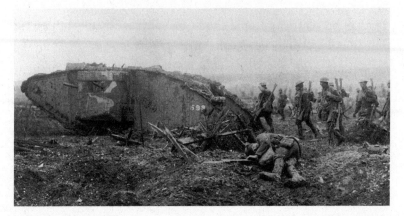

The price of victory. A dead soldier lies in the foreground of this
photograph taken on the 2nd Division's front as the Canadians storm Vimy.

was a curious feeling of bewilderment and helplessness and the
stifling smell of powder and smoke," he remarked.[31] As far as
Burrell could see, platoons and sections of Canadian infantrymen
shot and clawed their way forward, some soldiers dropping periodically while others were spun around and flung to the ground
as a bullet or piece of steel found flesh. The force of a single bullet
was so powerful that soldiers standing next to a man who was hit
sometimes felt the thud in their own bodies. The grisly wet-smack
sound of bullets penetrating flesh was luckily lost within the
shrieking of shells.

Seeking to help the wounded in this lethal battlefield, Burrell
described the first man he encountered, noting, "I found him suffering from fright more than anything else. He was a big husky
looking chap & I told him to get up & come along." Burrell's firm
encouragement allowed the soldier to regain his composure and
plunge ahead into combat. The terrified rifleman would not be the
last Canadian who dove into a shell crater and found that his legs
would not carry him out of it. "My next casualty," wrote Burrell,

"was a lad of the 2nd C.M.R. [2nd Canadian Mounted Rifles] who had a bad wound, being shot through the right lung. Then I attended to a man who had had his left hand shot off at the wrist & the member was just hanging by a thread or two and his eye was also injured. Poor fellow he was in great agony but set a splendid example in his stoical endurance. He begged for a cigarette & wanted to know my name."[32] Burrell responded to both requests before racing on, drawn to rifles stabbed bayonet first into the mud as informal signals of where the injured lay. The pungent smell of powder and smoke sent him reeling, and this sensory overload was only intensified by the stunning noise of continuous bombardments that left him and other soldiers with throbbing headaches. Burrell found other men and bandaged wounds that steamed in the cold air. When he encountered two stretcher-bearers, he led them to the plucky soldier from the 2nd CMR who had been shot through the lung. The man was in a bad way, hacking up blood and froth, although still alive. The two bearers looked at him and shook their heads. "There were other cases who were more likely to live," Burrell wrote in his diary, and they left the Canadian to die.[33]

With several thousand soldiers wounded in the first hours of combat, those who could walk were forced to make their own way to the rear. The extra stretcher-bearers who were pooled from the field ambulances had also sprung forward to carry out the wounded. They were given some basic tips such as to avoid giving water to men with intestinal wounds and to place a man with a face wound on his stomach so that he did not asphyxiate on his own fluids, but most importantly they were instructed to carry with haste. Many of the 4,000 German prisoners were also pressed into service, with Sergeant Robert Kentner of the 46th Battalion writing that "numerous German prisoners were utilized as stretcher bearers bringing the wounded from our forward positions, a very unpleasant and tiring task."[34] As strange as it was to use the enemy who only recently had been doing their best to kill Canadians, the Germans saved Canadian lives. Combat and care in war has always led to strange contradictions.

———

Many Canadians at Vimy would have echoed Corporal Jim Connoy, who, when writing to his mother in St. Thomas, Ontario, marvelled, "How I came through without getting hit I don't know."[35] The thousands of wounded who were not so lucky walked, crawled, or were carried from No Man's Land into the forward trenches and regimental aid posts. A few hours into the battle, these sites of care were already a shambolic mess of groaning, screaming, dying men on bloodied stretchers, a place of torment where too few medical officers were called upon to treat man after man. Many of the walking wounded bypassed these areas entirely, still trekking to the rear, some having lost their boots in the glutinous mud, continuing in their stockings as they followed wooden signs pointing to the advanced dressing stations that were connected to the field ambulances.[36] Situated in the deep caves to protect them against shellfire, the advanced dressing stations were places of refuge for the wounded, who could wait for a medical officer or one of his senior stretcher-bearers to see them.

Joseph Harrison MacFarlane, who had enlisted at age twenty as a student from Montreal and who would twice be awarded the Distinguished Conduct Medal, confided to his diary about the frantic day at No. 9 Canadian Field Ambulance, noting, "Worked

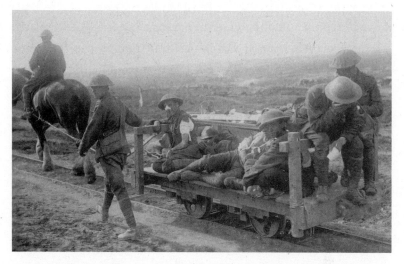

A horse-drawn light rail car takes wounded Canadians to medical care.

all night at Ambulance Corner loading ambulances + unloading tram trucks of wounded. Terrible experience."[37] The main dressing station for the stretcher cases from the 1st to 3rd Divisions, staffed by those divisions' medical personnel, was located in the southern centre of the battlefield, at les Quatre Vents, while the 4th Division, in the north, had its wounded treated at la Haie. Protected somewhat by enemy fire, the station on the northern front had heated tents and even a few temporary wooden structures. All were full. Some patients lay comatose, others raved with feverish visions, and many screamed in agony between gibberish pleas.

Demonstrating another medical technological innovation, at Vimy the forward medical units were also issued the Thomas splint for the first time. This invention consisted of a padded ring that fit around the upper thigh, and from which two stabilizing rods ran to the ankle to immobilize the leg. It would save lives by reducing the suffering of soldiers with broken legs.[38] Not many splints were available at Vimy, however, and it was never easy to move men with compound factures along the porridge-like roads. The journey was long. It was a five-hour bumpy trip by motor ambulance from the main dressing station to les Quatre Vents, for example—and it was absolute torture for those patients who were thrown about in the horse-drawn ambulances. At Vimy, however, another innovation emerged in the form of clearing the battlefield with hand-pushed trucks and horse-pulled trams that ran on narrow-gauge rails. This eased the suffering of some soldiers and took pressure off the road system.

The capture of most of Vimy Ridge by late on April 9 forced the enemy to retreat. Unlike the Somme, with its unsuccessful and see-saw battles making it difficult to remove the wounded from No Man's Land, the clear-cut Canadian victory at Vimy ensured that much of the enemy artillery and machine guns were captured or drawn back. Had the Germans been able to counterattack and retake the ridge as they had planned to do if they had kept even a small remaining toehold on their original line, not only would the Canadian infantry have suffered heavily and possibly been forced into retreat, but the thousands of wounded who lay on the battlefield during the 9th and 10th, as well as the many thousands in the immediate rear areas, would have been caught in the fighting as the counterattacking forces swept over them.

By the end of the second day of combat, during which the Canadians continued to drive forward down the eastern slope of the ridge or consolidate enemy trenches, almost 6,000 injured soldiers—Canadians, British, and Germans—were funnelled through the medical system, for a total of 14,018 wounded to that point in the battle.[39] The 11th saw little direct fighting, with the Germans in retreat but still shelling the Canadians on the ridge. Major

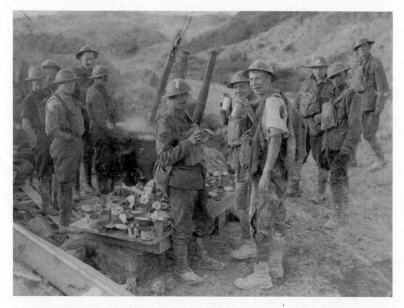

Wounded and mud-splattered Canadians enjoy drinks behind the lines.

Stanley Graham Ross of No. 6 Canadian Field Ambulance wrote in his diary that day about the "beastly weather. Snowing most of the afternoon."[40] As Canadian riflemen and machine-gunners dug in to prepare for German attacks, behind them small groups of stretcher-bearers searched the craters for the wounded throughout the day, while others took brief rests in the cave system. A final push on the 12th captured a strongpoint to the north of the ridge called the Pimple, with three Canadian battalions overrunning the enemy positions in a blinding snowstorm.

With the clash for the ridge over, ongoing bloody campaigns continued in the medical units. It was a heartbreaking time as the stretcher-bearers and medical officers encountered mangled soldiers whom they knew intimately. Brave and resolute, happy and joking only days earlier, these men were now writhing in

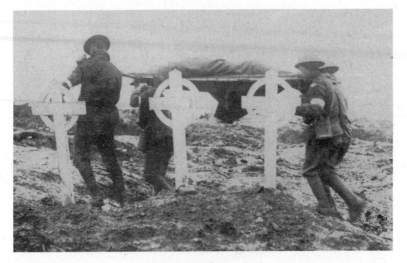

Not all could be saved.

agony with a yawning stomach wound or a broken femur bone jutting through torn flesh. Some of the worst-wounded soldiers, delusional with pain and thrashing about, had to be tied to their stretchers. Morphine and cocaine were issued while supplies lasted, and then the doctors turned to overproof rum. Soldiers recounted seeing hypothermic men who had lain in the mud for hours and whose teeth were chattering so loudly that they were in danger of breaking. The snapping of jaws and gnashing of teeth summed up the horror along the ridge.

Private Sydney Amyas Winterbottom, a student from Kamloops, British Columbia, told his father in a letter, "I have often heard you say how you longed to be a soldier, old man. Well all I can tell you is that longing would surely fade away if you could see a battlefield after an advance. Little heaps of blood and bones here and there, a shoulder and head there, a couple of legs somewhere else."[41] Winterbottom survived Vimy only to be killed at Passchendaele later in the year. A staggering 3,598 Canadians were slain during the four-day Vimy operation, with another 7,004 listed as wounded. Despite the successful driving of the Germans from the ridge, the smothering of enemy artillery batteries, and the effective clearing of the wounded, the biting cold contributed to the death of many soldiers who rapidly succumbed to shock. In fact, the ratio of 1 killed to 1.95 wounded was the second worst in the war for the Canadians and almost on par with the slaughter of the Somme. And even more soldiers would die in the battle's aftermath, with the official fatalities counting the dead only from April 9 to 14.[42]

———

"I would not have missed that attack for all the money in the world," wrote Private Edison Blue from Cobourg, Ontario, even though he had been knocked out with shrapnel in the chest and hip.[43] He survived to know that the victory at Vimy was immediately signalled as a significant and recognizable Canadian achievement. Its meaning would continue to gather in strength for Canadians and, increasingly, the battle was fused with the memorial that was unveiled on the ridge in 1936 to create the Vimy legend. A sacred place of sorrow and of pride, it was a symbol to Europe of Canada's service and sacrifice.[44]

By examining Vimy through the lens of the medical services, we see the important role of force protection before the operation to ensure that the Canadian Corps was not shorn of strength and endurance before the battle was even fought. The incredible contributions of the medical services were also essential in supporting the victory at the sharp end. However, April 9, 1917, a clear-cut

CHAPTER 11

CARE AND RECOVERY

"Some of the wounds are so dreadful that one's most vivid imagination couldn't even faintly picture them," wrote Nursing Sister Sophie Hoerner, a Montreal-born nurse who was superintendent of a hospital in Saranac Lake, New York, before the war.[1] While soldiers with recoverable injuries that would rapidly heal usually remained at hospitals in France, most of the trauma to the body that involved the tearing of flesh, the ripping of muscles, and the shattering of bones required a longer recovery. Those patients were sent to hospitals and convalescent homes in England to free up the beds in France for the steady flow of mangled men from the front. The patients were "dirty, disheveled, unshaven, with their clothes in tatters," remembered one Voluntary Aid Detachment worker at No. 1 Southern General Hospital in Birmingham. The VADs, as they were called, were women, usually without nursing experience, who came from Canada to serve in Canadian and British hospitals. VADs were also involved in the care of patients and the upkeep in hospitals, even though the nurses guarded their professionalism with vigour. By war's end, some 2,000 Canadian and Newfoundland women cared for the sick as VADs, and some even drove ambulances at the front.[2]

Those patients sent directly from the battle front were almost always crawling with lice, which were sometimes passed on to nurses and doctors. Experienced medical practitioners also learned to check the pockets of soldiers' battle jerkins for grenades. It was less worrisome to deal with patients who had been treated and cared for in Western Europe as they wore "hospital blues," a formal-looking pyjama that replaced their cut-away, blood-stained uniform.[3] Occasionally a soldier retained a good luck charm, clutched desperately by the patient through all the pain and misery. Surgeons were increasingly aware that all soldiers carried talismans and charms, and they tried to find them on their patients—worn around the neck, tucked into a pocket, sewn into a uniform—before an operation, to be returned to their owners later.[4] Moreover, the extracted metal from a soldier's body—a deformed bullet, a twisted piece of shell splinter, an iron marble-sized shrapnel ball—was also handed over to the patient, a dark object of service that was often kept for the rest of the men's lives as a symbol of survival. These "grim souvenirs," as one Canadian called the bullet fragments removed from his chest, back, and arm, represented the tenuous but tangible link between life and death on the Western Front.[5]

The evacuation, care, and recovery process was experienced by many soldiers, as the total number of Canadian cases admitted to a medical unit or facility in all theatres of war was 539,690. While different statistics were compiled during the course of the war and afterwards, one set revealed that 144,606 cases were battle casualties and the remaining 395,084 cases were due to accident, disease, or illness.[6] As the total number of soldiers in the

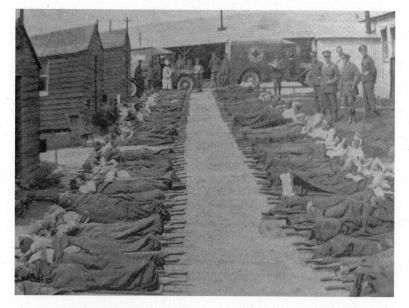

*Canadian hospitals were always moving wounded men from
France to England to clear space for more injured soldiers.*

Canadian Expeditionary Force deployed overseas was formally
counted at 418,052 (although this did not include sailors, some
airmen, and those in British units), with about 350,000 Canadians
serving along the Western Front, the statistics indicate that most
soldiers had more than one visit to a hospital during the course of
the war. The hospitals were both congested sites of care and places
of negotiation where soldiers interacted with nurses, orderlies,
doctors, and other patients as they underwent treatment with the
goal of returning to their units.

———

The *massive* expansion of the CEF from 1914 to 1916 required
new medical units at the front and behind the lines. Many

hospitals had over 1,000 beds and a staff at full strength of 30 medical officers, 70 nurses, and 205 other ranks. For example, in early 1917, No. 6 Canadian General Hospital, originally formed from Laval's medical school, consisted of a 1,400-bed hospital. In its first three months, when it cared primarily for soldiers of the French Army, the staff dealt with 2,350 medical cases, conducted 1,450 surgeries, and carried out 11,948 treatments and dressings.[7] The CAMC would eventually have 37 medical units overseas with a bed capacity of 14,000, a count that included specialist hospitals or wards that focused on diverse issues ranging from shell shock to orthopedic care, from venereal disease to tuberculosis.[8]

Hospital trains moved the wounded from the forward medical units to the French coast along fixed rail lines, picking up patients from casualty clearing stations and hospitals en route. Hospital trains were not in use at the start of the war, but they were soon found essential for the transfer of mass casualties. Within a year several dozen British-run trains were operating, eventually rising to a total of 63, with each one having at least a dozen cars and carrying up to 400 patients. Those soldiers that succumbed to their injuries before reaching their destination were buried in the many cemeteries along the coast, while hospital ships ferried the survivors of battle or disease across the Channel to British soil. Contributing to the staggering statistics from the war, the ambulance trains eventually carried 3,443,507 sick and wounded soldiers.[9]

After surveying the ghastly injuries to soldiers, one Canadian VAD wrote, "One wonders if it would not be more merciful to let the men die."[10] While many must have entertained this thought with a shudder, all struggled to save the lives of the broken soldiers from the front. However, the physical and emotional effort of dealing with hundreds of mangled men in great rushes was particularly trying for nurses, VADs, orderlies (privates in the CAMC), and doctors. Staff at civilian hospitals in Canada never had to deal with these unending waves of dying men—save for the once-in-a-century disaster of the Halifax Explosion of December 1917 that killed about 2,000 and injured at least 9,000 more. A Canadian nurse described the chaos in her military hospital, writing, "We have been dreadfully busy, seven hundred patients. As I sit here in my little hut, ambulance after ambulance bringing in the wounded, it's too terrible to watch and hear, and it goes on all night, too. The wounds caused by the bursting shrapnel are most severe. It rips, tears, lacerates and penetrates the tissues in a horrible manner. The doctor tries to repair and make good the best he can, but our best is often of little avail. One man completely blind, another with a knee joint blown open. . . . A weary road these men have trod."[11]

Canadians from the front were dispersed throughout the many Canadian and British hospitals and convalescent homes. Patients received state-of-the-art treatment and therapeutic care to support their return to good health. The goal was to get the soldiers back to the front or, if this was impossible for men with a debilitating injury or amputation, to transfer them to Canada to begin a long period of rehabilitation. Soldiers who had already faced surgery in France often had more operations scheduled in England, especially since it was not uncommon practice for surgeons along the battle front—who were always rushed and harried—to leave bullets or shell fragments in the body of a soldier, to be dealt with later if he survived.

Lance-Corporal Charles Savage, while recovering from a leg wound in an English hospital, was in a ward with a soldier no more than sixteen years old. A bag of grenades had detonated near him and he had endured the breaking of almost every major bone in his body, along with countless lacerations to his skin. The boy-soldier had been recovering for months, and he would proudly show the other patients the metal that had been removed from his body. "Each day the Doctor picked out a piece or so of shrapnel that had worked its way close to the skin and gave it to him to add to the collection which he kept in a bag tied to the head of his bed," recounted Savage.[12] By the time Savage left the hospital to return to the front, the scarred boy had over 105 pieces of jagged metal in his bag, although he was cheerfully healing, with some feeling returning to his extremities even though he was not likely to ever walk again.

———

"If the dreaded gaseous infection has made itself known, by reason of subcutaneous emphysema, brownish discolouration of the skin, bubbles of gas in the brownish red discharge or by the character-istic odour of this, the wound must be more widely opened . . . to stop the spread of the infection," wrote Major Thomas Archibald Malloch, a surgeon in the CAMC.[13] The gas gangrene infection came from a life-threatening bacterium that was difficult to treat. In France and Belgium, the physicians in uniform had found that almost every shrapnel and splinter wound became infected. Cut-ting away the flesh and muscle was the only hope for preventing disease from running rampant, which was done in tandem with irrigating the deepened gash in the body with chemical solutions. "Some of the smells of the wounds are awful," recounted a Canadian surgeon in his diary, "and the necessary incisions are ghastly."[14] Most of these debridement operations were carried out

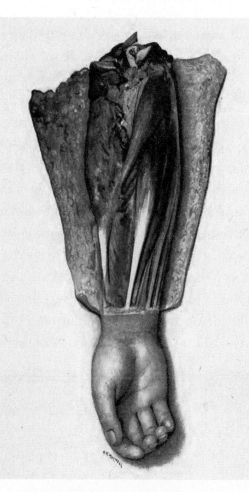

An amputated arm revealing gas gangrene.

at the casualty clearing stations and general hospitals, but new interventions were sometimes necessary during the recovery phase as deep holes in flesh took months to heal, poorly mended bones needed to be rebroken, or infection returned again and again.

In the age before antibiotics, several saline solutions were employed to keep wounds clean of infection. Most of these solutions used a combination of salt and a small dose of chlorine of

lime and bleach, although in the first two years of the war experimentation with many chemicals took place as the horrific wreckage of battle created hundreds of thousands of cases upon which
to try new methods. By mid-1916, the Carrell-Dakin hypochlorite
fluid approach proved the most effective, and it became standard-
ized within the CAMC.[15] The treatment required constant irrigation of the yawning cavities in the body, usually via a series of
tubes through which the saline was dispersed as often as every two
hours. The Carrell-Dakin solution was one of the groundbreaking
medical innovations of the war that saved the wounded from an
amputation or an agonizing death by infection, but it created horrifying scenes of wounded men with multiple tubes running into
their weeping sores, packed in place with gauze and bandages.

It fell to the nurses to check the irrigation tubes to ensure they
were not choked with pus and clotted blood. Without this medical

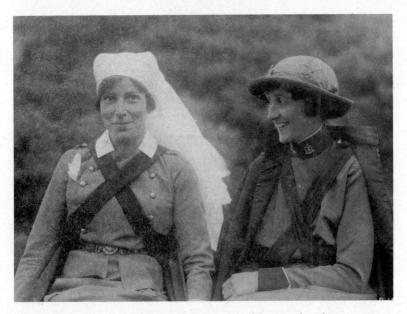

Nursing sisters played a key role in assisting soldiers in their long recovery.

surveillance, blocked hoses could lead to festering infections. Of course, such examinations by nurses came with no little pain to the patients as their open wounds were probed, studied, and threaded with tubes. The dressings that were packed into the cavities to keep the tubes in place and to prevent foreign material entering the area also had to be changed regularly. This was excruciating and the task usually fell to the nurses, although occasionally doctors performed the work to study the progression of healing. "After breakfast the surgeon appeared and the dreadful ordeal of dressing the wounds began," explained one eyewitness in a ward. "The orderly would cut the bandages and lay bare the great wound. The surgeon, equipped with sterilized gown and gloves, would pull out all the old packing and tubes, often having to probe deep with the points of his instrument."[16] The howls of the patient resounded through the ward.

———

"This is all the heart could desire," wrote Private James Herbert Gibson from Perth, Ontario, who was recovering from a bullet to the left arm at a convalescent home. In case his loved ones did not get the point, he added that it was "a regular soldier's paradise."[17] Another Canadian officer at a convalescent home described the estate as having "all the means necessary to render a holiday pleasant."[18] This was indeed the best of Blighty and many soldiers savoured these bucolic experiences in the stately mansions turned convalescent homes. Canada had eight convalescent hospitals in Britain, with a bed capacity of 7,456 in 1918, although thousands of Canadians were sent to recover in British-run manors and institutions.[19] The spacious grounds included outdoor areas for sports and indoor reading rooms with newspapers and musical instruments. Much of this care was funded by the local community or patriotic associations in Britain and Canada, and many plaques and posters noted that a specific rehabilitation or leisure area was donated by the people of a particular community.

Whether in a hospital or one of the many convalescent homes, the men participated in a vibrant ward culture. Away from the misery and dirt, and even though they were suffering with pain or the uncertainty of an infection, many soldiers had their minds eased by the white sheets and conscientious care. On the firing line, soldiers had banded together and coped with the strain of

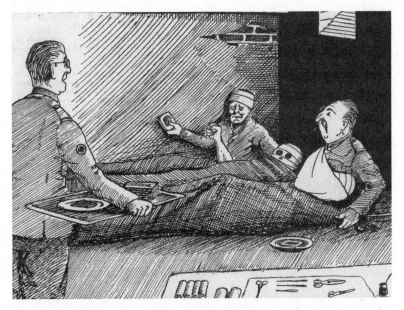

To endure the strain, soldiers turned to gallows humour at the front and in the hospitals. This cartoon pokes fun at an older private in the CAMC who stupidly chastises wounded soldiers. The caption reads, "Orderly (to badly wounded infantrymen who has complained of the bully [beef]): You guys don't seem to know that there is a war on!"

service by singing songs and spreading rumours, or by creating trench art and publishing newspapers.[20] Together, these cultural acts and products were a shield against the terrible strain of the war, drawing the soldiers together, forging bonds of comradeship, and allowing for group expression. As part of the recovery process, and often as a pushback against the constant control over their bodies, soldiers continued with these cultural expressions.

In the hospitals, gramophones played the latest patriotic or frivolous songs while film nights provided escapist moments and group singalongs brought the patients together in shared experiences.[21] Civilian lecturers moved from hospital to hospital, frequently paid for by the Red Cross, offering informative talks using lantern slides, some moralizing in tone and others featuring distracting adventures in foreign lands. Talented soldier-patients—entertainers, singers, poets, and even jugglers—put on shows, with one recovering soldier, Roderick Anderson Todd, writing from No. 2 Military Hospital in Exeter, "There is always some fun going around the wards here."[22]

Patients also played pranks on one another, kidded with their doctors, and chided the nurses. Guided by a unit's talented writers, editors, and poets, some of the hospitals, clearing stations, and field ambulances produced newspapers, too, in which recovering men occasionally contributed poems, jokes, or prose. *The Iodine Chronicles* (No. 1 Canadian Field Ambulance), *The McGilliken* (No. 3 Canadian General Hospital), *Canadian Hospital News* (Granville Canadian Special Hospital), and several other papers were venues for this distinct cultural expression.[23] *The Stretcher*, a paper produced at the Ontario Military Hospital at Orpington, published a jokey list of "don'ts" for patients, which included, "DON'T shave more than twice a week. Your visitors are more likely to believe your sob-stories if you look the part," and "DON'T get up when you're called. The Night Sister will enjoy tipping you out."[24] Others wrote lightly of their painful experience, using humour to frame their journey from the front to the hospitals, joking about stopping a piece of metal or being taken out not by an ambulance but on the ammunition wagon because they were so full of bullets. One British soldier scoffed at the surprising over-care at McGill's No. 3 Canadian General Hospital in a humorous story: "I was helped out of the ambulance, the Colonel took my hand, then three lieutenant-colonels took my pulse, four majors hurried to take my temperature, and some blighter took my watch."[25] It was not for nothing that abbreviation RAMC was often sourly said to stand for "Rob All My Comrades." And a similar idea held that some members of the CAMC, especially those further from the rear, treated themselves to the vulnerable soldiers' valuables, such as wallets and watches.

In the hospital wards and in the convalescent homes, these soldier-patients were encouraged and taught to create inventive arts. They learned to sew and to make baskets, or to forge sweetheart jewellery for those who waited at home. One of the Canadian orderlies enthused in a letter, "You'd die to see some of the results. . . . It is great fun."[26] These decorative arts revealed the soldiers' creativity, whiled away the time, and were useful in restoring some fine motor skills. The war had reduced the soldiers to patients, but some refused to let their wounds crush their spirit.

Not all recuperating soldiers were cheerful, of course. Injured young men brooding over debilitating injuries and a future filled with uncertainty were not always the best patients. Arthur Gamester, who served with a siege battery on the Somme, described his convalescent hospital in Berkshire, England: "These are bad

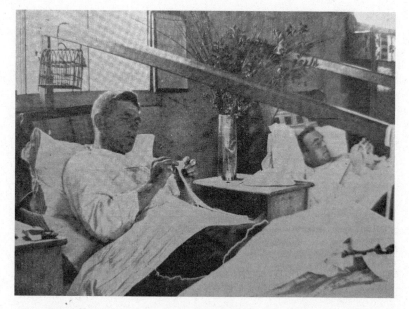

*Canadian patients knitting and engaging in art therapy as part
of the recovery process at Queen's University hospital. Note their
fractured legs attached to a pully for better recovery.*

days, for the shells and bullets of the enemy have laid claim to a
heavy toll of our men. I have seen sights within the walls of this
hospital calculated to draw tears of sorrow and sympathy."[27]
Elmer Bowness was nearly knocked out several times at the front
by shot or shell before his number came up. He wrote to his father
from a hospital in Wales during his long recovery, noting, "If the
people at home could see the real horrors of the battle-field they
would be worried to death."[28] For many of these devastated men,
with their nightmares and distant shell-shocked stares, laughter
had long died away.

"Every bed was occupied, and the nurses were working practically day and night," observed an admiring Private William Millar of the 52nd Battalion, a former plumber who enlisted at age thirty-three and who was shot in the thigh in August 1916. "Far too little is heard of the great work done by these noble women."[29] The soldiers in the wards admired the nurses for their professionalism, caring attitudes, and hard work. After months or years of all-male company, many privates' deep affectation for their female caregivers turned to love, but the rank of lieutenant for Nursing Sisters ensured no fraternization could take place with the rank and file. Nurses were officers and usually older than soldiers, and they often referred to the patients as their "boys," although they were still forced to fend off many amorous advances with a lighthearted laugh or a stern word.[30] It was a different story with patients who were officers; forming relationships, friendly or intimate, with these men was more acceptable, and many marriages were begun during the war.

Attesting to the charged relationships in hospitals, soldiers continued to pen letters to the nurses after returning to the front or when they were discharged back to Canada. During their time of convalescence, many of the soldiers also left their mark by contributing to nurses' autograph books. Women in uniform often kept these souvenir journals as memory objects to mark the relationships of patients and nurses, and they functioned a bit like modern-day yearbooks. In contrast, few soldiers compiled records in this same way. In the autograph books, some soldiers simply signed their names, but many drew cartoons and offered cheeky comments, irreverent jokes, gushy phrases, and sentimental poetry. Patients might also include sexually veiled comments, like this one in Nursing Sister Margaret Reilly's autograph book: "There was a young girl named Bess / Who treated the boys in our mess / to a jolly good time / and it wont be a crime / her name forever to Bless—A. E. Piper 25th Battalion / 5th Brigade / 2nd Canadian Division / Military Hospital Hastings."[31] Nurse Georgina Beach McCullough's autograph book contains many of the typical soldiers' scratchings, including the 2nd Battalion's Private George Macdonald's poem, "Carry On":

> When the Bosche has done your
> Chum in,
> And the Sergeant's done the
> Rum in,
> And there ain't no rations
> Coming
>   Carry on.[32]

The poem captured the common theme of soldiers in the line or recovering in the wards having to find ways to endure.

Nurses also wrote in each other's books, sometimes in a farewell statement since they were often transferred among multiple units and hospitals, with many having a goal of getting to the Western Front. A fellow Canadian nurse added to Nursing Sister Gertrude Mills's book a poetic aphorism: "It is easy enough to be pleasant / when life flows along like a song. / But the sister worth while, / is the one who still smiles / when everything goes dead wrong."[33] These books and other aspects of ward culture reveal a very human side to the nurses, as they struggled to save lives, winning and losing, feeling grief and frustration. Patients often described their nurses as angels; indeed, they often carried out angelic care work, but the emotional toil could be high on them.

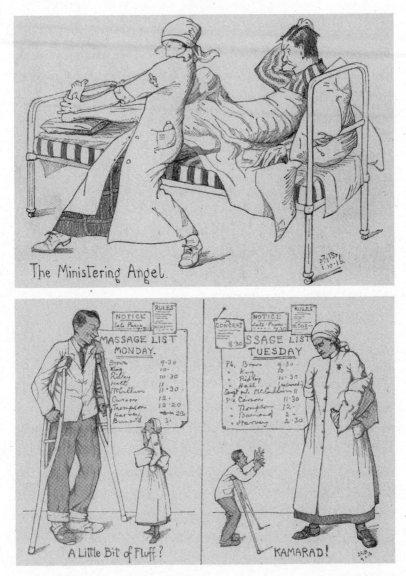

Two postcards from the Bliss series that reveal ward culture and the
contested role of the nurse. In the first cartoon, the "Ministering Angel"
is engaging in physiotherapy with a patient who is in obvious pain. The
second postcard is a commentary on the power imbalance in the hospitals.
Both postcards use humour to question the notion of nurses as angels.

Sisters who broke from the overwork and the relentless bloodshed were sent to recuperate at the Northwood Hospital for Sick Sisters. However, most survived the unyielding strain, even as they gave unstintingly of their time as lifesavers.

———

Not all wounds were created equal. Katherine Wilson-Simmie, a nursing sister who served in the Mediterranean, France, and England, described the many injured patients she encountered in her care: "Perhaps the head cases were the most harrowing. A boy would come in with all his senses, and suddenly I would hear a scream, and would find that he had gone absolutely insane, often with all his bandages torn off, and his wound haemorrhaging, with particles of his brain oozing out of the open wound."[34] These distressing injuries were trying for even the most experienced of doctors and nurses. Soldiers with facial injuries typically did not survive the bullet or shrapnel that broke skulls, exposed brains, pulped eyeballs, or ripped off lower jaws. However, those who did suffered frightening disfigurement, periodic seizures, and partial or full paralysis. Attesting to the nearly unthinkable losses that numbered millions of battlefield killed, there was a chillingly large number—some 208,000 French, German, and British soldiers— who survived a form of maxillofacial injury, as these face wounds were known.[35] Called *les gueules cassées* (the broken faces) in France, these men had many operations in front of them, requiring surgeons with a speciality in the slow process of rebuilding faces.[36] It was an art much advanced by the traumatic effects of this war.

Many of the facially mutilated were prioritized for removal to a special surgical centre at the Queen Mary's Hospital at Sidcup,

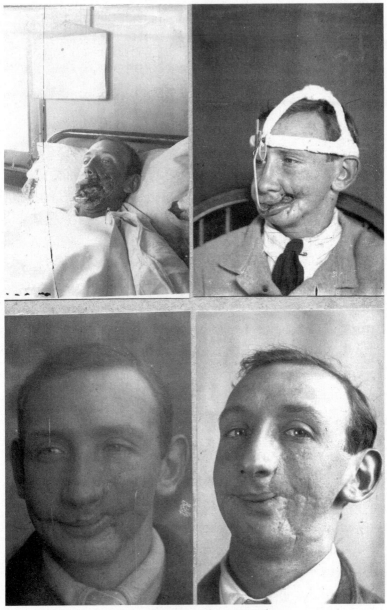

The wounds of war were shocking.

So, too, was the related art of remaking soldiers' faces.

where they underwent operations. There, Dr. Harold Gillies, a New Zealand–born pioneer in the field of plastic surgery and facial reconstruction, brought together a small team of experts that included dental surgeons to help rebuild sheared-off noses, crushed facial bones, and shattered jaws.[37] For men with deep gouges in their face, skin and bone grafts were required as noses, eyelids, or ears were fashioned from flesh harvested from other parts of the body.

In the CAMC, Major Joseph Napoleon Roy, formerly of the Hotel-Dieu in Montreal and serving during the war with No. 4 Stationary Hospital, was a trailblazer in facial reconstruction. He wrote about his pioneering work in the pages of the *CMAJ*, describing a Canadian officer, known as Captain E.C., who was twenty-six years old when he was shot in the face on April 16, 1916. The man had survived his grave wound, but his jaw had been shattered and his nose torn off; in Major Roy's words, he had suffered "considerable disfigurement."[38] The doctor carried out three reconstructive operations—on May 10, September 23, and October 31 —rebuilding the bone that had been hacked away and creating a new prosthetic nose, all of which was held together by an elaborate splint.[39] Incredibly, the officer returned to duty in a brigade headquarter at the end of 1917, growing a moustache to partially hide the scars.

Major Roy also noted that the work of dental surgeons was "almost indispensable."[40] While dentists had enlisted in the CAMC from the start of the war and were put to good work in pulling rotten teeth to allow many men to enlist at Valcartier and other camps, the Canadian Army Dental Corps was established in 1915 when Sam Hughes appointed his own dentist, Lieutenant-Colonel

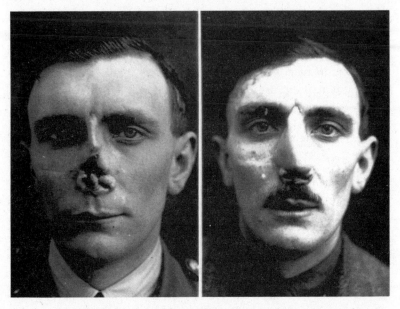

A facially disfigured soldier with a new nose that was created
from skin extracted from another part of his body.

J.A. Armstrong. Eventually the Canadians would have one dentist for every 1,000 men, while the British had only one dentist for every 10,000 soldiers.[41] Stationary dental clinics were created in Western Europe and Britain, and roving teeth-pullers visited units in the field. A significant need for mouth care developed in the dentally challenged army, with many men never using a tooth-brush. Almost all soldiers were missing teeth when they came into the ranks, while many more broke them on the rock-hard biscuits. About 70 percent of all soldiers needed dental work, and Canadian dentists performed a staggering 2,225,442 procedures during the war. One of the hidden wartime legacies was that a generation of veterans emerged, as the army put it, "dentally fit for peacetime."[42]

The CEF saw so many cases of facial wounds and fractured jaws that a special CAMC clinic was established at the Ontario

Military Hospital at Orpington, which was 10 kilometres from Sidcup. Mirrors did not adorn the walls. In addition to the reconstructive surgery provided by the flesh artists, special facial masks were created to cover untreatable injuries. They were constructed out of tin or plastic and painted to match skin colour, although they often had an uncanny, doll-like quality. After multiple operations, some of the patients were able to shed their prosthetics. A gradual return to normalcy occurred for most of the war-maimed in a stunning revelation of how medicine slowly undid the war's trauma.[43] One visitor to the special clinic at Orpington watched the reconstructive surgical work in the "beauty parlour," as the patients called the surgical area, and believed it was "the difference between regeneration and a living death."[44]

The survivors of amputation were treated at several specialized orthopedic centres. The first such Canadian facility, established at Ramsgate in November 1915, was, in the words of one Canadian nurse, "the hospital of empty sleeves and crutches and well-chairs."[45] Hundreds of Canadian amputees passed through its wards to be fitted with artificial hands and legs. They underwent training in the use of their prosthetics and it was not uncommon for men to suffer through additional operations if wounds healed poorly. To soothe raw stumps, massage therapists used their trained hands to work atrophied muscles, reduce scar tissue, and try to ease chronic pain. While one Canadian patient described the therapy in a letter home as "torture business," he finished by noting that it was "cruel treatment but of course it is necessary."[46]

———

Medical personnel devoted themselves day and night to mending broken bodies and defeating rampant infections, with the successes far outweighing the failures. And yet still thousands died in hospitals. Nursing Sister Elizabeth Paynter recounted the agony of caring for young men with terrible wounds, hoping they would recover and then seeing infection end their lives: "Another patient died, and another still was very low, while there were at least four other delirious head cases, who seemed to take turns pulling off their dressings or getting out of bed."[47] Nurses and chaplains sat with the dying soldiers, bringing succor in the final hours. "Many times in the night to come," wrote one Canadian nurse, "I would wish that the parents had known that their boy had at least the comfort of a decent bed, and a Padre standing by for his last hours."[48] This was an emotional load for the caregivers and they bore it within this shared kinship of suffering as part of a sacred bond that few outsiders will ever understand.

It was not just the nurses or doctors who offered a kind word, a steady hand, or a cheerful smile. Soldiers tried to comfort one another in the wards when they were low. The able-bodied fetched cigarettes and books, stoked up the central oven, and even sometimes helped in changing dressings. "The boys look after one another," observed one Canadian VAD. "The lame lead the blind and the man without an arm wheels the man without a leg."[49] Harry Morris, whose leg was shattered by shrapnel fire on the Vimy front, spent some of his recovery time offering comfort to a dying comrade. Morris communicated by letter to his own family that the "poor fellow died in the next bed to me this morning. He was literally riddled with bullets; he was a Canadian from Toronto. Just before he died, he asked me the question 'Am I reported wounded, dead or missing?'"[50] Morris was shaken by the experience and had a better understanding of soldiers' loved ones' dread of their fighting family member or friend being reported missing while they agonized at home, never knowing for certain if he was killed, and forever aching for news of his fate. Morris recovered and went home to his family in Montreal in early 1918, his war over but the experience at the front and in the hospital searing deep.

Private Archibald John Polson was serving with the 5th Canadian Machine Gun Company when he was wounded before the Battle of Vimy Ridge. A series of savage injuries to the right side of his body meant that an arm had to be amputated at the shoulder. He slowly recovered from his multiple shrapnel gashes, and several padres and nursing sisters from British No. 16 General Hospital sent written updates to his concerned parents about his fragile health. Within a few days of his amputation, one nurse wrote a letter on his behalf, saying, "I don't want you to worry. I have every hope he will recover."[51] His mother sent a reply from Gimli, Manitoba, which a nurse read to the gravely ill Archie: "My Darling Boy Oh how will I commence this letter. . . . I want to be worthy to be a mother of a brave Soldier Boy. Oh how Proud we all are of you my own Brave Boy."[52] Another letter went out from a Red Cross volunteer, Annie Paine, to Archie's mother, with the hopeful message "He looks much better than many of our men who I have seen after amputations."[53] Archie continued to recover, passed through various hospitals, and learned to write awkwardly with his left hand. But a tetanus infection took hold, and despite months of treatment, operations, and irrigation of the wound, the infection could not be overcome. The twenty-one-year-old soldier died on September 1, 1917, at Princess Patricia's Red Cross Hospital in Ramsgate. One of the condolence letters sent to Mrs. Polson noted that a funeral had been held for Archie and a "decent grave" placed in England, contrasting his end to those of so many Canadians who "die on the battlefield" and whose bodies were lost.[54] Perhaps that was a comfort.

While the primary goal of the medical staff was to restore the wounded to health, they were also ordered to return as many soldiers as possible to their units. This duty weighed heavily on the healers as they examined their patients to determine if they would ever again be fit for service. Like their counterparts along the Western Front, the doctors were placed in the Jekyll and Hyde role as they balanced the army's demand for more soldiers with that of the well-being of patients, many of whom pleaded openly not to be sent back to the front. Some doctors were sympathetic to the soldiers' belief that they had done their bit, especially when there were tens of thousands of other soldiers in England and about a million men of military age in Canada who were not in uniform. But rules and regulations had to be followed, and the process of determining a soldiers' fortune began by studying, examining, and interrogating the recovered man, much like the regimental medical officers' sick parade, although now conducted by a panel of three older doctors who had likely never been to the front. Questions were asked about the patients' physical injuries, pain, and mobility. Statistics indicate that about 80 percent of the battle casualties were returned to the Western Front, and while not all were fit for combat, therefore being assigned to positions behind the lines, this figure suggests an emphasis on manpower rather than the soldiers' concerns.[55] It was agonizing for some doctors to be responsible for sending healed and still recovering soldiers back into the line for another sustained tour at the front. One senior Canadian medical officer struggled with the heavy responsibility of determining a man's fate, lamenting, "So many soldiers look to me wistfully but never utter a word when I recruit them towards the front." He worried deeply about ordering soldiers to battle, but steeled himself because "necessity is great."[56] As always, the relationship between soldiers and doctors was complex and threaded with trying choices.

Those who were injured wore a wound stripe perpendicularly on the left sleeve of their service jacket—a two-inch gold braid that showed a man's fighting experience at a glance.[57] A number of classifications were created to determine a soldier's level of fitness, with those who were crippled but able to serve in some capacity kept in an administrative role in England or Western Europe. They

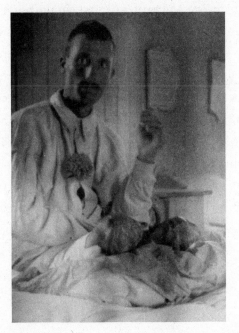

Badly wounded Canadians who had no chance of returning to the front were sent back to Canada, where they would fight new battles in the long recovery process.

might thus free up a healthier man for the front, and this type of position was generally acceptable to patients who could continue to serve. Those too far gone—due to gas-corrupted lungs, a mangled or missing limb, or one of the many other debilitating injuries—were ordered back to Canada, usually travelling on a hospital ship and under the care of Canadian doctors and nurses. One officer involved in the process wrote of those going home who were "badly mutilated," and yet many, he felt, revealed "what endurance the human frame has, and what one can go through and still retain a cheerful smile."[58]

These soldiers who returned to Canada eventually passed out of the care of the CAMC and began a rehabilitation process with the civilian-run Military Hospital Commission. Established in 1915, this organization evolved through a number of name changes but was the precursor to the Department of Veterans Affairs. In 1917, almost 9,000 Canadians were returned to the Dominion, while in 1918 before the armistice, another 13,481 crossed the Atlantic.[59] Across Canada, dozens of hospitals and convalescent homes were built for these soldiers, to aid in their recovery from physical and mental injuries, to retrain them, and to have them return to their communities as productive members of society. This largely state-run system was an important legacy that recognized the debt owed to the citizen-soldiers who had answered their country's call and now deserved the care and compassion of all Canadians.

———

At the end of the war, No. 3 Canadian General Hospital calculated that from August 7, 1915, when it first stood up as a unit, to its last day, on May 12, 1919, the hospital had treated 143,762 patients, had performed 11,395 operations, and had recorded 986 deaths from all casualties. Overall, the hospital's death rate was 1 in every 135 patients treated.[60] And this was but one of dozens of Canadian medical units. Closer to the front, at the casualty clearing stations, the field ambulances, and the carnage-ridden regimental aid posts, the death rate was higher, though more than 90 percent of soldiers survived a wound if they were treated by a medical doctor.[61] However, survival of course did not always mean that soldiers were able to carry on with their lives as before. Many veterans would suffer physical and mental pain long after the guns went silent, living with disabilities as they carried the war with them. The weight of the wounded was also borne by the medical practitioners, with the ordeal imprinting itself on doctors, nurses, and caregivers who, though trained in their profession to deal with such experiences, nonetheless were worn down by the relentless orgy of suffering. Reflecting on the hospital experience, Lieutenant-Colonel G.E. Armstrong wrote, "On the whole it is depressing to go through our hospitals day after day and week after week, observing the thousands of wounded, many of them sadly mutilated. It brings home to one the cruelties of war, and when at leisure one thinks of the homes of these men—of their dependents, their father, mother, brothers, wives and children, sisters and lovers, and a feeling of horror comes over one."[62]

CHAPTER 12

A TOXIC PLAGUE

"Gassing weakens the morale of troops," observed Canadian medical officer Robert James Manion. "Men do not fear to stand up and face an enemy whom they have a chance of overcoming, but they do hate dying like so many rats in a trap."[1] Poison gas was uniquely terrifying. Virtually unnoticeable amid the chaos and din of an artillery bombardment, chemical weapons struck with little warning. The Canadians had withstood the chlorine attack at Ypres in April 1915, and afterwards many soldiers described gas as a wicked weapon, even though shells and bullets killed and maimed far more soldiers. It was the ethereal quality of the chemical agents that contributed to the fright. Private John Lynch of Princess Patricia's Canadian Light Infantry, a young American serving with the Canadians, described the experience in vivid language: "From the first velvety phut of the shell burst to those corpse-like breaths that a man inhaled almost unawares. It lingered about out of control. When he fired it, a man released an evil force that became free to bite friend or foe til such time as it died into the earth. Above all, it went against God-inspired conscience."[2]

The Canadians had encountered poison gas sporadically since the chlorine clouds in Flanders fields, although after that surprise strike, the British had scrambled to manufacture respirators for the exposed soldiers. The first attempts consisted merely of a cloth padding that was to be wetted with a solution and tied around the head. Research continued at a desperate pace, with increasingly effective gas masks being produced until, in the Empire's forces, the process culminated in late 1916 with the small box respirator. This device offered effective protection via a bug-like facemask attached with a rubber hose to a charcoal-filled canister that filtered out the lethal chemicals. While it was an exhausting apparatus to wear for any extended period of time because it restricted breathing, it generally kept the user safe if

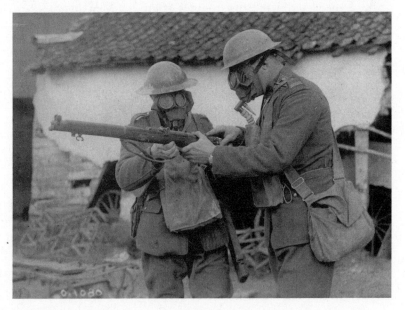

Two Canadian soldiers wearing small box respirators try to master the Lee-Enfield rifle while almost blind. Everything was made harder while wearing a respirator.

the wearer engaged in little movement except in the highest concentrations of gas.

Accompanying the distribution of respirators was the need for experts to assist with training in their use. As soldiers had an average education level of grade six, the subject of chemistry was foreign to many of them, further adding to their distress. As a result, all of the armies established specialist gas formations to train regimental officers and non-commissioned officers, and Canadian gas experts were engaged at the corps, division, brigade, and battalion levels.[3] These chemical specialists, usually university-educated men, instructed soldiers in how to get their respirator on with haste, how to identify the gasses by their smell, and how to fight while wearing the debilitating masks. And yet even as an anti-gas doctrine emerged, more noxious chemicals were being introduced through new delivery systems.

By 1917, two categories of war gases had been developed—lethal and harassing—and both sides in the war used chemical agents in increasing numbers to kill or wound, or to attrite enemy strength. The harassing agents were not very effective on the battlefield, as these non-lethal "tear gases" were meant to force the enemy to put on respirators that would interfere with their work. These gases were often fired amid high explosive and shrapnel bombardments, concealed among the eruptions and employed against enemy gunners to slow their rate of fire. Gas that affected the lungs was more toxic, particularly after chlorine had been superseded by the much more lethal phosgene. Nearly odorless and colourless, phosgene was difficult to detect and insidious in its effects. The victims often did not know that they had been poisoned. After a few hours, and with a growing heavy feeling in the chest, sick men began to cough up fluid. The amount of pus-filled and blood-tinged frothy liquid expelled was appalling, with a typical phosgene victim hacking up to four pints of liquid from his damaged lungs for several hours.[4] The afflicted became cyanosed as they slowly suffocated. One Canadian sergeant who instructed in protecting against gas—and who was himself later gassed—said of phosgene, "A very deadly poison, breathed for 3 minutes will cause death . . . the lungs begin to fill, breathing becomes harder, and the patient slowly suffocates, drowned within himself. A horrible death."[5]

With gas shells filled with phosgene from early 1916 and used at the Battle of Verdun between the Germans and the French that same year, this weapon sparked new dread among soldiers. Unlike the gas clouds created by opening hundreds of steel canisters to form a cloud to blow over No Man's Land, chemical shells landed with little warning. As the sentries rang alarms with horns and sirens, soldiers raced to put on their respirators and worried they hadn't donned them in time to protect against the unseen killer. Officers reported on large groups of men becoming hysterical after the release of gas, believing that the nearly imperceptible poison had penetrated their masks and that they were doomed. How would one know until it was too late? In August 1916, the British medical services issued a pamphlet to all front-line commanding officers stating that "no man suffering from the effects of gas should be allowed to walk to the dressing stations," since activity stimulated the effects of lungs filling with fluid.[6] Unfortunately, the "phosgene-rule," as one British colonel called it, resulted in "trenches packed with men who considered themselves gassed and thought that further movement would be fatal."[7] The medical services were further burdened as stretcher-bearers carried out the soldiers who often lay stiff with terror, afraid to move or speak.

While the shell-delivered gas rarely killed significant numbers of soldiers due to the challenge of building up a thick density of lethal gas before respirators could be put on, even a few hundred well-placed phosgene shells could cause casualties and could be psychologically dispiriting and physically exhausting for a large number of men forced to wear their masks. All of the available gases, however, lasted at most a few hours, and they were even less potent in strong wind or rain. But the chemical war changed on July 12, 1917, when the Germans released a new agent that burned, blinded, and killed. Mustard gas—the chemical dichloro-diethyl sulphide—took its name from the mild aroma of mustard that alerted victims to its presence. Marked with a yellow cross, the mustard gas shells contained an oily liquid that was transformed into a vaporous gas when the shell burst. This gas affected

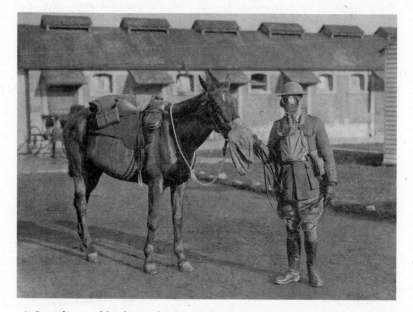

A Canadian and his horse, both wearing respirators. Gas shells were often used against the lines of communication to slow the movement of supplies.

14,000 British soldiers in the first three weeks of its use, with about 500 of them dying.[8]

The mustard gas vapours that were spread over a wide area when the shell detonated did not immediately burn the skin or irritate the eyes as chlorine did. "It affects the eyes and nose, but not at first," wrote one CAMC surgeon who encountered these new gas casualties, "so the men don't put on their helmets till the damage is done."[9] Eyelids soon swelled up and then shut, as men looked like boxers bashed in the face. Skin became red and then blistered. "The vile mustard gas that turned lungs to fluid, and burned skin from the body," wrote one soldier, "now permeated the light summer clothing, and the men writhed at the scorching touch."[10] A harsh cough with a wet rattle set in, men vomited uncontrollably as the body shook in convulsions, and they lost their sight. The blindness usually lasted two to three weeks, although some unlucky men never saw again through their clouded eyes. Badly exposed soldiers began to die on the second day—their seared lungs unable to draw in breath. They expired in agony as if they had breathed in fire.

Phosgene and chlorine were dispersed with wind after a few hours, but the mustard gas settled into the soil, mud, and water. Labelled a persistent agent, it retained its ability to burn and blind for up to two weeks, and the infected soil clung to uniforms and boots. Like a chemical plague, the gas had "contagious" effects: when a soldier entered a closed space such as an underground dugout, the gas fumes from the despoiled mud were released and began to poison those next to the victim.[11] One Canadian stretcher-bearer wrote home about the mustard gas, noting, "You can absorb it through the skin by rubbing your clothes with your hands; in fact, any old way."[12] Mustard gas caused many minor burns and temporary blindness, and it was most effective as a casualty-causing agent that frightened and maimed while clogging the medical system. In fact, captured German artillery plans indicated that one of the acknowledged uses for mustard gas was to fire it against "infantry strong points and billets to cause large numbers of slight casualties."[13] A secret British assessment of chemical agents confirmed that mustard gas was "in a class by itself so far as casualty producing power is concerned," and the Germans sought to overload the Allied medical system with a large number of casualties rather than with slain soldiers, who were more easily dealt with as part of the burial system.[14]

———

The Canadian Corps emerged from the victory at Vimy in April and fought across the Douai Plain, with additional successful engagements at Arleux and Fresnoy in late April and early May. After that, throughout the summer, the Canadians aggressively raided the enemy trenches on the outskirts of German-occupied Lens in increasingly sophisticated and large-scale operations involving hundreds of soldiers supported by complex machine-gun and artillery barrages. But the primary British campaign was in the Flanders region, to the east of Ypres, where Sir Douglas Haig launched his offensive on July 31. It would commonly be known as the Battle of Passchendaele and the field marshal hoped that a successful assault there would achieve the two-fold result of diverting German attention from the French army that was suffering from shattered morale due to horrendous casualties in fruitless campaigns, and cutting off German U-boat bases along the north coast when the enemy was driven into retreat. These were not unsound goals, although the operation failed almost from the start. Unseasonable rain poured down throughout early August, transforming the shell-pitted battlefield into a sea of mud. The obstinate Haig refused to call off the offensive, even as his soldiers floundered in unspeakable conditions, with the Germans keeping them at bay as they held the high ground of Passchendaele Ridge.

Further to the south, the new Canadian Corps commander Sir Arthur Currie was ordered to capture Lens to siphon off German strength and to ensure defenders were not sent to the Flanders front. Currie had taken over from Sir Julian Byng in June 1917, and the former land developer from Victoria, British Columbia, had a well-deserved reputation as the Canadians' best general. He had served from the first month of the war, first as an infantry brigadier and then as a major-general commanding a division. Able to absorb the hard lessons of war, the forty-one-year-old Currie impressed both Canadian and British generals. He was known for intricate planning and for prioritizing gunpower instead of manpower to achieve his operational goals.

Instead of charging into the heavily defended Lens, Currie decided to snatch Hill 70, a high point that dominated the city to the northwest. If the Canadians could capture and hold Hill 70, then the Germans would likely counterattack to regain it, ordering their troops to leave the protection of their trenches to advance into massed fire.[15] The complicated assault was launched on August 15 after several weeks of planning, with the 1st and 2nd Canadian Divisions swarming up Hill 70 while the 4th Canadian Division, to the south and opposite Lens, offered a diversion. A hurricane bombardment of artillery shells stunned the defenders, and after hard fighting the Canadians captured the hill within a few hours.

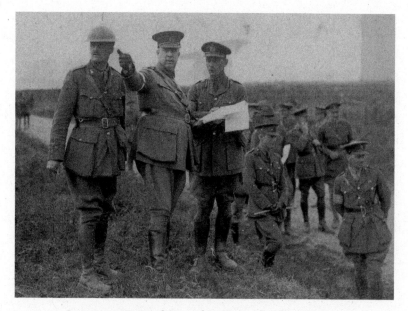

*Lieutenant-General Sir Arthur Currie faced his first test
as corps commander at the Battle of Hill 70.*

As expected, the Germans counterattacked, advancing across
No Man's Land into the mouth of the Canadian guns. The battlefield became a charnel house and the Germans suffered far more
losses than Currie's forces, although shells and snipers also took
down the Canadian attackers turned defenders. The stretcher-
bearers carried out their brave work as the trenches were filled
with the wounded, although one bearer from the 7th Battalion
was singled out for his awe-inspiring actions. Private Michael
James O'Rourke, born in Ireland and already a recipient of the
Military Medal on the Somme, carried men day and night from
the shattered slopes of Hill 70. According to his Victoria Cross
citation, for seventy-two hours, Private O'Rourke "worked
unceasingly in bringing the wounded into safety, dressing them,
and getting them food and water."[16] He did it as shells plummeted

down and riflemen fired on him, running from crater to crater, trench bay to trench bay. His comrades witnessed his utter disregard for danger and held their breath, assuming he would need to be carried out in pieces. And yet after each shell lit down, hurling him through the air, he would pick himself up and seek the next wounded man. When the injured lay vulnerable in forward positions, he cared for them no matter the risk, with a guardian angel somehow keeping him safe in the blizzard of steel. O'Rourke survived the battle and the war to live out his days in Vancouver, British Columbia, awarded the Victoria Cross not only for his eye-watering valour but perhaps for the inspiration he provided to others in showing that, indeed, some men were unkillable.

After mounting more than a dozen counterattacks, the frustrated German high command turned to gassing the Canadian

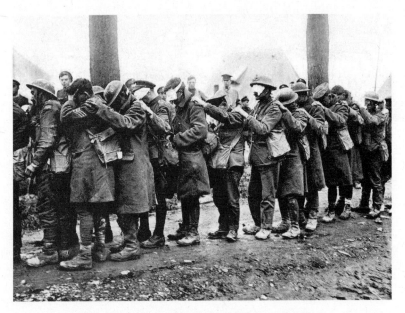

*Mustard-gassed soldiers being led from the front
with their eyes covered by bandages.*

front in the hope of demoralizing the infantry and slowing the artillerymen who frantically fed the guns. On the night of August 17, the Germans fired more than 15,000 mustard gas shells into the Canadian rearward areas, targeting the lines of communication and artillery batteries.[17] With the guns temporarily silenced, the German infantry struck again, although the Canadians held off the onslaught through tremendous sacrifice and tenacity. Many of the Canadian gunners, unable to see through their respirators, even removed their gas masks to keep firing and support their comrades in the front lines who were bearing the brunt of attack.[18] The gunners suffered within the swirling gas vapours, but they did not let down the infantry.

The medical services carried out their lifesaving work day and night, with forward stretcher-bearers and regimental medical officers straining to move the wounded through the system that stretched back to the field ambulance units and on to the casualty clearing stations. Before the battle, senior staff officers in the medical services had had time to plan for the clearing of the stretcher cases along narrow-gauge tramways, and this would save lives during the battle.[19] In the first forty-eight hours of combat, 3,580 Canadians and 330 captured Germans passed through the medical units in a mad rush of broken bodies.[20]

Private Clair Barrey was one of them. Serving with the 7th Battalion, Barrey took shrapnel in his right leg that eventually necessitated an amputation at the knee. "It must be a great shock to you, but I think it is all for the best," he wrote to his sister, Aggie. "I know you would think I was lucky if you could see some of the poor fellows here all shot to pieces."[21] Private Victor Wheeler of the 50th Battalion, who was in the firefight opposite Lens, wrote about the unending tension, noting, "There was no let up in shelling by either side, and our casualties continued to mount. . . . The strain on everyone's nerves in this scorching furnace of Lens became more apparent each day."[22] So bad were the conditions that some men shot themselves in the hand or stabbed themselves in the leg to escape the inferno. Others broke under the strain of the shellfire. Lieutenant-Colonel Agar Adamson of the Princess Patricia's Canadian Light Infantry wrote of stumbling through the trenches and encountering dismembered "legs and arms blown from some distance," and of witnessing many cases of shell shock, where twitching, raving soldiers were out of their minds from the trauma. "The men have to be held down," he noted, and the sight of them is "gruesome and horrible to see."[23]

———

The Battle of Hill 70 was widely seen as another Canadian triumph that came on the heels of the heralded victory at Vimy in April, but the Canadians once again paid heavily for the win. The Corps suffered 9,198 casualties from August 15 to 25, while another 2,000 were killed and injured during the previous two weeks of preparation.[24] Poison gas was responsible for 1,122 casualties—about 10 percent of the total Canadian losses—though the fatality rate among the victims of chemical warfare was very low.[25] The stretcher-bearers and medical officers could do little for men with mustard gas exposure in the forward zone, and the key was to rapidly evacuate tormented soldiers to stave off severe burns. The advanced dressing stations of the field ambulances, where many of the lightly treated were cared for, were bypassed and the gassed men—smelling of death and usually blind at this point—were guided to the main dressing station of the field ambulance and onward to the casualty clearing stations.

The knock-on effect of the mustard gas pestilence was another indication of how the war demanded constant innovation. The victims were a living weapon that burned the medical staff that touched infected bodies, and vapours were sometimes strong enough to cause nurses and doctors to go temporarily blind. Even corpses many days dead could poison the living. Given this danger, new procedures were implemented, including cutting off the soldier's uniform and washing him down even as he was bleeding from his wounds. Medical practitioners still suffered, with one Canadian nurse recounting the effects of the toxic plague: "[the] next day all the nurses had chest trouble and streaming eyes from the gassing. They were all yellow and dazed. Even their hair turned yellow and they were nearly as bad as the men, just from the fumes

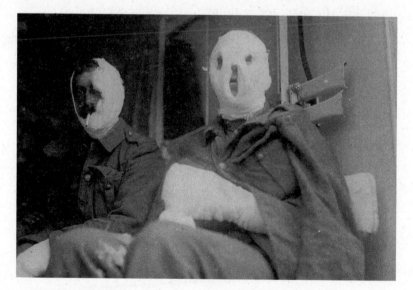

Canadian soldiers with full-body chemical burns.

from their clothing."[26] The lifesavers paid a price, and at least 115 members of the CAMC were gassed during the battle.[27]

Within these frightful conditions, the medical practitioners still found ways to ease the suffering and start the healing. Treatments varied, depending on the type of gas and the length of exposure. In response to the first chlorine attack, it was thought a good idea for patients to vomit, and while many were already retching uncontrollably, this purging was aided by various salts and castor oils. More pleasant for patients was the good dose of rum given to those making their way through the field ambulance, which calmed the nerves.[28] The commander of No. 8 Canadian Field Ambulance, Lieutenant-Colonel John Nisbet Gunn, wrote that oxygen "gave almost instant relief to the terrible pain and irritation, and was a very efficacious remedy for this hideous result of warfare."[29] For those who received it, oxygen acted as a psychological stimulant too, although most soldiers preferred receiving it orally instead of through the rectum, with both ways administered.[30] In cases where oxygen stocks were depleted or where it would not help, morphine delivered by pill or needle relieved the pain. It was remarked upon frequently that those with fatal doses of gas usually remained conscious almost to the end, beyond the care of nurses and doctors who watched with impotence as the victims clawed at their throats and thrashed about in agony from "air hunger."[31]

Mustard gas victims were usually blind by the time they arrived at the casualty clearing station many kilometres behind the front lines. Faces were puffy and had an unnatural shiny appearance. Eyes and nostrils streamed tears and mucus. The neck, ears, and even genitals were swollen. The massive skin blisters 15 to 20 centimetres in length often became infected. The more serious

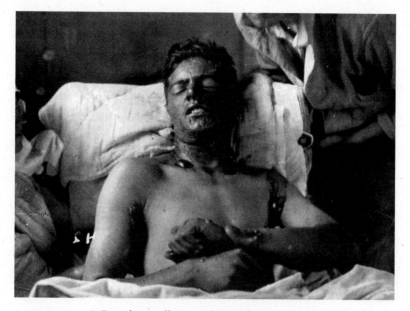

A Canadian suffering in hospital with his body
scorched and blistered by mustard gas.

cases hacked up blood-flecked sputum, and afflicted men took on the smell of rotting fruit. "There was nothing more horrible than to see men dying from gas," wrote Canon Frederick Scott, the much-loved poet and padre of the 1st Division. "Nothing could be done to relieve their suffering."[32]

Major Gilbert Peat, a doctor from Andover, New Brunswick, and one of the CAMC's gas specialists, wrote in the pages of *CMAJ* about treating the chemically wounded. Peat described the wards of blinded and burned men, gasping through ravaged lungs, their bluish lips and dark skin indicating oxygen deficiency. Many were delirious with fever and haunted by nightmares of being burned alive, and as Peat remarked, "The agony suffered by this group of cases was intense and the scene was the most gruesome one could imagine." While many wounded men took pride in presenting a manly demeanour and stifling the pain from conventional wounds, the gassed men visibly wailed and struggled, wrote Peat, "coughing, gasping and fighting for breath."[33] A British nurse observed that the "gas cases are terrible" and that they thrashed about, wheezing for breath, eyes wide in fear. "Their lungs are gone—literally burnt out. Some have their eyes and faces entirely eaten away by gas and their bodies covered with first-degree burns. . . . Gas burns must be agonizing because usually the other cases do not complain even with the worst wounds but gas cases are invariably beyond endurance and they cannot help crying out. One boy today, screaming to die, the entire top layer of his skin burnt from face and body."[34] It was the stuff of the worst nightmares in an already nightmarish war.

Methods were available to ease some of the pain and assist in healing. Bathing patients in a mild alkaline solution, for example, helped to aid in healing the blisters and reduce infections, and special preventative creams containing boracic acid diminished the severity of skin burns. However, as one medical report noted, deep chemical burns were "practically always infected."[35] By 1918, field ambulances were issued stores of bicarbonate of soda for early treatment, and medical officers sometimes ordered gassed men to snort the soda through the nose in the hope of relieving the chemical burns along the nasal passage.[36] It looked like cocaine, and that too was a pharmaceutical that was occasionally given to stimulate patients who had trouble breathing.

The treatment for gas-induced blindness involved daily washing of the eyes with warm water and sodium bicarbonate. Bandages were wrapped around the head to allow the eyes to heal in darkness. About two thirds of the mustard gas casualties were relatively minor in nature and those soldiers returned to their units within eight weeks, but reports of ghastly wounds from gas proliferated, with patients having their bandages removed to reveal opaque eyes that would never see again.[37] No cure existed for those with phosgene or mustard gas poisoning of the lungs, and the best solution was that which had been recommended for countless years for tuberculosis patients: rest, little movement, and fresh air.

Frustrated medical officers studied chemically burned soldiers throughout the war, hoping that an analysis of their wounds might provide a clue to effective future treatments. Patients were prodded and interrogated, while post-mortem autopsies led to an examination of corrupted organs. A series of manuals, pamphlets, and lessons-learned documents highlighting new treatment was issued to the British, Canadian, and other dominion medical services. Word was also passed in official and unofficial exchanges, including lectures at the front and temporary secondments of specialists to medical units. One wartime communiqué from the British observed that sharp objects should be kept away from patients with failing lungs after a dying British Tommy cut his own throat with a pair of dull scissors to end the misery.[38]

In the late summer of 1917, the medical services, in their search for better treatments, even turned to the old practice of bleeding victims. As patients struggled for breath, the bleeding was thought to relieve pressure on the gas-affected heart, which autopsies had revealed to be enlarged.[39] It was, unfortunately, quackery. Bleeding sometimes helped patients by initially leading to a flushing of the skin, but the worst cases still died within a few days. By December 1917, Canadian medical officers at No. 1 Canadian General Hospital recommended its disuse as a treatment because it was "considered a useless measure."[40] The medical innovations at the front were not always successful or helpful, but the doctors had no shortage of patients upon whom to test new treatments.

———

Writing about gas victims, one Canadian medical officer observed that the "cough they have is like no other cough you ever heard—not dry or hard, but as if their throats were full of froth of some sort. It is fearful."[41] The otherworldly nature of poison gas added to soldiers' terror, contributed to battle stress, and exhausted the men who were marooned in the gas environment. The many minor gas cases also put a strain on the medical system, drawing doctors' and nurses' attention away from other wounded men. The threat to the lifesavers from their own gas-corrupted patients was also deeply concerning and added to the burden faced by medical staff. And the losses to chemical weapons were not insubstantial, with 11,572 recorded cases in the Canadian Corps by the end of the war. Even more instances occurred as it was widely acknowledged that soldiers often toughed out multiple minor gassings, especially in 1918 when chemical shells were unleashed daily along the front.[42]

"The bronchitis often goes on to a broncho-pneumonia and this is the commonest cause of death," wrote Major George S. Strathy, an experienced Canadian medical officer.[43] While the lethality rate of mustard gas was 19.5 percent among serious cases, it fell to a low of 3.2 percent of the total number of cases throughout the war.[44] Most soldiers did not die from the chemical plague, but many sustained irreversible lung damage, making them more vulnerable to chronic bronchitis and pneumonia, and in late 1918 to the lethal pandemic virus. As Canadian infantry-man Robert Clements noted of his comrades who survived the chemical assault, "many men were condemned to months of lin-gering illness and early death."[45]

CHAPTER 13

DISPLAYING HUMAN REMAINS

P rivate William Gerald Arthrell of the 25th Battalion was shot through the head on March 25, 1916, while serving in the trenches on the Western Front. Born November 24, 1897, Arthrell gave his trade as a miner when he enlisted at Glace Bay, Cape Breton. He was unmarried and his parents, William and Alice, who lived in Stellarton, Nova Scotia, were his next of kin. He was a giant of a man for the time, standing six foot two and a half inches, with brown eyes, fair hair, and a light complexion. Like his fellow soldiers on the Western Front, Arthrell had not yet been equipped with a steel helmet, an important protection that might have deflected the bullet that smashed his skull. Despite a shattered cranium and exposed brain matter, Arthrell clung to life for thirteen hours but died the next day at No. 1 Canadian Casualty Clearing Station. The nineteen-year-old was buried at Bailleul Communal Cemetery, although without his brain.

While Arthrell's medical personnel records make no mention of the post-mortem performed on him, the records related to Colonel George Adami's body-snatching medical initiative make note that the young man's bullet-furrowed brain had been removed as a prized pathological sample. His headstone at Bailleul bears the inscription "John 15.13," which reads, "Greater love has no one than this: to lay down one's life for one's friends." Indeed, many soldiers believed that sentiment, though Arthrell's Christian parents chose that epitaph under the assumption that he was buried in full, having died for King and country, and that he now lay, intact, with his comrades. The sanctification of the fallen was an important part of dealing with the grief over sons and daughters killed in war and of making meaning of the losses. The idea that an unknown doctor had extracted Arthrell's brain for scientific advancement and public display would have been an unthinkable horror that traversed all boundaries of societal norms and decent behaviour towards the dead.

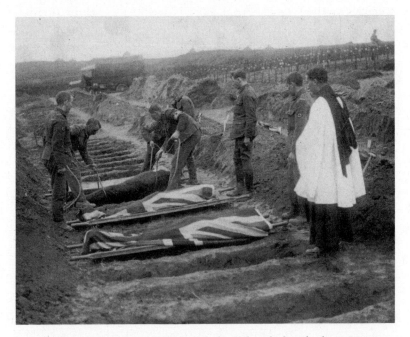

Not all of the Canadian dead were buried with their bodies intact.

A Christian burial for the fallen was a tradition in Canada and Britain, and one much embraced by the soldiers' overseas.[1] Even though the mass killing at the front and the shocking battlefield conditions led to the dismemberment of bodies and the inability to properly bury many of them, it was clear from both army policy and the letters of soldiers that the men sought to give their mates a proper burial whenever possible.[2] While Canadians became callous to the unknown dead around them—those left rotting on the battlefield or jutting from trench walls—they often risked their lives to go into No Man's Land to bring in the bodies of chums, driven by a duty to comrades and their families, and by a desire to ensure that their mates were properly buried in accordance with societal and religious norms.[3] A Canadian staff officer in England wrote of the importance of proper burials and the need to "ensure that the last resting places of these soldiers, who have died far away from their homes, may realise the wishes of their relatives and kinsfolk overseas and be not unworthy of the cause in which they died."[4] Canadian units, like the 28th Battalion, reminded their soldiers that the burying of their comrades and providing a proper grave was "a source of consolation to the relatives and friends of the deceased."[5]

This tradition mattered to the soldiers and was not easily squared with the collection of body parts that was an aspect of the long medical practice of using corpses as teaching tools. Though families would rightly grieve and mourn, it was felt in the medical profession that doctors needed to use the body after death to assist in saving future patients. And yet during the war these were not just the corpses of those taken by accident or disease. These were soldiers who had enlisted in a time of great need, who had been asked to leave behind their loved ones and communities to do their duty in what many believed was a war against an aggressive nation, to support Canadian national interests, and to stand at Britain's side. Society-wide messaging that focused on the service of Canadians in a just cause against German militarism seemed incongruous with the actions of the medical services' personnel who believed they had the right to take the body parts of killed citizen-soldiers and that the service required of them extended beyond death.

————

The gathering of soldiers' body parts was not well known to the general public in Britain or Canada, but on October 11, 1917, the Royal College of Surgeons in London opened its exhibition on the Army Medical Collection of War Specimens.[6] Sir Alfred Keogh, the director-general of the British Army Medical Services, spoke at the event about this new medical collection that was presented in three large curatorial spaces at the Royal College. With several hundred body parts and pathological samples on display, Keogh described the soldiers' deaths at the front as not only a sacrifice for their country but a sacrifice for knowledge. "Men will be able to learn from each other's ingenuity, and to avoid each other's errors," he declared. "There cannot be any doubt that in our former wars we have been too apt to attend to the medical exigencies of the campaign, and when it closed to bury our experience instead of consolidating it for the use of a future time and generation."[7] In short, the harvesting of body parts for study would result in more soldiers being saved in this war and in wars "for many generations to come."[8] The Canadian military medical community was in lockstep with this idea, and the *Bulletin of the*

Canadian Army Medical Corps, a new journal expressly created to document the medical wartime breakthroughs at the front in the interest of better treating the wounded, noted in its first issue that the exhibition, with a special section devoted to Canadian soldiers' body parts, would be the basis for a future military medical museum in Ottawa. The exhibition was "most instructive, containing material which, both from a surgical and medical point of view, is of first importance." The sanctioned journal encouraged "officers of the C.A.M.C. on leave in London . . . to visit the general war exhibit."[9]

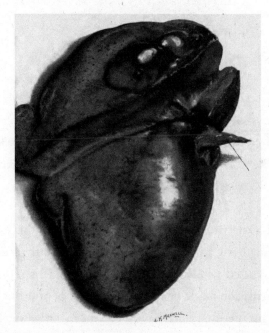

An example of one of the pathological specimens extracted from a British or dominion soldier. This one illustrates a lung that was speared by a rib fragment that had been broken by a shell splinter, leading to death. It was part of the Royal College of Surgeons collection.

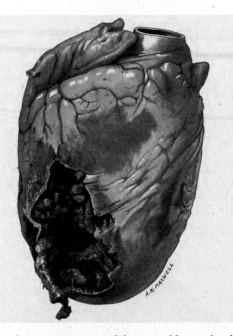

Pathological specimen extracted from a soldier and published in a
postwar surgical history that illustrates a wound to a heart.
This specimen's supporting text reads, "Represent[s] immediately
fatal injuries, and illustrates the amount of destruction which the
missiles of war are capable of producing."

A wide variety of war wounds was depicted at this exhibition, and the many body parts in their dismembered state could be seen in a reconstituted whole. "Each of these specimens represents an exact investigation made in such a way as to permit the visitor to gain at a glance results which have taken the investigators laborious pains to elucidate, and adds the value of research into the course and treatment of wounds," wrote an enthusiastic Canadian doctor in the *CMAJ*. "The main characteristics of modern gunshot wounds can be studied also in great numbers of other specimens, those of the chest, lungs and pleura with their sequelae being especially interesting. Other series of much interest show the lungs of men who suffered from the first poisonous gas sent over the British-Canadian troops at Ypres in 1915."[10] With specimens, organs, and bones extracted from hundreds of slain soldiers, there emerged under glass a Frankensteinian whole that provided a glimpse into the effect of war weapons on the collective soldiers' body.

Osteological material was arranged so that femurs, ribcages, spines, clavicles, and skulls provided evidence of the devastating effects of bullets or shell fragments. One traumatized cranium had been carefully reconstituted, with the bullet hole and splintered bone revealing the fatal damage. Another exhibition area was filled with "wet specimens," as they were called: the brain, lungs, and the vascular system preserved and arranged for optimal viewing, sometimes with organs flayed open. Cases of trench foot were represented via an amputated gangrenous foot, and several specimens revealed the corrupting effects of chemical weapons on the esophagus and lungs.[11] Some of the displays featured pathological samples that had begun to heal before the soldier succumbed to infection or sepsis, and these organs offered other insights into the body and the spread of disease. Canadian medical officer Andrew Macphail, a fierce imperialist and public intellectual who had returned to England after serving as a captain for over a year amid the gore of a field ambulance, believed that "the whole was a collection unique in the history of war, and a brilliant example of the triumph of personal skill and intelligent collaboration over serious difficulties."[12] No mention was made of the men to whom these organs and bones once belonged, and who had given no consent to this act of dismemberment. From the perspective of the military medical authorities it was probably better left unsaid, especially if wounded or sick soldiers might wonder if the medical

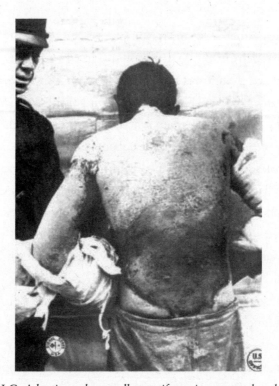

Colonel J.G. Adami sought to collect artifacts, images, and pathological specimens that illustrated wounds and medical work. He would have been interested in this rare photograph documenting a soldier with extensive mustard gas burns to his back and shoulders.

officers treating them were also at the same time eyeing them up as potential museum pieces in waiting.

———

Colonel Adami had been much impressed by the Royal College exhibition, which contained dozens of body parts from Canadian soldiers. He was not alone. A report on the display appeared in the January 1918 issue of *CMAJ*, which declared, "Probably no event in the evolution of the present War is of greater scientific value, or more productive of lasting benefit to this and later generations than the remarkable exhibition of War specimens at the Royal College of Surgeons in London."[13] In fact, an editorial in the same issue of *CMAJ* argued that, given the success of the exhibition in London, the Canadian body parts should be sent to Ottawa: "The importance to us here in Canada of such an Army Medical collection, if properly preserved, studied, and displayed, can hardly be over-estimated, and constitutes an opportunity the neglect of which would be a criminal waste."[14] Adami needed no convincing, of course, and he almost certainly even supplied information to the editor of the journal, one of his colleagues at McGill, Maude Abbott.

After the exhibition opening, Adami redoubled efforts to secure the pathological samples by writing to advise the CAMC high command that, as of August 1917, 147 Canadian specimens had been collected at the Royal College, although he knew some Canadian units held additional pathological samples that had not yet been shipped to London.[15] He did not stop there. As a master of the paper war, Adami fired off letters to military and medical authorities in France, England, and Canada, and in October 1917 he proposed the establishment of a medical section in a yet unbuilt Canadian museum. Although Ottawa senior medical staff had agreed to Adami's earlier pleas for a new medical museum as an ideal place to keep alive the memories of service, showcase war-related artifacts, and present to the Canadian public the hard-won wartime medical breakthroughs, the energetic doctor was eager to circulate this new proposal that was perhaps more realistic. As opposed to a stand-alone medical museum, a medical gallery would be developed in a Canadian war museum, which Adami

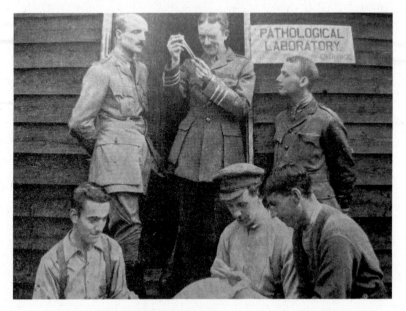

The staff of the pathological laboratory at No. 3 Canadian
General Hospital, along with pet rabbit.

had discussed with Lord Beaverbrook and other prominent Canadians who were also talking publicly of postwar museum and art gallery.[16]

Armed with the official title of medical historical recorder, Adami was, as he indicated in one document, already collecting in five broad areas: "war hygiene"; preventive medicine; "war treatment"; statistics, models, and diagrams; and pathological samples.[17] War hygiene and preventative medicine had ensured that the armies did not waste away from diseases in the static trenches, and the artifacts, images, and historical papers that illustrated this success were being gathered. The collection plan also included a consideration of refuse from the Western Front, including tin cans and other garbage—all the things an army consumes, discards, or buries. The doctor also had his eye on medical artifacts related to preventative medicine—including rubber boots and whale oil that was to be smeared on feet to avoid trench foot—and information documenting the administration of vaccines, which had been controversial, but which Adami had energetically championed. Chemical warfare was of particular interest, and the material culture of protective devices like respirators, anti-gas blankets, and creams to reduce the effects of mustard gas burns were all to be saved. Adami also sought to represent the new war diseases, such as trench fever and, as he described them, "Three Day Fever (Salonika) and Dysentery."

His third category, "war treatment," was related to the structure of the medical system, from the front-line care through the chain of formations, including ambulance trains and hospital ships. He also planned to collect artifacts such as bandages, stretchers, and splints. In the fourth category, a breakdown of weekly casualty and sickness rates, as well as information on "different forms of wounds of different parts of body," were grouped under the heading of "statistics," which were important both for the future museum and the planned historical series. The final, pathological section would be populated with a "collection of wax, plaster, and other models of deformities induced by wounds; drawings of different forms of wound infection, gas gangrene, etc.; collections illustrating wound bacteriology," which was not surprising since the gifted Adami was also a watercolour artist. As part of this theme, the museum would also store and present a collection of "pathological specimens, bones, tissues, and organs."[18]

Colonel Adami's ambitious but calculated three-part plan was to rally support for a museum, to excite interest across the CAMC in collecting, and to ensure that the Imperials did not claim the Dominion's pathological samples. However, he had no place to store this material, a challenge also faced by Dominion Archivist Sir Arthur Doughty, who was at the same time cataloguing the staggering output of the paper war and gathering war trophies captured at the front for a museum at home. While Lord Beaverbrook had the physical site of the Canadian War Record Office buildings in London to archive historical records, photographs, film footage, and completed works of art, the safest place for medical artifacts and pathological objects remained the Royal College of Surgeons. And yet Adami believed, along with Doughty and Beaverbrook, that only an active collection policy would lead to the preservation of artifacts and body parts. They could not wait until after the war in the hope that these objects would find their way to a museum, and that was especially the case with pathological samples. In a letter to one medical officer at No. 10 Canadian Stationary Hospital in early 1918, Adami advised, "Just as units who have captured pieces of artillery are permitted to retain these pieces for presentation to their native towns, so medical war material taken by individual units, may be allocated to those units."[19] The artifacts and pathological prizes collected by Canadian doctors would not be lost to the Imperials under Adami's watch.

———

After the exhibition Colonel Adami continued with his communiqués to Ottawa, warning about the possibility of losing control of the pathological collection through apathy or Imperial deviousness, and urging that action be taken to get these priceless artifacts back to Canada. While he displayed a more collegial belief in the Royal College in his private correspondence, Adami reminded the authorities in Ottawa that the pathological samples should soon be sent to McGill University, which already had an established pathological museum. This institution was overseen by Dr. Maude Abbott, whom he described as "the leading medical museum curator in the Dominion."[20] While Adami had hired Abbott at McGill in 1899, she consistently faced sexist barriers in the medical profession and at the university. Throughout most of her professional life, she was denied key appointments, even as she took on extra duties beyond her work in the McGill Medical Museum, including developing a growing expertise in the study of heart defects that led to recognition in Canada and abroad. During the Great War, with so many McGill professors overseas, Abbott became temporary editor of the *Canadian Medical Association Journal*, although the position was never formally acknowledged in the publication. Kept informed by Adami and other McGillites in uniform about the emerging pathological collection, Abbott hoped to work at the Royal College to prepare the Canadian pathological samples for their eventual transfer to Montreal. She wrote several letters to Arthur Keith, the curator of the collection, but she was blocked from going overseas by military authorities in Ottawa.[21] Like other women doctors who might have sought to enlist and who formed about 3 percent of the medical profession, she was denied the opportunity to serve. Professor Abbott would have to wait for the body parts to come to her.[22]

Anxious to hurry the process, Adami pressed Keith in early January 1918, advising him that Abbott planned a temporary exhibition in Canada to showcase the pathological samples and that material had to be sent immediately.[23] The Canadian colonel had some leverage since he had already lent a skilled pathologist to work with Keith. A professor at the University of Alberta, Morton Hall was building a reputation as a young scholar who had published about the pathological changes in the left temporal bone in patients with cranial syphilis.[24] Enlisting with most of the medical staff and professors from the university, Captain Hall was assigned to the Royal College in 1917 to work on the specimens being returned from the front. He was a bit of an eccentric character, with his uniform in disarray, his hair longer than most, and his face often stubbled, but his work was much praised by Keith. Hall and Keith would eventually co-author four illustrated articles about pathological samples, all published in the *British Journal of Surgery*.[25] Far from the front, Hall, like everyone in and out of uniform, was not untouched by the war. One of his closest friends, Lieutenant-Colonel Heber Havelock Moshier, a fellow University of Toronto medical school classmate and a professor of physiology at the University of Alberta, was killed at the front in the last months of the war at the age of twenty-nine when a shell exploded over him.[26]

At the Royal College, Keith agreed to Adami's request, and by mid-February 1918 Abbott reported that she had received the first batch of fifty specimens of Canadian soldiers' body parts, many of them having been prepared by Hall. They had been packaged up rapidly with little contextualizing information, other than the soldier's name to whom the body part once belonged. Abbott noted that, disappointingly, they were missing the "pathological diagnosis." She also observed that the specimens were stunningly good for educational purposes, "but in nearly all the colors are badly preserved or absent."[27] Another problem was that a number of preserved organs "wrapped in cotton or lint" were imprinted with the fabric. Nonetheless, they were a significant addition to the established McGill museum, and the bone specimens, Abbott stressed, were a particularly "beautiful collection."[28]

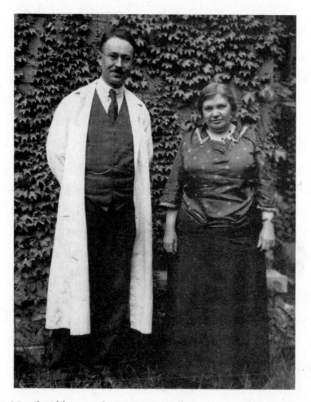

Dr. Maude Abbott with a museum colleague at McGill University.

Other shipments arrived over the next month, shepherded across the Atlantic by Captain Arthur Butler Chandler, a pediatrician from Perth, Ontario, with 181 prized possessions coming in this first tranche.[29] Abbott, Chandler, and an assistant scrambled to organize, catalogue, mount, and display pathological samples for a small travelling exhibition to be opened in Hamilton, Ontario, in late May 1918. As part of another transfer from London, and left to us in history through insurance notes on the collection, was a series of wax and plaster models of soldiers with shattered skulls whose faces were made by plastic surgeons.[30] These came from the Ontario Military Hospital at Orpington, with one document noting, "We have a collection of water colours, coloured photographs, war masks, also gelatine masks for trial operations, and plastic moulds showing the wounds and deformities of the face, limbs, and body . . . during the process of treatment. These will eventually be placed in the New Museum which is being built by the Dominion Government in Ottawa."[31]

The first Canadian public display of soldiers' body parts occurred in Hamilton from May 27 to June 1, 1918, at the Hotel Connaught. This was the site of the Canadian Medical Association's annual meeting, where some 1,200 doctors were attending full days of lectures and presentations. The *Hamilton Spectator* also reported on "scientific exhibits" that "were crowded with spectators."[32] University professors showed their own specimens removed from civilian and animal dead, as well as microscopic preparations of bacteria and culture swabs. However, the overseas soldiers' bones and organs were the highlight of the exhibition. "Keen enthusiasm in the examination and study of these, the first war specimens to reach Canada, was displayed not only by the many military surgeons and civilian practitioners who visited the exhibition, but also by a continuous procession of the general public," noted one correspondent.[33] The *Hamilton Spectator* echoed the observation and highlighted how curious doctors and the gawking public waited in long lines to view the thirty-five specimens from the Western Front. They were not for the faint of heart. One doctor wrote, "In the series the specimens of intestines showing multiple wounds of entry and exit produced by a single bullet traversing successive coils, and brains showing impact from the opposite side of the cranium were especially noteworthy."[34]

These body parts were not a state secret. Presented in publications and then exhibited for doctors and members of the public in

Hamilton, this first transfer of soldiers' organs and bones excited much commentary, with a *CMAJ* editorial arguing that the interest in the pathological samples were evidence that they should be on permanent display: "The value of a Canadian War Museum to the country at large and to the Army Medical Corps in particular, and the wisdom of the military authorities in initiating this, was universally felt and warm appreciation was expressed on all sides."[35] These sentiments were echoed by the Ontario Medical Association, which wrote to Ottawa and sent a copy of its resolution drawing attention to the "collection of specimens from the C.A.M.C. Museum" that "have aroused great interest both among Military Surgeons, Civilian Practitioners and the general public." The association of physicians publicly called for a military medical museum, stating its belief that the artifacts and pathological samples of soldiers would be a "fitting memorial to the future generation of sacrifices of our troops overseas."[36]

———

Throughout 1918, Colonel Adami kept Ottawa apprised of the ongoing collecting at the front, doing so, as he noted, "with the intention of having a magnificent War Museum at Ottawa."[37] The doctor rallied support at every turn, which included meeting in April 1918 with an American medical officer, with whom he discussed the importance of gathering artifacts and pathological samples. Adami duly informed the authorities in London and at home that the Americans were keen to start their own program of gathering pathological objects, chiding his superiors for being less organized in the work than their counterparts south of the border, despite the fact that U.S. troops had only recently begun to arrive overseas in strength.[38] The nationalistic sting of the Americans galloping ahead of the Canucks compelled the senior CAMC command in Ottawa to agree by mid-1918 that they would demand of the Imperials that the medical specimens would go to McGill at war's end, while other collected material would be housed at 12 Emmett Street in Ottawa, which was described as "the old medical quarters."[39] This was an important step towards the creation of a medical museum, and it was followed in July by the assigning of Captain Lloyd Philips MacHaffie of the CAMC to No. 3 Canadian (McGill) General Hospital in France to fulfill Adami's plan of aggressively gathering body parts.[40]

Captain MacHaffie was a pathologist by training who worked at hospitals in Boston and Montreal and believed strongly in the body-snatching program. Beginning in August 1918, he gathered 315 organs and 663 bone specimens, along with 724 artifacts such as crutches, bandages, splints, and gas masks.[41] Medical officers at Canadian units in the field also continued to bring together artifacts for Adami, with, for example, Lieutenant-Colonel Gunn's No. 8 Canadian Field Ambulance saving captured German bandages made of "assorted cloth fabrics, and even of woven paper." These were a tangible sign of the Royal Navy's blockade that was strangling Germany of raw material and supplies, the success of which was revealed in many ways, especially via the discovery of substandard medical supplies. These bandages, wrote Gunn, "were brought away, and forwarded to the Canadian medical museum."[42] Collecting work continued along the front and in England. For instance, at Taplow in England, a notable grouping of lantern slides of X-ray plates depicting broken bones was being curated for eventual transfer to the museum.[43] In Orpington, models of face wounds were collected, with these sculptures, as

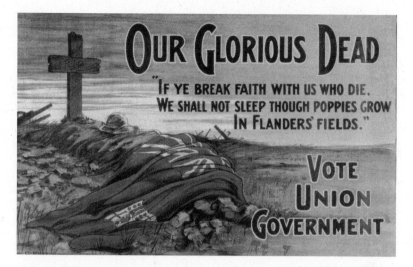

This poster draws upon John McCrae's famous poem and the imagery of the country's "glorious dead." It was a common sentiment expressed by Sir Robert Borden's Union Government (a wartime coalition party with the primary goal of winning the war). There were no posters that drew attention to soldiers' bodies being harvested for future medical specimens.

one doctor noted, providing evidence of the advanced process of reconstructive facial surgery in which "the surgeon, dentist, artist, and sculptor were collected to try and restore not only the functions destroyed by the ghastly wounds, but also to so bring back the appearance of the man to so near normal that he could re-enter the society he left on enlistment."[44]

With British soldiers treated in Canadian hospitals—and the opposite also true, as Canadians moved though Imperial or other dominion medical units—the CAMC's harvesting of body parts, especially that undertaken by the medical officers who were collecting in addition to Captain MacHaffie, did not always draw exclusively from the Canadian slain. Private Alfred Charrett of the Royal Irish Rifles (posted to the 1/18 London Regiment) was exposed to mustard gas on November 30, 1917, and he died in agony on December 3 at the age of nineteen from ghastly chemical burns to his body and infected lungs. A Canadian surgeon performed an autopsy, collecting his trachea and lungs, with both of them, a report noted, "covered with a very thick layer of yellow pus, which extends from the larynx into the bifurcation."[45] Charett's removed lungs and trachea were eventually sent to Ottawa, even as his parents were requesting the inscription on his headstone to be "Oh For a Touch of a Vanished Hand," a line from a poem about grieving. Given the importance of the Christian burial and the comfort brought by the knowledge that loved ones were provided a grave, what would his mourning parents have felt had they learned that his organs had been extracted from his corpse and carried off to Canada? Records collected by Adami also note that Gunner W.J. Pullen's thoracic viscera scorched by mustard gas was selected for the future museum, and Private R. Becket's "neck wound," which was likely a cast of the lethal injury, was a good example of trauma and was sent to Canada. These soldiers were all British, with Pullen having served with the 182nd Siege Battery, Royal Garrison Artillery, and having died on September 28, 1917.[46] Just as British, Canadian, and dominion soldiers fought together and died together in common cause, they would be displayed together in a new cause to advance medical knowledge—albeit without their consent.

———

A remarkable visitor arrived at the Royal College of Surgeons on August 14, 1918, when Prime Minister Sir Robert Borden was received there as an honoured guest. It was an astonishing visit from Borden, who from late 1915 was the driving force in encouraging Canadians to serve in the war as part of the nation's duty to the Empire. The visit to the college by the sixty-three-year-old Borden, handsome in bearing, with his large moustache and grey parted hair, was all the more surprising since he had demanded during previous trips to England to visit wounded Canadians in hospitals. He did not shy away from the grim effects of combat and he sought out the young heroes, always expressing the greatest interest and care in their recovery and also noting that they had sacrificed much for the war effort. After conferring with and talking to hundreds of Canadians in visits to fifty-two hospitals and convalescent homes, he said publicly "it was the most deeply-moving experience of all my life" and that one "could not return from such a visit without a renewed courage and strengthened determination."[47]

A year after his trip to those hospitals, Borden made this visit to the Royal College to, in Adami's words, "formally inspect and inaugurate the Canadian collection of medical war specimens there on exhibition, which comprise a sample of the different forms of material being collected for the proposed National Medical War Museum at Ottawa."[48] The Canadian prime minister studied the contents of the display cases, which consisted of, as one medical journalist noted, "a remarkable series of head wounds, drawings, photographs and models." Guided by curator Arthur Keith, Borden was told of the specimens' value to science, and it was reported that the Canadian prime minister "expressed his interest in the collection."[49] Borden had not changed his attitude towards the soldiers he had met in hospitals, whom he continued to fervently support and respect, but like Adami and the other medical officers, he did not see a contradiction in sending

CHAPTER 14

MEDICINE IN THE MUD, 1917

After marching out of the swirling gas fumes and away from the brutal combat at Hill 70, infantryman John Alexander Bain wrote that "a great many of the boys had to report sick and quite a few had to go to hospital. . . . This was due to the great nervous strain which we had undergone in the last battle. I was low spirited, could not sleep at nights, and suffered considerably with pains in my legs. . . . I just felt that I never could go up into the line again, or bear the sound of a shell."[1] Bain, a prewar travelling salesman, regained his health and continued to serve in the 21st Battalion, as did many of his comrades who had passed through the trial at Lens. None would ever forget the trauma, however, although Hill 70 would soon be overshadowed by the horror of Passchendaele, where the Canadians would fight from October 1917.

The Canadians had secured another victory at Hill 70 in August, grinding down the enemy forces and building on the success of Vimy, but the Corps had been battered with about 10,000 casualties. The Germans endured even heavier losses, although they retained Lens. Lieutenant-General Arthur Currie was preparing for a new offensive to dislodge the enemy from the city when Sir Douglas Haig, the British commander-in-chief, ordered him to the forlorn Flanders battlefield. While the Canadian general pleaded with the field marshal to let the Canadians finish the job at Lens, the British army needed a victory. If the Canadians could capture Passchendaele Ridge, a key position still in German hands after months of battle, at least the British forces could consolidate the ground won at such a terrible cost in that slow-moving offensive that had been launched on July 31 and that, after three months, had made few gains amid mud and massacre.

——

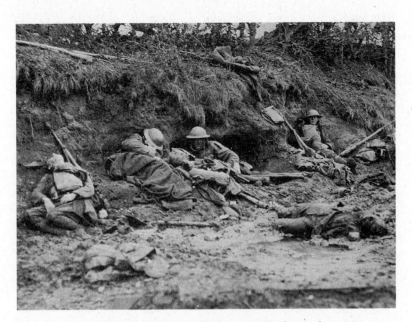

A ghastly image of soldiers resting in the mud
with a dismembered body in close proximity.

Earth-shattering, terrain-destroying bombardments from millions of high explosive shells had broken the water tables and the irrigation system to the east of the ruined city of Ypres, which, when combined with the deluge of unseasonable heavy rain, created a sea of mud. Within this quagmire, soldiers struggled to avoid being pulled under in the thick sludge that was also corrupted with mustard gas and tens of thousands of rotting corpses. On the high ground of Passchendaele Ridge, the Germans were dug in on drier terrain, with barbed wire protecting irregular trench systems centred on concrete pillboxes bristling with multiple machine guns.

British, Australian, and New Zealand forces, unable to advance very far through the well-prepared German defences and the nearly impassable muck from early August to mid-October, had absorbed grievous losses, and, as winter loomed, they were in danger of a massive defeat that might lead to a widespread collapse of morale across the army and on the home front.[2] The French army had been badly shaken earlier in the year by crippling casualties and indifferent leaders, with about a fourth of the force in revolt as of June. The French had slowly recovered by employing a series of punishments and rewards—executions and more frequent leave— and by slowing the pace of battle, but Passchendaele was a similar trial for the British and dominion soldiers who suffered plummeting morale, especially with the temperature dropping as fall turned to early winter. No victory seemed possible in such unbelievable conditions.

The Canadians marched into the cauldron in early October, and no one in Currie's headquarters was under any illusion as to the severity of what they faced at Passchendaele. Deputy director of medical services Colonel Arthur Edward Ross, a prewar physician from Kingston, Ontario, who commanded the medical units in the Canadian Corps, was part of an advance guard to survey the open cesspool of the battlefield. By this point in the war, the medical services were integrated into the planning of operations, with significant focus being directed on the logistics of clearing the battlefield. Ross warned that the "the evacuation of the wounded will be a matter of extreme difficulty. Owing to the almost complete absence of shelter of any kind, it will be impossible to keep cases under cover; and in consequence the wounded will suffer hardship."[3]

After the bulk of the Corps arrived at the front in mid-October, the Canadians began the difficult work of laying new roads, digging gun pits with solid foundations to ensure the artillery pieces did not disappear into the filth, and seeking out the few dry pieces of ground. Often medical units were grouped there, although this made them vulnerable to enemy shellfire. While the Germans also suffered in the mud, they had the benefit of drier ground due to their location further up the ridge. They also had the advantage of observation into the Canadian lines that were laid out before them. German artillery fire raked the Canadians during the daylight hours, with gunners and those working on the lines of communication targeted and taking frightful losses. In fact, during the battle the gunners' losses jumped from about 4 percent in previous operations to 12 percent of total casualties.[4] Lieutenant Wilfred Kerr of the Canadian Field Artillery lamented, "We stayed and endured and paid the price."[5]

As the Canadians filtered into the battle zone, hardboiled soldiers stared in disbelief at the mud; others wept and swore at the callous nature of their commanders who had sent them into this wicked arena. The nauseating odour of the unburied dead lay heavy over the front like the mist that emerged from the shattered earth most mornings. The apocalyptic battleground was littered with abandoned and shattered equipment. Medical officers looked at the thousands of corpses lying in shell craters and wondered how long it would be before a disease ravaged the Corps. Even though soldiers stood in sludgy water, sometimes up to their knees or thighs, every drop was contaminated, necessitating horse-drawn water trucks to move tens of thousands of potable litres to the front every day, which then had to be hand-carried in jugs and cans into the forward positions. It was an arduous task and soldiers in their water-filled craters or the few dissolving trenches stared into the sea of scummy water with burning thirst. Rum became the saving grace for almost all soldiers, and even con-firmed abstainers abandoned their temperance beliefs.

Currie's Corps headquarters worked with the divisions in planning several short, sharp attacks, supported by as many guns as possible. Despite the preparation, all knew that success could be delivered only by the "poor bloody infantry," who would be pushed to the limit of their stamina. The medical services also prepared for the coming campaign, taking over British field ambulance positions but being hamstrung by the lack of roads and rails.[6] Only wooden duckboards, narrow and slippery with slime, connected the front to the rear through a spider web of walkways, and all soldiers had been warned of the danger of falling off them, as heavy kit and hobnailed boots would drag men to their death. Evidence of such a fate was everywhere, with decaying soldiers in the mire, their blackened limbs protruding, beckoning the living to join them.

The mud was shocking, but it also unexpectedly reduced the number of casualties caused by the rain of enemy shellfire. "I believe it was only the depth and softness of the mud that saved us from being practically wiped out," stated one Canadian. "The shells would plunge deep into the mud close beside us and by leaning away from the burst as it shot skyward you got nothing worse than a mud and water bath with a bit of shaking up from the concussion."[7] However, with boots sodden, all units saw a return of the plague of trench foot, as toes and feet were chilled and reduced to a fish-belly-white bulbous mess. After a few days at the front, a Blighty wound began to look appealing.

A British medical study of a single day of battlefield losses—on September 21, 1917—revealed the nature of injuries in 10,789 casualties. Of these, 35.8 percent received wounds from high explosive shells, 19.9 percent from shrapnel, 27.2 percent from bullet, and less than 3 percent from bayonet, hand grenade, and gas. Another 14 percent of wounds could not be ascribed to a particular weapon.[8] It was clear that shells and bullets accounted for the vast majority of injuries to soldiers, although mustard gas would affect more Canadians when they fought intensely from late October onward, as the Germans used their stocks of chemical weapons more freely. In the two weeks of preparation before the first Canadian phase of the battle, soldiers were killed or maimed every day, as snipers, machine guns, mortar bombs, poison gas, and shellfire claimed some 1,500 Canadians killed and wounded. Sergeant John Williams, a machinist from St. Thomas, Ontario, wrote to his wife from a hospital bed about how he had been knocked out before the operation began in earnest: "The shell that got us blew one of the stretcher bearers all to pieces—we did not see a thing of him. The other stretcher bearer was shell shocked, which is an awful thing to see, and I just got a piece of shell in my left thigh."[9] Williams felt he was lucky to escape with only that injury.

———

In staring out at the morass, everyone from the staff officers to the privates understood the importance of increasing the number of stretcher-bearers before the first battle. Soldiers' morale would plummet even further if they believed that they would be abandoned in the mud after being wounded. But even with an extra 100 men per battalion and another 1,150 bearers pooled and ready at the divisional level to be allocated where necessary, there was little hope of a timely clearing of the battlefield once the full-scale assault began on October 26. It was estimated to take six men, spelling off each other, at least six hours to haul in an injured man. Anticipating heavy casualties, three field ambulance units were crammed into the limited space, although divided into three sections to give them more flexibility and to enable them to sufficiently operate a series of advanced dressing stations. Just as the infantry would attack forward in stages, the medical services were similarly echeloned in stages leading back from the front to accommodate the waves of wounded that would wash over them.

General Currie held off his British superiors who demanded that he hurry the assault, refusing to attack until the logistics were ready and the guns in place. The first offensive would be a limited bite into the enemy line using five first-wave battalions along a 3,000-metre frontage, which, if successful, would pull the infantry out of the worst of the mud and up the ridge between 550 and 1,100 metres along an uneven trench line. About 3,000 Canadian infantrymen swept forward at 5:40 A.M. on October 26, backed by 587 British and Canadian artillery pieces. It was a staggering bombardment that deafened the attackers and pummelled the enemy positions, killing hundreds of Germans caught in the water-logged trenches that had few deep dugouts. It did little damage, however, to those defenders who crowded into the concrete pill-boxes, with their one-foot-thick concrete walls. As the creeping barrage of shells smashed over the lines, moving much slower than previous battles to accommodate the infantry struggling forward, the German infantry emerged to fight. Muddy men on both sides, their uniforms so slathered in filth that the combatants had few distinguishing marks other than the shape of their helmets, engaged in ferocious close-range combat, throwing grenades, shooting, and stabbing.

Along with the trained stretcher-bearers who acted as battle-field medics, the additional bearers set to carrying out the wounded. Some were equipped with rope to pull stuck men out of the swamp. With soldiers' uniforms soaked, it was a significant challenge even to lift a prone man. They cut off all the kit they could, including greatcoats, although the cold and wet weather meant that the wounded had to have something to keep them warm during the long journey back to medical care. The stretcher-bearers some-times laid their own battle jerkin over the exposed soldier, or, if a corpse could be found with a somewhat dry coat, they used the dead man's uniform to warm the living. "The stretcher bearers worked heroically and to their noble efforts many a man owes his life," wrote one wounded Canadian from the 26th Battalion, who noted further that the bearers "seemed not to know that the air was alive with shells . . . and their only thought was to answer the pitiful groan of a wounded man lying helpless in that sea of

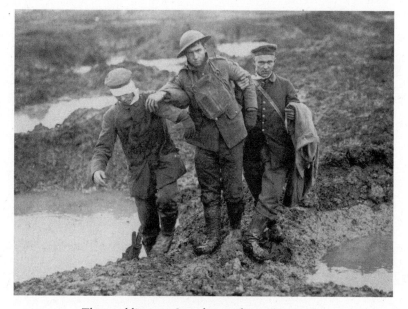

Three soldiers—a Canadian and two Germans—
help each other through the Flanders mud.

mud."[10] Another Canadian medical officer, Captain Norman Guiou, believed that the way the bearers fearlessly sought out those helpless Canadians through the hurricane of fire was nothing short of inspiring; in his opinion, "the Regimental Stretcher Bearers all deserved the Victoria Cross."[11]

"Hun prisoners were pressed into service, some of them at the point of the pistol," wrote Major George McFarland of the 4th Canadian Mounted Rifles. "It is certain, however, that many of the wounded sank into the morass, and were drowned or suffocated before they could be reached."[12] And yet a mass of bleeding soldiers journeyed on stretchers or stumbled back for medical treatment. No. 8 Canadian Field Ambulance handled 3,270 wounded Canadian, British, and Germans during the course of the frenetic day. Each man was studied and his injuries catalogued;

tea and coffee were dispensed, and sometimes a bit of food; and surprisingly gentle care, comfort, and occasional succour were given as soldiers died, with bearers, privates, and even doctors sometimes holding a man's hand as he called out for his mother and slipped from this world.[13]

———

"A dreary waste of shell-torn earth and mud," wrote Sergeant J.A. Bryce of the PPCLI, describing the scorched terrain. "For over six miles in depth the land is nothing but a sea of shell-craters, the majority of which are full of water."[14] Into this mouth of madness a second Canadian offensive was launched on October 30, with some 420 Allied guns supporting six Canadian first-wave battalions. They set off at dawn under a crimson sky and immediately encountered hard fighting, with the Germans ready and laying down sweeping fire. And yet the Canadians drove them back in countless acts of bravery, courage, and self-sacrifice, capturing their objectives and advancing another 600 metres up the ridge.

All along the front lay the freshly wounded and slain. As men were hammered to the ground by bullets and splinters, adrenaline kicked in rapidly or numbness spread from the wound, and even grave injuries were sometimes initially unnoticed by the wounded. Private Donald Fraser of the 31st Battalion, a long-service veteran of the front, punched his ticket in the sludge when he was taken down by a shell splinter on October 30. After the shell detonated near him, flinging him down as a geyser of filth shot skyward, he dragged himself to his feet and continued about 20 metres towards the enemy before he noticed he had blood on his tunic and pants.

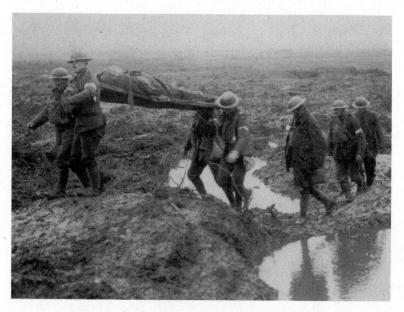

Four stretcher-bearers and three replacements carry a
wounded man through the shattered Passchendaele landscape.

On closer inspection, he noted, "My right arm was shattered at the shoulder, completely twisted around and dangling."[15]

By the end of the day, the Canadians suffered 2,313 casualties—884 killed and 1,429 wounded, including 130 gassed soldiers—about four men lost for every metre gained. The ratio of killed to wounded was usually about one to four, but it was much higher at Passchendaele, at about one killed for about every two wounded. Many of the injured soldiers died in the muck, especially those who crawled into shell craters to escape the shellfire and found the water rising around them. Lieutenant-Colonel Agar Adamson offered a literary shudder in one letter, writing that "the battlefield beggared description," with evidence of soldiers "drowned in shell holes for want of strength to pull themselves out."[16] Another Canuck, John C. MacEwen, who served with the Royal Canadian Regiment, recounted how "lots of poor fellows were bogged in the mud and if wounded never got out."[17] This was a fate that many soldiers commented upon, along with the haunting dread of being pulled under, their bodies lost and their status listed as "missing."

———

The Germans saturated the front with mustard gas to add to the Canadian soldiers' misery, with the chemical agents polluting the slurry of water and leaving many with painful blisters. Infection frequently took hold in the chemical burns, leading to septic wounds. Aware of the coming blindness, some of the gassed soldiers set off to the rear, alone or in small groups, as their eyesight dimmed, hoping to reach a doctor before they lost all sense of sight. Others were grouped together, one sighted man leading a winding column of the blinded, who stumbled forward wearing bandages wrapped around their heads to protect their eyes. For hours and hours, these men were exposed to shellfire as they shambled along the slippery wooden mats. By battle's end, 843 cases of Canadians being gassed at Passchendaele were recorded, forming about 5 percent of the total casualties, with many other Canadians continuing to fight as they suffered minor inhalations that left them hacking and coughing through raw lungs and seared throats.[18]

The personal observations of medical officers at the front also provide a glimpse into the devastating situation. Major George S. Strathy, who was sent forward from a field ambulance to relieve the regimental medical officer of the 47th Battalion in this second phase of intense combat, described the scene he encountered:

"Outside the aid post I found lying on the stretcher about 9 or 10 very severe stretcher cases, chest and abdomens, compound femurs, spinal injuries. They were quite unprotected from shellfire, the night was cold, almost freezing, and many of them had no great coats."[19] Another twenty-five dying soldiers were inside a captured German concrete pillbox about 9 metres long and wide, with a 3-metre ceiling. Amid screaming men wallowing in their own gore, Strathy discovered the medical officer cowering under a table, his head covered in a groundsheet, his will (and possibly his mind) broken. A concerned Strathy relieved him and the doctor fled to the rear, a moment that underscores physicians' lack of immunity to shell shock as they bore witness to ghastly sights. Strathy worked his position for the next three days and nights, with shells falling so close to the position that candles were repeatedly blown out from the blast. He organized stretcher-bearers to carry out some of the wounded, including a group from the 50th Battalion "in spite of the fact that they were exhausted, having had no sleep for 5 days." The plucky bearers carried out a few of the patients who had a chance of surviving the long journey, and Strathy was eventually relieved, having survived a gas attack and still suffering from a case of trench foot.

On another part of the front, Private Herbert Burrell of the 1st Canadian Mounted Rifles, a stretcher-bearer who roamed the battlefield saving lives, found all the regimental aid posts "choked with the wounded, some perishing from the cold, others lying in painful positions and no one apparently paying them [the] slightest attention." With men dying of exposure for want of being cleared, Burrell appealed to a group of exhausted infantrymen who were holed up in water-filled craters, clutching groundsheets around their shivering shoulders as they watched for an enemy

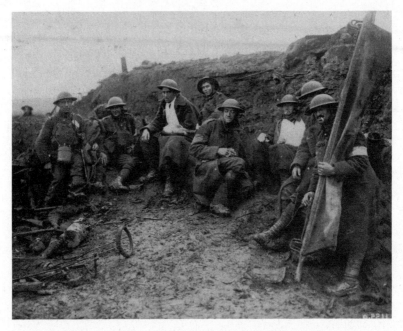

Exhausted stretcher-bearers and wounded soldiers in the mud.
The bearer on the right holds a canvas stretcher.

counterattack. A few of the infantry agreed to carry out some of the injured. However, to remove four or more infantrymen from the forward trenches to transport each wounded man was not sustainable and would leave those defences even more precarious. Some of the casualties who were judged to have a fighting chance of surviving were carried to the rear, but, as Burrell scribbled in his private diary, of those who remained, "many died before the end of the day."[20]

In such pitiless circumstances, it often fell to the wounded soldiers to struggle for their own survival. Soldiers set off for medical care when they should not have been on their feet, let alone walking several kilometres along narrow duckboards as blood pooled in their boots. Infantryman William McDonald of Glen

William, P.E.I., who was shot during the battle, bandaged up, and directed to the rear with another wounded soldier, noted, "The mud was actually up to my waist, and several times I sank right down in it but there was a lad (about seventeen) helping me, and a good fellow he was." The pair had been told that the dressing station was about 3 kilometres away, but they wandered about, lost, in great pain, and increasingly panicky that they would collapse from shock before they got there. Enemy shelling crashed down around them, and the two chums, leaning on each other, periodically threw themselves down on the duckboards or in the sludge as they heard the incoming shells. Eventually they had to stop dropping down for fear that they would not be able to get back up to their feet. Adrenaline and fear drove them as they continued to stumble and shuffle onwards, passing chilling sights of dying men who cried out for assistance, with shells exploding around them and leaving them spasming from the blasts. "What gruesome sights, pieces of bodies scattered around just like leaves," continued McDonald. "One landed a few yards away [and] a piece of shrapnel hit me in the right shoulder and knocked me down. I thought all was up but the lad lifted me. . . . It's wonderful what one is able to do when it's [a] matter of life and death." Through the agony and exhaustion, the two men finally arrived at a dressing station, where they both collapsed, destined to survive.[21]

The CMAC orderlies set to work as the wounded staggered into the dressing stations and main aid areas of the field ambulance units. Dressings were cut away, jagged gashes examined, and new bandages applied. "Like most dressing stations it was a medley of sounds—the groans of suffering, the wheeze of those hit in the lungs, the call for stretcher bearers and requests for something to drink," recounted one medical diarist. "There was seldom

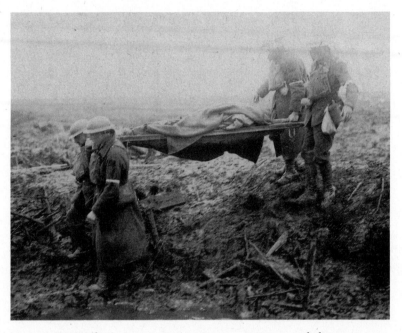

*It was always a race against time to carry a wounded man
to medical care before he died from shock or his wounds.*

any respite for the M.O.s and dressers during a push of the magnitude of Passchendaele. The business of evacuating wounded in
such cramped and dangerous spots taxed the body, mind and
soul."[22] If a man was slipping into shock and crashing, emergency
surgery could be carried out, but a new round of triage was conducted to determine who might be operated on with a chance of
saving them. Cigarettes were handed out to the shivering patients,
with a positive nod and a few cheery words reassuring them that
they were the lucky ones off to Blighty, even as a man's life ran out
of him. One commander of a field ambulance remembered the
"desperately awful" visions as the wounded writhed in agony and
feverishly whispered for loved ones before their death rattle.
"Passchendaele," he wrote, "is a story of hardship unparalleled,

of circumstances without comparison, of endurances that would not be believed . . . an experience of very hell upon earth."[23]

In the third major push on November 6, more than 3,300 Canadians from seven front-line infantry battalions wearily drove forward at 6:00 A.M. The Canadians encountered less mud as they moved up the ridge, but the enemy was defending the front with dozens of machine-gun teams and hundreds of infantrymen in defences in depth. The corpses piled up. The Canadians fought on, assaulting in small groups against the enemy strongpoints by pinning them down with Lewis machine-gun and rifle fire, while other infantrymen bravely stalked their way forward, throwing grenades and finally unleashing a bayonet rush. But despite these refined and effective tactics, most destroyed German machine guns left a semi-circle of Canadian bodies around them. By the end of the day, the Canadian losses would rise to 2,238—of which 734 were killed. The Germans had nonetheless been decisively driven back and the charred carcass of Passchendaele was in Canadian hands.

"The road in horrible state—strewn with bodies horribly mutilated—many of them almost naked," wrote Lieutenant-Colonel Robert Pierce Wright of the 1st Canadian Field Ambulance, a prewar militia man and specialist in otolaryngology at the Jeffery Hale Hospital in Quebec City, who went forward to try to aid the wounded on November 9, 1917.[24] The naked dead had been blown out of their uniforms by the force of high explosive shells. In the final phase of the battle, the evacuation of the wounded remained no easy thing and the last attack on November 10—a limited push over a murky, shell-torn field beyond the village—saw two battalions, the 7th and 8th, push north of the ruins, supported by the 10th and 20th Battalions. Even though the Germans were ready for the Canadians, the attackers hurled them back, captured four German 77mm field guns, and removed the enemy from a high point that looked down into their lines. Another 420 Canadians were killed and 674 wounded, an extraordinarily high ratio of killed to wounded that resulted from an inability to carry the injured to medical treatment in a timely manner due to widespread exhaustion and the shattered terrain after weeks of intense combat.

———

The operating rooms at the casualty clearing stations and general hospitals ran day and night. Soldiers arrived with holes in them and the doctors tried to seal them up, usually after cutting away dead and dying skin to lessen the chance of infection, extracting metal and foreign objects, and repairing that which was gouged, torn, and shredded. Grey-skinned, feverish, and with desperate eyes, the conscious patients prayed there would be time for a doctor to see them before they took on the look of those too far gone and were triaged out, never to return. The advances in surgical treatment and the immediate cleaning of wounds at the clearing stations reduced the number of gas gangrene cases in comparison to the first half of the war.[25] This reduction was further evidence of surgical advances, although it may also reveal that those soldiers with gut wounds, the type of wounds most lethal and likely to be infected, never made it off the battlefield, being triaged in the mud and left to die so that others could be saved.

Nursing Sister Isabel Davies was assigned to a surgical team at No. 2 Casualty Clearing Station, about 15 kilometres from the front. Between August and November, her team worked on Imperial, Canadian, and other dominion patients, as well as

Germans, performing over 870 operations. Around the big pushes, like those on October 26 and 30 and November 6 and 10, the team performed up to twenty-six surgeries a day.[26] Davies survived the war and became an operating room supervisor at the Montreal General Hospital, although nothing she faced there would ever match the intensity of the Passchendaele campaign.

While those with physical wounds worked their way through the medical system, being shifted gradually away from the front toward the rearward hospitals, those with mental injuries were usually kept at the field ambulances that established rest stations for soldiers who had been pushed beyond the point of endurance. Passchendaele broke many men. Vacant-eyed soldiers with twitching faces whimpered under the fall of the shells, as the cold and wet further sapped their energy. Corporal Will Bird of the 42nd Battalion lived through the nightmare in the mud, and one sight haunted him for his whole life: that of a soldier, still standing, "rigidly, feet braced apart. He had been killed by the force of the blast, and his body was split as if sliced by a great knife." Another mate was working beside Bird during the battle, digging a hole in the soupy ground for safety: "he straightened to say something to us, and the next instant a shell cut the top of his head away, leaving but the jaw and neck." Bewildered and lost, not knowing who was alive and who was dead, Bird took shelter with a young soldier, and the two of them hugged each other as they shivered from the cold and shuddered from the horror.[27]

Bird survived the appalling events with his body and mind intact, but others were broken. They dribbled out of the line during breaks in the battle and shelling, and were often cared for at the rest stations. Here, the soldiers were cleaned, offered a warm meal, and given several stiff shots of rum. Sometimes pharmaceuticals were added to the mix, with the hope of rendering the shattered men unconscious for at least twenty-four hours. Warmth, rest, and sleep allowed many to return to their units after a few days. The medical services, as in all battles, but especially at Passchendaele, sustained and restored the fragile morale of the soldiers caught in the vice of combat and inconceivable conditions from which there was no escape.

———

"The Ypres sector was ever the deathtrap of the Canadians and Passchendaele seemed the culmination of it," said Lieutenant-Colonel John Nisbet Gunn, who commanded the Calgary-raised No. 8 Canadian Field Ambulance and was awarded the Distinguished Service Order.[28] While the medical services had improved and evolved since their arrival on the Western Front in early 1915, they faced brutal conditions at Ypres two and a half years later. Without horse-drawn ambulances or light rail, only manpower could be relied on to clear the wounded. This was not enough, and wounded soldiers died for want of timely treatment. At the same time, the cold conditions hastened the death of many, and thousands of unburied corpses were mute testimony to the cost of fighting through the mud.

The capture of Passchendaele village and much of the ridge allowed the British to claim a victory of sorts within the sea of defeat. The victory—real, pyrrhic, or imagined—allowed the Canadians to limp away from the otherworldly battlefield. It would be weeks before the corpse counters sorted out the casualties from the many who were lost in the mud or who would die of infections once the microbes took hold in their injuries. When the two weeks of losses during the preparation phase were added to the bloodletting during the four-phased operation, the final total for the Canadian shock troops was 16,404 casualties. The ratio of dead to wounded was very high at about one to two, which reflected the large number of wounded who never escaped the muck.[29] In a letter home, Gunner Gordon J. Morrisette told his future wife, Marjorie Reed, "The Canadians have been in some bad places but this beats them all. The mud and weather conditions themselves are enough to drive a mortal crazy."[30]

CHAPTER 15

ADAPTING MEDICAL CARE IN THE WAR ZONE, 1918

"It was hell that's all," wrote Herbert Irwin, from Weston, Ontario, who served with the 41st Battery of the Canadian Field Artillery at Passchendaele. "We had 17 killed & 63 wounded, gassed and shell shock[ed] so you can judge for yourself. That's in one battery and we were considered lucky. . . . It was just a case of sit and take it. I've seen big strongmen cry like babies after things quieted down."[1] The Passchendaele campaign gutted the Canadians, with more than 16,000 casualties taken. The survivors were strung out and despondent, and few would disagree with Sergeant Frederick Noyes of the CAMC, who described the battle in the bog as a "long, weird terrible nightmare."[2]

Bidding good riddance to the Flanders front, the Canadians marched southward to Arras, where General Arthur Currie's Corps took over Vimy Ridge and the surrounding area. The winter months of late 1917 and early 1918 saw no major offensives, although active raids and patrols were waged against the enemy across No Man's Land, which saw men wounded and killed. These operations contributed to the Canadians' losses of the three previous years, and by the end of January 1918, the Canadians had suffered a total of 147,009 casualties on the Western Front:

Killed in action	25,367
Died of wounds	8,492
Died of disease	1,787
Wounded	103,669
Prisoners of war	2,753
Presumed dead	3,694
Missing	1,247[3]

There were 40,587 dead (including those missing and presumed dead), although without the medical services the number of slain would have been much higher. The CAMC doctors, nurses, and enlisted men had undergone continual training, learning, evolution, and adaptation from 1915 to 1917, struggling with new wounds and diseases, seeking to navigate the moral and ethical challenges of medical care within the confines of military discipline, and showing courage and resilience as they faced enemy attacks and sought to support their comrades along the Western Front. The year ahead, 1918, would prove one of the costliest in the war, a period of great sweeping battles during which the trench systems were finally pierced, although never fully broken, and the carnage was unimaginable.

———

The natural fortress of Vimy, with its commanding heights over the Douai Plain, was riven through with deep caves and established communication trenches. During this quiet period on the

Western Front, soldiers and nurses voted in the December 1917 federal election. But only one issue was on their minds: should conscription—the state's forcing of young men to serve in the CEF against their will—be enacted to fully prosecute the war? In broad terms, anglophones were pitted against francophones, and farmers against those in the cities, but Canadians across the country held passionate views on the subject. Old and acerbated fault lines grew deeper in one of the most divisive elections in the country's history. Following the lead of a few provinces that had enfranchised women, the Borden government had given the federal vote to women who had a husband or son in uniform.[4] Nurses overseas were also among those who proudly cast their ballot. In what was called the "khaki election," the vast majority of service personnel supported conscription—thought to be at 90 percent—and a number of military officers were elected as members of Parliament.

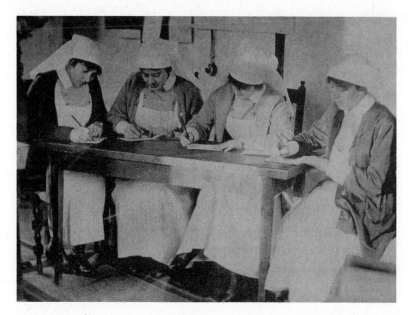

Canadian nurses voting overseas in the 1917 federal election.

Lessons had also been learned from the disaster at Passchen-daele—for example, too many patients in the medical facilities there had died from shock as they lay in the mud and their bodies shut down as a result of blood loss and cold. Over the winter, the medical services distributed hot water heaters and blankets, and even built stove piping to disperse warm steam in the field ambu-lances and casualty clearing stations.[8] Evolutions took place in medical care to prevent deaths from conventional physical wounds, but the soldiers' destroyed morale, a problem exacerbated by the horror of Passchendaele, was not easy to restore in the fourth year of the terrible war.

———

William Curtis, a First Contingent soldier who survived a shrapnel wound to the back and then returned to the front to keep fighting until he was killed in battle, wrote to his mother before his death, telling her, "It is nerve shattering to be under shell fire. No matter how strong a man's nerves are they are affected. I have seen many a poor fellow break under the strain."[9] Soldiers who spent any length of time in the trenches took on a haggard appearance, being affected both physically and emotionally as they developed visible ticks and tremors. Others stared off into the distance, lost—or trapped—in thought. The mud and slush that led to trench foot, the unending illnesses, and the revolting dead-flesh-eating rats all wore down soldiers. The snipers that killed the careless and the shells that wiped out the unlucky wrenched the survivors out of their temporary false complacency and sent hearts racing, stom-ach acids churning, and bowels liquifying. Passchendaele had accelerated this debilitating process as the war was etched deeply into bodies. It was widely acknowledged among the senior command that the fighting men needed a break, and yet there was no easy way to remove soldiers at the front from the war zone. Perhaps those on the edge might be shuffled off to a "bomb-proof" job behind the lines, but how were medical officers to distinguish between the bone-tired and those who were on the verge of a breakdown when they all looked like red-eyed, grey-skinned, walking corpses?

With no end to the war in sight, some soldiers felt compelled to seek a wound so they would be removed from the firing line and sent to a hospital. These desperate men sometimes deliberately exposed themselves, waving a hand or arm so that a sniper might put a bullet through it. While they wished for a through-and-through, more often bones were shattered, tendons cut, and hands permanently disabled. For other desolate men, cordite was chewed to induce illness; a bayonet could be lodged securely into a wall in order for the soldier to throw himself on it; or a man might close his eyes, screw up his courage, and hurl himself down a forty-foot flight of dugout stairs to land in a broken-boned heap at the bottom.

It was important for these injuries to look like accidents, because self-inflicted wounds were punished severely. Next to suicide, which appears to have been rare in the forward trenches, occurring most often behind the lines or after the war, a self-inflicted wound was the most serious manifestation of malingering, and for the high command it was evidence of a breakdown in morale.[10] The army command feared that if soldiers were allowed to escape the front through illness, or, in this more serious case, through a self-administered injury, the army would disintegrate from the cancer eating it away from inside.[11] It was the medical officers at the front who were primarily responsible for these distressed soldiers and for determining who had been injured legitimately in combat or suffered an illness and who had taken matters into their own hands. The search for these wounds further pitted the medical officer against the rank and file, and it was a part of the process whereby, as one historian has noted, the war was increasingly medicalized but the profession of medicine, in turn, was militarized.[12]

With the high command on the prowl for self-inflicted wounds, the medical officers at the front were ordered to examine any soldier with a suspect injury that took them out of the line, especially those resulting from poison gas, venereal disease, and shell shock. These were all stigmatized wounds that were generally seen as a result of carelessness, lack of character, or an intentional dodging of one's duty. However, in the front lines or rear areas, soldiers could be hurt in all manner of ways, whether in the course of the war or by accident, any of which might appear to be a self-inflicted wound. Horse and mule kicks disabled and even killed, sporting matches left men with broken jaws and hands, and the countless shell craters could lead to tripping in the dark, which broke ankles and legs. But all injuries were investigated. Private J.G. Sproule from Toronto, Ontario, wrote nonchalantly in a letter home in July 1916, "We had two fellows die recently. One got hit behind the ear with a bouncing baseball & never regained consciousness. The other died as a result of a clot of blood in the heart. He died in some agony."[13] While the clot was not an accident, it was another example of how the soldiers of the CEF—tired and exhausted, armed and dangerous—could be put in hospital or have their lives claimed by a wide variety of injuries and illnesses. A worrying number of soldiers were killed by grenade accidents or in cleaning rifles with a round in the chamber. The case of Private E.A. Stonebridge of the 46th Battalion revolved around his action in picking up an unexploded shell behind the lines, examining it, and then tossing it away.[14] The shell detonated, gravely injuring Stonebridge and two other men. The private was charged with administering a self-inflicted wound, which, in this case, was perhaps short-hand for exhibiting stupidity. Soldiers suffered cuts and punctures on rusted barbed wire and corrugated tin, or sustained more severe injuries, as in the case of Private J.E. Vienneau of the 87th Battalion, who fell in a shell crater in April 1918 during a working party in the dark. The unfortunate private landed on a discarded bayonet that speared his testicles.[15] Even his case was examined for a potential self-inflicted wound, although it was deemed an unfortunate accident, and perhaps the medical detective believed it beyond the bounds of what men might do to themselves in the dark to escape the front.

Shell shock continued to alarm the high command, who worried that it would provide a medically sanctioned exit from the front lines.[16] As of 1916, it was medical policy to keep most of those soldiers with "nerves" and anxiety-related wounds in Belgium and France. The renaming of shell shock as Not Yet Diagnosed (NYD), and other measures, including policing the medical officers who some in the high command felt were too sympathetic to the soldiers, all led to a drop in the official number of shell shock cases—although a rise occurred in other wounds related to exhaustion and nervousness.[17] The medical officer was responsible for assessing these injuries and, of course, for treating the injured at rest stations or special hospitals in France.

The rising number of gas wounds was also viewed with dismay by the generals. With so many non-fatal chemical casualties—about

97 percent of the total—both the medical officers and the special-ized gas officers were instructed to look out for malingerers. To add complexity to the issue, the medical services found frequent cases of soldiers who falsely thought they were gassed, developing psy-chosomatic symptoms as they coughed violently, had troubles with their eyes, and wailed at their imminent deaths. They were not faking it but suffering a hysterical reaction to the terror of gas, as the psychological dread physically affected the body.[18] Determining a legitimate wound in such conditions was no mean feat, and yet by the end of the war, the CAMC had recorded 729 cases of self-inflicted wounds—though more surely went undetected or were recorded under other categories of injuries.[19]

The medical officers' most repugnant task was to be a part of a firing squad. A number of offences could lead to death, including mutiny, cowardice, desertion, striking an officer, and murder—although this last offence was also punishable by death in civilian life. The harsh discipline was meant to strike fear into the soldiers and to reinforce the army hierarchy. Most often it brought only dismay to the mass of citizen-soldiers. "It was a nasty, beastly business and generally speaking quite useless," said Gunner Ernest Black of the death sentence.[20] During the course of the war, 222 sentences of death were passed on Canadian soldiers, although about 90 percent of these were commuted. The high rate of com-mutation has been interpreted by scholars as a strategy employed by the high command of inflicting the punishment to scare soldiers into submission and then offering clemency at the last moment, but the death sentence was carried through enough times—with 272 executions completed in the British Expeditionary Force, including those of 25 Canadians—to be understood as more than just an empty threat.[21]

After a last meal and counsel with a padre, the condemned prisoner was marched to a public spot, offered a blindfold, and told to await his fate. The executioners—usually six to eight infantrymen from the man's own battalion who all fired simultaneously—were informed that one of the rifles contained a blank and were ordered to shoot for the heart. A blank shell did little to assuage the disgusting nature of the act. The terrible task was no easier for the medical officers, who, while usually understanding the need for discipline, were repulsed by the act of meting out death to a Canadian volunteer. Medical officer Captain Andrew Macphail took part in one firing squad for nineteen-year-old Private Elsworth Young of the 25th Battalion, who was executed for desertion on the Somme. On his day of death, October 19, 1916, Young was bound to a chair and a fitted with a gas mask. Alone and with only his panicked breathing in his ears, Private Young was shot by his comrades, taking five bullets to the chest. Macphail pronounced him dead and felt that the entire act was "without dignity—a hangman's spectacle."[22]

———

Germany knocked Russia out of the war in late 1917, imposing a draconian peace on the Bolsheviks, who had risen up with the wartime conditions that undermined the nation's monarchy and created the unrest to fire a revolution. While a civil war raged, Russia abandoned its alliance with France and Britain against Germany, allowing the Kaiser's generals to transfer several dozen battle-hardened divisions to the Western Front to prepare for a last offensive before the Americans arrived in strength. On March 21, 1918, the Germans struck in Operation Michael behind a hurricane bombardment of shells and heavy saturations of poison gas. Trained stormtroopers surged forward around areas of resistance in a proto-Blitzkrieg style of warfighting that plunged deep into the Allied lines. On the first day of battle, over 38,000 British soldiers were killed, wounded, or captured, and by the third day of the offensive the Germans had advanced some 20 kilometres and were closing in on Amiens, an essential logistical centre for the British, whose loss would be disastrous.[23]

The front had been static for nearly three years, but now all of the roads, rail lines, supply dumps, and even medical units were threatened by the enemy's deep penetration. Although the field ambulances were meant to be mobile, many of the casualty clearing stations and all of the hospitals had become fixed structures. Now those formations close to the front were forced to gather up their voluminous hospital supplies and retreat from the battle zone. With so many of the medical units on the move, finding treatment for the wounded became more difficult. Nursing Sister Pauline Ivey, who had served in the Western University Hospital in England and at a British casualty clearing station in 1918, described the chaos in her overcrowded ward, writing, "I could see that the floors were covered with field stretchers on which the men were lying." Ivey was ordered to care for over sixty soldiers, and, afraid of stepping on them, she did so by crawling on her knees from patient to patient, changing bandages, offering sips of water, giving morphine. "The men are horribly wounded," she commented, "some were dying, some paralyzed, others insane strapped to the stretchers, all suffering horribly. War is certainly hell."[24]

From early in the offensive, No. 3 Canadian Stationary Hospital outside of Doullens—about 30 kilometres north of Amiens—had thousands of casualties diverted to it since all the clearing stations

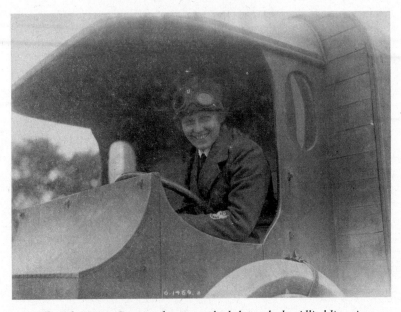

*The advancing German forces crashed through the Allied lines in
March 1918, driving medical units to retreat. A number of Canadian
women served as VADs (from the Volunteer Aid Detachment), and
some drove ambulances behind the lines.*

in advance of it were in retreat. Nursing Sister H.V. Petrie wrote
from the hospital during this hectic period, remarking, "All day
there was continual noise of the guns and thousands of wounded
pouring in, and the ambulances lined up the Amiens road for
miles, one line on one side coming in, and the other returning,
and the 'walkers,' some of whom had walked 12 and 14 miles
from the field ambulance." Petrie, like so many nurses and doctors, worked day after day to the point where she noted, "I could
barely hold up my head."[25] Over a ten-day period, for example,
Petrie and two other nurses were involved in 291 surgical operations. Throughout late March, with the Germans seemingly
unstoppable, admissions at the hospital jumped from 50 a day to

over 2,000 a day, and some 36,000 patients passed through the hospital from March 21 to May 30.[26]

In the ongoing medical war for survival, the loss of blood by patients during the agonizing journey from the battlefield to the operating table meant that many died from wound shock before they could be treated. In 1900, the main blood groups had been discovered through the Nobel Prize–winning work of Karl Landsteiner of Vienna, but the idea of blood transfusion had found little purchase in the Royal Army Medical Corps before the war. The Western Front forced these conservative views to change, and the Canadians were at the forefront in transfusing life back into patients on the threshold of death. One of the pioneers was Captain Lawrence Bruce Robertson of the CAMC, a prewar Toronto surgeon who spent his early career caring for children at Toronto's Hospital for Sick Children. On the Somme in 1916, he had conducted transfusions in No. 3 Canadian Field Ambulance at Albert. Forgoing the British technique of using saline, Robertson used a syringe to directly draw blood from a donor and then manually inject the blood through tubing into the recipient. He refined his technique on the constant flow of patients, experimenting in tracking blood pressure, noting when it dropped, and then infusing the patient with fresh blood.[27] Captain Robertson had remarkable success in restoring crashing men with life-giving blood.

From 1917 onwards, a more common and less laborious method was developed, using tubing to allow for direct blood flow from the donor to the patient. The incision was made in the donor's arm, the tubing attached, and blood was flowed into a glass cannula—to avoid clotting—and then into the patient. Captain Norman Guiou, a young doctor from Ottawa and another innovator in the CAMC, experimented with transfusions at field ambulances. Some doctors still voiced pigheaded resistance to the practice, and Guiou was accused more than once of killing patients with his radical interventions. Shaken by the charge, he nonetheless continued to try to save the grievously wounded. In April 1918, with thousands of soldiers wounded during the intense fighting, Guiou encountered a young soldier brought in on a stretcher, his upper arm shattered and several jagged bones jutting through the skin. The wounded man unblinkingly stared off into the distance, although he would periodically thrash around in his delirium. The soldier was close to death and Captain Guiou found a donor who gave 750cc of blood. The infusion dramatically improved the soldier's condition, and he calmed down, regained colour, and even had the strength to raise himself to drink some tea. His arm was cleaned and the bones set, and he was fit enough to be moved to a hospital. Captain Guiou did not know if the young man survived, but it was certain that he did not experience his pre-transfusion fate of dying in the field ambulance.

———

As the Kaiser's infantry thrust deeply into the Allied positions in March and April, the Germans also added bomber strikes against the lines of communication. During the last two years of the war, fixed-wing airplanes replaced the slower and less nimble Zeppelins. Armed with high explosive and incendiary bombs, enemy planes could do significant damage against ground targets, although the result was a far cry from the massive aerial bombardments' total devastation in the next war. Even though the Allied hospitals far behind the lines were clearly marked with large red crosses to alert aviators, the buildings were dangerously close to the road and rail networks that were often the targets of some of these bombing operations.

In May 1918, several Canadian hospitals were struck by enemy bombs in night attacks. A raid against No. 1 Canadian General Hospital on May 19 in the crowded area of Étaples caused tremendous destruction when, during the two-hour raid late in the evening, high explosives landed directly on a number of structures. The flames consumed the buildings and threatened several wards, including one in which over 300 patients with fractured femurs were strapped to their beds. The nurses and orderlies evacuated hundreds of patients while other caregivers stayed at the side of those who were immobile, comforting the ensnared soldiers and fighting off the flames. Not all could be saved. "The poor chaps didn't have the smallest chance of escape," wrote Sergeant-Major A.P. Reid. "Many of them were burned to death in their beds, while others had their legs blown off and were dependent upon the other boys carrying them out." Sixty-six Canadians were

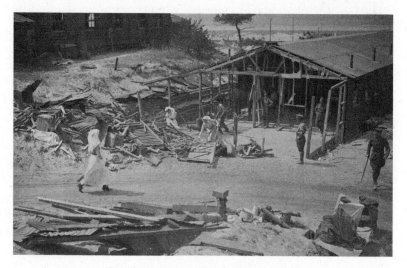

After the bombing of Canadian hospitals.

killed, including three nurses and a medical officer, and 73 more were wounded. Reid noted that in the coming days, "they were all buried in trenches in the military ceremony at Étaples, and each grave is marked with a cross."[28]

One of the dead was Katherine Maud MacDonald, a nurse born in Brantford, Ontario, who had worked at the Victoria Hospital in London, Ontario. Enlisting in March 1917, she served in several hospitals in England before being transferred to the Western Front in February 1918. Nursing Sister MacDonald sent letters home regularly to her "Mums and Sis!," with one from March 24, 1918, stating, "Have not written in two or three days but have been so busy that when I got off duty I was too tired to write." She shared some of her experiences, especially her acts of comforting patients with frightful injuries: "Here at night poor fellows[,] they have some awful wounds. We have one very sick man. Amputation of both legs above the knee[;] he lost so much blood that I am afraid for him. We had to send him to the O.R. again tonight and when he came back he would not rest unless he had my hand [and] there I sat and thought that every minute my back would break." In a letter on May 18, 1918, MacDonald assured her mother that she was "far from harm."[29] The twenty-five-year-old nurse was killed the next day and was buried in Étaples Military Cemetery in France. Her headstone epitaph, as picked by her parents, reads, "Killed in Action."

The bombing of No. 1 General Hospital was not an isolated event, and additional attacks were mounted on hospitals on May 21, 30, and 31. On the 30th, the target was No. 3 Canadian Stationary Hospital at Doullens, where bombs struck after midnight. Despite the late hour, several operations were in progress due to the mass of wounded that poured in from the fighting fronts, and two surgeons, three nursing sisters, sixteen orderlies, and four patients were killed.[30] Canadian infantryman John Harold Becker witnessed the bombing and the "shambles" of blackened iron cots, charred clothing, and congealed blood, recalling, "I saw every possible form of destruction of both life and property but there was certainly nothing that compares with this wrecking of hospitals and the thought of helpless bed-ridden wounded who could not escape explosives even at this point miles back of the trench line."[31]

Just as medical units were targeted behind the lines by bombers, hospital ships were threatened by marauding U-boats. The German U-boats (submarines) sought to sever Britain's essential lifeline across the Atlantic, its source of food, supplies, and soldiers from North America. The U-boats had been unleashed in February 1915, when the German admiralty ordered them to engage in unrestricted warfare on all ships—military and civilian—but they had been demonized after the sinking of RMS *Lusitania* in May 1915, which killed almost 1,200 civilians. While the U-boats had been pulled back to avoid further condemnation, after the terrible German losses of 1916 at the Somme and Verdun they had been let loose again to hunt with no restrictions. From February 1917 onwards, submarines sank hundreds of civilian ships.

In the work of evacuating the wounded to Canada, the Canadian medical services employed five hospital ships, which made 42 voyages during the course of the war, carrying over 28,000 patients.[32] They were the blind and the mangled, those suffering from mental injuries or wheezing through gas-scorched lungs. All were sent back to Canada to engage in the long process of rehabilitation and training. *Llandovery Castle* was one of the hospital ships used by the CAMC, and it was therefore marked with

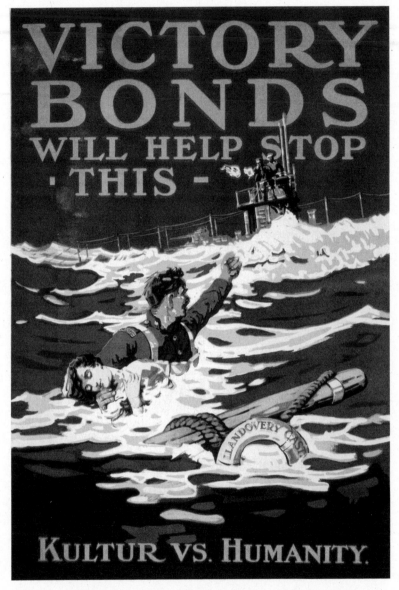

A Canadian poster encouraging the purchase of Victory Bonds
to support the war effort by demonizing the Germans for the
sinking of the Llandovery Castle.

enormous red crosses. Nonetheless, on the night of June 27, 1918, some 185 kilometres southwest off Fastnest, Ireland, a German torpedo ripped through the ship's hull. In a shudder of steel, the mortally wounded vessel listed, took on water, and went down within ten minutes. Although the hospital ship had no patients on board, many of the crew and CAMC personnel were killed in the initial blast, torn apart by the explosion, or engulfed in the subsequent fires. Others were unable to escape the sinking liner, with dozens in the water being pulled into the suction as *Llandovery Castle* went to its final resting place in the dark waters.

Of the 258 onboard, only 24 survived. More would have returned home to their loved ones if *U-86* had not circled the vulnerable lifeboats in the water and rammed them. In an attempt to kill everyone to cover up the attack on a hospital ship, the malicious U-boat captain even ordered that machine guns be turned on the survivors. For two hours the U-boat carried out its war crime, killing and maiming, sinking the lifeboats, and forcing survivors into the water, where many of them drowned. Fourteen Canadian nursing sisters died in the strike. Even as their families grieved them, the medical staff, but especially the nurses, were martyred in propaganda and journalistic accounts declaring that their sacrifice and courage would "serve to inspire men and women throughout the Empire."[33]

———

Despite the reversals all along the line from March to May, the Canadian Corps escaped the worst of the German offensives. Three of the four Canadian divisions were pulled from the line in

April and had the summer to recuperate and engage in open warfare training.[34] The German army's innovative, if costly, tactics of rapidly advancing and moving around areas of resistance provoked the Allies to study and further refine their own all-arms training, which saw combat formations—primarily the infantry, artillery, tanks, and machine-gun teams—support one another and fight together more effectively. "The modes of warfare have changed greatly since I first came out," wrote Private Frederick Robison in a June 1918 letter when he returned to the 58th Battalion after being wounded at Passchendaele. "I could scarcely recognize it as the same war."[35]

In anticipation of the static trench lines being broken in future operations, the medical services were also integrated into these combined-arms operations, with one official Canadian report noting that by 1918 it was "impossible to divorce the Medical Service from the rest of the military machine which it serves."[36] The CAMC officers studied the problem of advancing with the forward units, especially the issue of field ambulances likely being left several kilometres behind the newly established front lines on the first day of battle if all went according to plan. In such conditions, stretcher-bearers would not be able to carry the wounded many kilometres back along ever-lengthening routes, and so the medical services would have to rely more heavily on motorized ambulances and on increasingly mobile field hospitals.

This vigorous training was slowed in late May 1918 by a strange virulent flu. "Several of our men have been attacked by a mysterious sickness," noted Private Arthur Lapointe of the 22nd Battalion. "They are seized suddenly with a violent headache, accompanied by other pains and a swift rise of fever."[37] Initially misdiagnosed as trench fever or PUO (pyrexia of unknown origin), the virus was highly contagious and knocked men off their feet for three to five days, hitting the Corps in strength in June and July.[38] This flu was not yet the deadly mutated strain that would lay waste to millions a few months later, especially civilian populations already malnourished from years of war, but it struck many soldiers. While few Canadians in uniform initially died from the flu—other than those with tuberculosis or gassed men who, because of their weakened lungs, were susceptible to broncho-pneumonia—the medical services dealt with the rush of sick and created isolation wards in the medical units.[39] This controlled some of the spread of the virus and provided lessons that would be applied in a few months' time as the flu returned with a charged lethality.

Private Cecil Moody of the No. 8 Canadian Field Ambulance wrote to his girlfriend at the end of June 1918 about the many sick soldiers who were felled by influenza, although he also observed that the worst effects passed after a few days. "I think Fritz's army is also suffering from the plague from the reports of the prisoners taken lately," he noted. "In fact, it is rumoured that that was the reason their offensive was given up."[40] The transmissible virus indeed struck Germany with severity, with a sizeable number of the 1,966,000 total soldier-casualties lost to the flu from March to July.[41] German commander Erich Ludendorff lamented, "It was a grievous business having to listen every morning to the Chiefs of Staff's recital of the number of influenza cases and their complaints about the weakness of their troops."[42] The unexpected flu was a factor in slowing the German offensives as of mid-summer, exacerbating the horrendous battlefield losses since March, although few in the Allied command predicted the end of the war before 1919 or perhaps 1920.

General Currie's Canadian Corps had delivered three major if costly victories in 1917, but they had come off lightly from the fighting since March. "Never has our training been more severe," remarked Sergeant L. McLeod Gould of the 102nd Battalion in the summer of 1918. "Every day makes it clearer that when we move it will be to enter the bloodiest fight in which we have yet taken part."[43] The more experienced soldiers like Gould warned the new men that they would likely go into combat soon. Starting in August at Amiens, the Canadian Corps would indeed be ordered to spearhead some of the hardest and costliest battles of the war in withering fighting that would eventually break the back of the German army. The losses were gut-wrenching for both sides, the wear on the soldiers unending, and none of it could have been endured without the medical services adapting to support the soldiers at the sharp end.

CHAPTER 16

CARNAGE IN THE VICTORY CAMPAIGN, 1918

T he British, French, and dominion forces struck back on August 8, 1918, east of Amiens in France. After five months of battling the Kaiser's armies, from March to July, the Allies had defeated the multiple German offensives in grinding combat that bled the enemy white. Having rolled the iron dice and failed to end the war before the Americans arrived in strength, the Germans were now weakened and vulnerable. Sir Douglas Haig ordered two of his best formations, the Australian and Canadian corps, to spearhead a strategic counterattack. It was a secret operation in which hundreds of thousands of Allied soldiers gathered, along with the largest mass of tanks in the war—more than 600 metal beasts that would be unleashed—and all without alerting the enemy. The offensive was known among the Canadians as the LC Operation, in reference to the sunk hospital ship *Llandovery Castle*, signalling that Lieutenant-General Arthur Currie's Corps was coming for revenge. The Canadian assault was planned as an all-arms battle, with the infantry, artillery, machine-gunners, engineers, and armour entwined to fight more effectively and supported by air power and supply units. And, of course, the medical services were ready to deal with the wounded, having long been a part of this integrated system of combat.

The Battle of Amiens and the subsequent major battles east of Arras that sought to capture the key city of Cambrai were a series of stunning victories. But the war featured no bloodless campaigns, and these three successive operations would form the costliest period of fighting for the Canadian Corps. The 100,000-strong corps would suffer over 42,000 casualties in 60 days of intense combat.[1] The Canadian soldier would be pushed to his limit during these three campaigns that formed the milestone battles of what has come to be known as the Hundred Days campaign, which ultimately led to the German defeat on November 11, 1918. The price of victory would have been higher without the Canadian medical services.

———

At 4:20 A.M. on August 8, 1918, a stunning artillery bombardment from 646 artillery pieces opened up, illuminating the darkened battlefield. "All hell let loose all at once," remembered twenty-eight-year-old Lieutenant Albert George Lunt of the 4th Battalion, who would be shot in the hip later in the day but would survive the severe injury to make it home to Hamilton, Ontario.[2] This was heavy-metal warfare. The creeping barrage moved fast, tearing through the enemy lines as the Canadian ground-pounders tried to stay 100 metres behind the appalling shriek of shells that passed overhead and crashed down in advance of them. An obscuring wall of fog and smoke offered additional protection to the advancing forces, although they met little opposition in the first couple of hours as the front was only lightly held by the Germans and there was a deep buffer zone. However, secondary lines of defence several kilometres to the east were increasingly well defended by dug-in infantry supported and situated around machine guns. "The Germans were never cowards," wrote one Canadian. "They fought hard but could not resist the weight and speed of the attack as it rolled over them."[3]

The crimson tide of the first wounded soldiers was seen at the dressing stations within an hour of the battle's start, just as dawn was breaking. Of those who could not walk in, some knew enough to drag themselves to the primary routes running through the area, especially the Amiens-Roye road. They lay there like bloodied rags, hoping that a horse-drawn or motorized ambulance would pass by, pick them up, and take them to the surgeons. In anticipation of open warfare and a breaking of the enemy trenches, no regimental aid posts had been set up on the first day of the assault, and the medical officers were instead ordered to move forward with their stretcher-bearers to aid the wounded as they lay in the farmers' fields. With three divisions spread over 8 kilometres and advancing an astonishing 11 kilometres on the first day, the front ranged across 88,000 square metres, and so the stretcher-bearers dragged or carried their injured comrades to collection posts, creating small nests of the bleeding men in shell craters or in folds in the ground. In these positions, the wounded were better able attend to one another and were easier to find later in the day to be cleared to the field ambulance units where care was administered under tents.

"Distances were now considerable," observed Captain Norman Guiou, a medical officer attached to the 6th Canadian Field Ambulance but who spent the 8th roaming the front on a horse he acquired from a wounded cavalryman to more effectively treat injured soldiers.[4] As the front was increasingly pushed forward from the initial jumping-off areas, the motorized ambulances played an essential role on the battlefield. Six field ambulance units were echeloned across the front and they also pooled some resources to maintain a large corps-wide dressing station at the White Chateau, about 7 kilometres southeast of Amiens. From that position, another fleet of British motor ambulances assisted the Canadians and drove the injured to the casualty clearing stations, which were positioned far behind the lines as a result of both the rough terrain and a new wariness after the German offensives in March had overrun hospitals. Although three Canadian clearing stations were in operation, at 17 to 28 kilometres from the front they were too far from the action, which would prove a disaster later in the day as the wounded were stuck at the field ambulance units. Sergeant Frederick Noyes, serving at a Canadian ambulance, wrote of the hundreds of patients who overwhelmed the doctors, leading to a "shortage of blankets, stretchers and medical supplies."[5]

Even as Allied field and siege guns suppressed many German batteries with shrapnel and high explosives, enemy shelling still claimed soldiers and medical personnel along the front. Captain Thomas Hazel Whitmore served as a regimental medical officer with the 5th Battalion. After hours of treating the injured, and even carrying out emergency surgery, he was mortally wounded later in the day when shrapnel tore through his body. A week later, his unit received a letter from a Canadian private who was grateful to Captain Whitmore for saving his life and who wrote, "I shall never forget you. I should very much like a photo of yours to keep

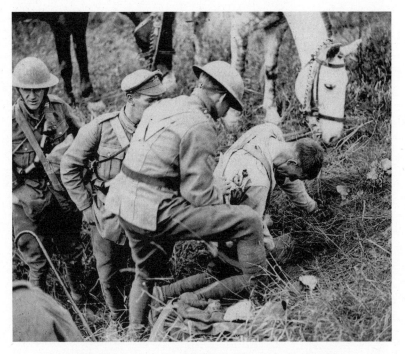

Battlefield care for a Canadian shot through the shoulder.

as a souvenir to say to my people that it was you, who saved my life, may God always have you safe."[6]

A few hours into the offensive, a No. 3 Canadian Field Ambulance vehicle was moving towards the front to pick up the wounded when it was caught in a bombardment. One driver was killed, four were injured, and several horses were torn apart,[7] but the shaken survivors regrouped, unlimbered the dead animals, and continued their work on foot. By the end of the day, most of the ambulances and cars pressed into service were perforated with shrapnel, the large red crosses painted on their sides scarred and lashed. As the sun went down on this costly day of victory, an emergency injection of an additional ninety cars from a number of Canadian units helped to ease the congestion at the field ambulances as the wounded were ferried to the clearing station operating rooms.

On the outskirts of Villers-Bretonneux, Private Clifton Cate of the 12th Battery, Canadian Field Artillery, witnessed how "the bodies of men and horses were strewn all about, mangled in every possible manner."[8] Despite the triumph on the 8th, the losses were staggering, with 1,036 Canadian dead and 2,803 wounded. The ratio of killed to wounded was 1 to 2.7, a higher rate of death than might have been expected considering the depth and speed of the advance, but the great surge into enemy lines had slowed the evacuation of the wounded. Many died in those farmers' fields.[9] Because of the Canadians' success, soldiers assumed that the casualties were not heavy, but the statistics reveal that the limited view of the soldier is not always accurate.

To deal with the trauma and to take pressure off the field ambulances that were congested with the dying because of a lack of transport, an additional Canadian clearing station was hastily established closer to the front in a psychiatric hospital outside of Amiens. Here and at other sites, surgical teams set up makeshift overflow operating tables outside, with doctors and nurses operating in the sunlight while cooled by a gentle breeze. Working assembly-line style, orderlies and nurses prepared the next patients, cutting off uniforms, disinfecting wounds, and whispering encouraging words to the men who waited for their turn under the scalpel.

The massed armoured strike, with 168 tanks on the Canadian front, rocked the enemy. The faster, smaller Whippet tanks advanced deep into enemy lines, while the more heavily armoured Mk V lumbered through machine-gun strongpoints.[10] But the Germans were ready for the tanks and had modified their defences,

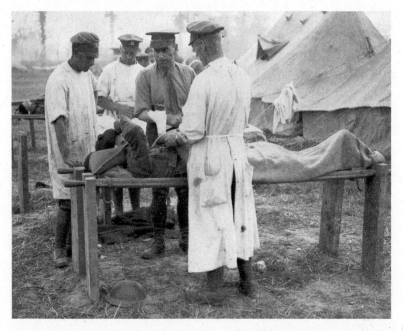

Canadian surgeons operating outdoors at a casualty clearing station.

bringing forward field artillery pieces and mortars and deploying them in a direct-fire anti-tank role. Armour-piercing shells reduced many tanks to charred ruins, incinerating the crews. Passing two smouldering tanks, Private Harold Becker of the 75th Battalion, who would be wounded later in the fighting, recalled, "The crews were probably burning to a crisp inside but we could do nothing for them."[11] Another stretcher-bearer looking for surviving troopers recorded that they had "died horrible deaths inside their steel pyre."[12] Those who escaped the cauldrons often had ghastly burns and would face plastic surgery and multiple skin grafts on their long road to recovery.

The battle continued into the 9th, but it was a day of confusion, especially for medical units as stretcher-bearers, spread over the large field of combat, were out of touch due to unreliable communications. However, the wounded were not abandoned. Along the wide front, medical officers took over enemy dugouts to treat Canadian and German soldiers. Horses were pressed into service as the motorized ambulances had no off-road capability, with the brave drivers and their beasts able to manoeuvre and carry back the wounded along the country clay roads and across the fields. Private James Robert Johnson, a young driver, recounted how the horses were distressed by the incessant shellfire, remarking of one that was badly injured, "It was pitiful to see him tremble."[13] The twitching and traumatized animals nonetheless saved many Canadians, as did most of the 5,033 German prisoners who were conscripted to carry the wounded. By the end of August 9, Currie's soldiers snatched another 6 kilometres from the enemy, which cost 2,574 casualties, adding significantly to the 3,800 casualties on the first day.[14]

Amiens was a grand victory, although the second and third day of battle saw hard fighting as the Germans reacted to the initial blow by rushing forward reinforcements, especially machine-gun teams. "There are dead men laying all through the standing crops around here, both the enemies and ours," wrote Private Victor Swanston from Saskatchewan, a First Contingent soldier who had survived many campaigns and who would make it back home to his loved ones.[15] To further add to the Canadians' misery, the Germans drenched the battlefield in chemical weapons. "A gas alarm had to be experienced to be appreciated," recalled one CAMC sergeant. "Cries of 'Gas!'—and a near-panic spread like wildfire."[16] High explosive shells could blow men around, lift them off their feet, and rip off respirators, thus exposing stunned soldiers to the hazy chemical mist. Even in the best of conditions it was common for soldiers to suffer from minor gas inhalations, leaving them hacking up sputum through raw lungs as they huddled in shallow craters or hurled themselves against the enemy. Even though many Canadians had minor chemical burns and deep coughs, most continued to stay with their unit and not abandon comrades, especially as every rifle was needed at the front. However, on day three of the nearly continuous fighting, combat fatigue washed over soldiers who were asked to do too much for too long. Writing in his diary, Private Andrew Coulter, an American who had enlisted in the CEF at age nineteen and who later became a doctor in Saskatchewan, described "dead bodies of both sides lying quite thick everywhere."[17]

The battle wound down on the 11th as both sides were bleeding out in vicious clashes. "The whole thing gave one the impression that a chunk of hell had broken loose," was how Private A.E. Smith of the 116th Battalion summed up his experiences.[18] General Currie and his Australian counterpart understood that the break-in had been blunted by the enemy and that no breakout would be achieved into the green fields beyond. They appealed to their British seniors, and most of the fighting ended on the 11th, although skirmishes continued for another nine days and the never-ending fall of shells claimed lives.

"At Amiens, for the first time after nearly three weary years, they had tasted complete victory," said Nova Scotian Captain Robert Clements of the Canadians. "Now they sensed the kill."[19] To quantify that success, the Corps' four divisions met and defeated elements of 14 German divisions, capturing 9,311 prisoners, 201 guns, 152 trench mortars, and 755 machine guns.[20] The Germans were badly shaken by the losses along the Canadian front, and by their equal failure against the Australians, leading to grave doubts among the German high command, who wondered if the army could hold out until the fighting season ended in a few months. But the victory came at a heavy cost in lives and in ghastly wounds: from the 8th to the 20th, the total number of Canadian casualties was 11,822.[21] Seven members of the CAMC were killed and another twenty-eight wounded,[22] and a far greater number of stretcher-bearers attached to forward units were cut down, although they were counted as losses to their units rather than to the CAMC. Following the stunning success at Amiens, the battle-hardened Canadian Corps was ordered to the Arras front near Vimy Ridge, to take part in another hammer-blow offensive against the Germans.

———

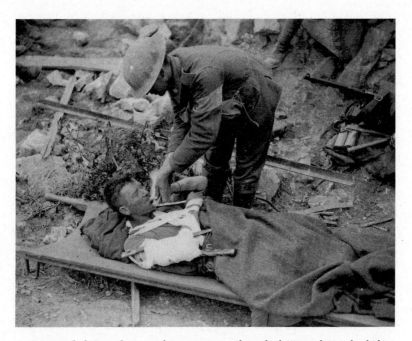

A wounded Canadian smokes a cigarette for relief. Note the makeshift splint consisting of two bayonets to stabilize his broken right arm.

After the surprising success at Amiens, Allied supreme commander Ferdinand Foch, the French general who loosely coordinated the war effort that involved American, French, Belgian, British, and dominion forces, ordered a new series of offensives along the Western Front. The goal now was to hit the Germans repeatedly, force them to spread their dwindling reserves to defend multiple fronts, and attrite their armies through unyielding combat. As part of these large-scale operations, the Canadian Corps would lead another attack against the fearsome and fortified Hindenburg Line. Foch said of Currie's formation, "The Canadians are the force on which I can rely to clean up between Arras and the Hindenburg Line."[23] While the Canadians knew the terrain around Vimy, they had only a few days to prepare for the coming battle, but the First British Army assisted them with artillery and logistical support and they were lucky to take over established lines of communication.

The medical services had faced grave challenges at Amiens because the casualty clearing stations were located too far from the front, and so in this operation—called the Second Battle of Arras, although more often known as the assault on the Drocourt-Quéant Line—they were moved closer to the fighting. Canadian medical units took over buildings and chalets and prepared for the influx of wounded. The approach to clearing the battlefield would be similar to that at Amiens, with each division handling its own wounded, but instead of a single corps-wide dressing station, there were now three, with collection points established along the front to which bearers would drag the wounded.[24] This reorganization, a tangible response to a lesson learned from Amiens, would aid in the bottleneck of the expected thousands of injured soldiers passing through a single point. A railway was also laid from Arras to the front, which would allow for the evacuation of soldiers more efficiently and, for the benefit of the wounded, more smoothly.

The Canadians faced the strongest part of the German line for their attack on August 26, with multiple trenches extending 18 kilometres in places and more than 1,000 machine-gun positions prepared in hardened strongpoints with overlapping fields of fire, all of which was protected by deep rows of tangled barbed wire. No one should have expected another Amiens-like advance of 11 kilometres on the first day through this fortress. The battle would be a dog fight.

At 3:00 A.M., 762 Allied guns opened up on the enemy lines under a bright moonlit sky. Overwhelmed German batteries were smothered by shrapnel, high explosives, and poison gas, while the creeping barrage led the Canadian infantry through the trench system. The severe fighting on the 26th bled into the 27th and 28th, with few breaks. In the see-saw combat that saw units engaged in attack, defence, and then counterattack, often the wounded were overrun as they lay helpless in No Man's Land, with Canadians pushed back and forced to leave their comrades behind, hoping the captors would treat them decently. But over the course of hours of fighting, a section or platoon would drive forward and sometimes encounter their own wounded, allowing men to be cleared if they had not already succumbed to their injuries. The three forward field ambulances were busy during the heavy fighting, with No. 8 Canadian Field Ambulance caring for 64 officers and 2,039 other ranks over a three-day period.[25] "The country around here is terribly cut up," penned one stretcher-bearer in his diary. "Lots of prisoners coming down and was glad to see them, using them as stretcher bearers."[26]

Despite heavy enemy shellfire, the stretcher-bearers were effective in clearing the battlefield, as one CAMC report noted, and in the first couple of days of combat the "wounds were less severe than those we handled in the Amiens fight."[27] Horse-drawn and motorized ambulances transported soldiers by the primary route of evacuation, dispersing their injured cargo to five Canadian and Imperial casualty clearing stations where surgery had begun early on the 26th. As bandages were hardened with gore and uniforms caked with sweat, CAMC privates had to peel layers off the wounded soldiers before nurses and doctors could appraise their wounds. While the usual chaos reigned at the front, the Canadians' steady advance into the enemy lines meant that the rear areas were largely free of artillery fire by the second day. Furthermore, one of the new innovations in mass clearing was the introduction of ten specially fitted buses that could each accept up to thirty stretcher cases, thus aiding in getting the wounded more rapidly to surgery.[28]

The stream of mangled from the front kept coming and the drive on the 28th was a bloodbath as Currie and his generals were pushing the infantry too hard. The units in the firing line were down by at least 50 percent strength, meaning that instead of 650 going into an attack, there were only 300 or 350. They faced a hornet's nest as the Germans, also badly mauled, were nonetheless prepared for another clash of arms. On one part of the front, the 22nd and 24th Battalions, severely cut up after two days of battle, attempted to dislodge the Germans from positions around the Fresnes-Rouvroy Line. It was a frontal assault against impossible odds and it should not have been ordered by the divisional commander, although other battalions along the front achieved their objectives.[29]

The brave soldiers did their duty, with their few remaining officers leading them forward. One of the 22nd Battalion's still-standing leaders was Major Georges Vanier, an aggressive and courageous soldier from Montreal. In going "over the top," Major Vanier was struck by several bullets in the legs and chest. Even as he was immobilized and in tremendous pain, he continued to inspire his men by urging them onwards, rising up and falling again until he was carried off the battlefield. Pale and lifeless, he was close to death. Major Vanier later wrote, "A transfusion was done in direct contact with the donor. The immediate effect was a feeling of active physical resuscitation. I have no doubt whatever that the transfusion saved my life."[30] With a leg amputated, Vanier accepted that his war was over, but he survived to serve his country as a soldier and diplomat, and, from 1959 to 1967, as governor general.[31]

———

"We are now trying to break the hinge of the German position," scribbled General Currie in his personal diary, describing the coming battle on September 2. "For this reason the Boche will fight us very hard."[32] Captured prisoners and intelligence gathered from aircraft and infantry patrols revealed the strength of the German position, a series of trenches known as the Drocourt-Quéant Line. The Canadians had suffered close to 9,000 casualties since August 26, on top of the 12,000 losses at Amiens, and although they had crashed through much of the enemy trench system, they were now down to the bone. With these two great victories came shattering costs, and August 1918 was the deadliest month of the war for the Canadians. John Lynch of the PPCLI recounted a conversation among the few survivors of his platoon, where they talked about the long odds of survival and suggested their only hope was for a Blighty wound. "If a man keeps coming back, in battle after battle," said the dispirited soldiers, "he is bound to be killed."[33] Another Canuck, Lieutenant Joseph Sproston of the 10th Battalion, had led a company of 112 all ranks into battle and emerged with 23. He had told his commanding officer, "I can't take no more. This isn't war, it's murder. It's just pure bloody murder."[34]

After three days of aggressive patrols, raids, and skirmishes, the Canadians were in place for the final advance on September 2. The job fell to tired infantrymen, their dirty faces set towards the enemy with cracked lips and inflamed eyes exacerbated by lack of sleep and stinging gas. The barrage from hundreds of guns opened at 4:50 A.M., shattering the enemy trenches, but many of the German machine guns remained active and had to be knocked out along the front in battles hard fought by dwindling groups of Canadian infantrymen. "I could never quite understand how anyone survived at all in an attack of this kind, for it was over dead-level country with all the enemy in trenches firing all the machine gun bullets they could at us," remarked Company Sergeant Major Arthur Shelford of the 54th Battalion, a prewar farmer from the area around Wistaria, British Columbia. "The ground resembled a hail-storm, as the bullets hit all around us," he said of the fighting on September 2.[35] A few days later, Shelford would be shot through the shoulder, with the bullet exiting his back. He survived his wound as a result of timely and skilled medical treatment.

The Canadians fought their way forward with bomb, bullet, and bayonet, clawing and scratching, slowly making headway. In some sections of the front the attack was stopped dead, with platoons destroyed, companies decimated, and battalions driven into the ground. It was "the hardest scrap I've ever been through," said Lieutenant Clarence Gass of the 85th Battalion.[36] But other victories were achieved and the Canadians gained the upper hand throughout the day. As the sun set, the enemy line was broken in another devastating defeat of the Kaiser's forces.

In grim fighting throughout September 2, tremendous bravery was exhibited along the front. This extended to the stretcher-bearers and medical officers, two of whom were awarded the Victoria Cross. Captain Bellenden Hutcheson, an American serving with the CAMC, was recognized for his outstanding work under artillery fire, mortar bombs, and snipers. At one point in the battle, he evacuated a wounded officer to the rear through a storm of bullets and then returned into the fire when he saw a sergeant cut down. Disregarding the danger, Hutcheson dragged the unconscious sergeant into a crater and treated his life-threatening injuries.[37] Stretcher-bearer Private Francis Young of the 87th Battalion was recognized with the Victoria Cross for similarly exposing himself to danger again and again as he cared for the wounded under fire.[38] In another unexpected act, four captured German doctors assisted in caring for the wounded at a Canadian dressing station, where their skill, one report noted, aided in the "quickness of our evacuation."[39] In doing so, they helped to balance the loss of the fifteen CAMC officers and men who were killed in this battle, along with another sixty-one who were wounded.[40]

"The much vaunted Hindenburg Line was pierced," wrote Lieutenant R.J. Holmes in a letter home. "Of course, these glorious victories have their cost, and there are many familiar faces missing from our line-up of a month ago."[41] Despite sustaining some 14,349 casualties from August 26 to the breaking of the Drocourt-Quéant Line on September 2, the Canadians killed thousands of Germans, captured 10,492 prisoners, and snatched an astonishing total of 927 enemy machine guns.[42] According to General Currie, the Corps' success came from "the unparalleled striking power of our Battalions and the individual bravery of our men. . . . I cannot say any more and a lump comes in one's throat whenever you think about it."[43]

———

Leaving many of their dead, the Germans retreated from their fortress position and crossed to the east side of the Canal du Nord, anxious to protect Cambrai, a crucial logistical hub. The Canadian Corps slowly advanced to the western bank of the canal, but then waited as Americans, Australians, British, French, and Belgians attacked methodically along the Western Front. With the 40-metre-wide canal in front of them, the Canadians thinned out the front and spent time integrating new reinforcements from England, including conscripts and some of the wounded from earlier in the year.[44]

The unending wastage to units continued as the Germans dumped poison gas on the Canucks day and night. The nefarious chemicals added to the soldiers' war weariness after the two battles that had cost 26,000 casualties. Infantryman George Bell of the 1st Battalion, who survived the war, observed that his exhausted and sometimes dispirited comrades were succumbing to more illness, while others courted a self-inflicted wound. "They had seen so much death, bloodshed and suffering," he wrote, "that they were sick of it all."[45]

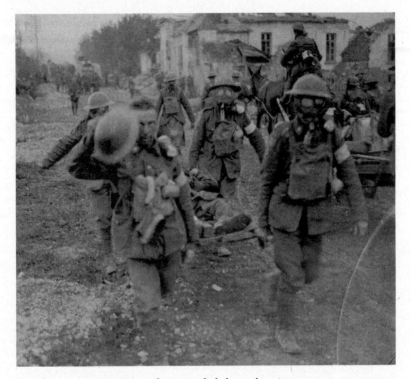

Carrying in the wounded through poison gas.

It was the medical services, especially the regimental medical officers, who monitored the worn-out soldiers at the front. Men who were near collapse were ordered to the rest stations at the field ambulances, especially when the tempo of fighting slowed in mid-September. While the medical services played a much-heralded role in saving lives, they also provided unsung support in ensuring that the fragile morale of the soldiers was not enervated by the ordeal of this hyper-intense warfare.[46] Rest stations afforded the warriors a day or two of respite, aided by rum-infused coffee and sedatives. In darkened tents soldiers slept deeply, although periodic moans and screams could be heard coming from the cots as soldiers fought battles of the mind that could not be won. As one medical officer remarked, "No one can quite appreciate what the strain means, unless they have been here."[47]

——

Launching a third Canadian set-piece battle within a space of less than two months appeared impossible, especially as the Germans had stacked some of their best divisions in depth on the east bank of the Canal du Nord, with multiple trench systems guarding Cambrai.[48] "Most of us have no illusions about the possible duration of the war," wrote Private Thomas Clarke Lapp, a former printer from Belleville, Ontario, in a letter written on September 20, 1918, as he recovered from a gunshot wound to the abdomen. "While we hope for an early finish we are not building any hopes on leaving the shores of France before the close of 1919." Nonetheless, he continued to believe that "we must win, and win we will, regardless of the time and price. I am writing this from a forward line where daily the price of blood is paid."[49] Lapp survived, although he likely would have died if he had suffered the gut wound at Passchendaele, Vimy, or the Somme, before advances had been made in abdominal surgery. What had not changed since these battles was that it was still and always soldiers like Lapp who paid for victory in blood.

The new offensive began behind a tornado of shellfire on September 27, catching the Germans flat-footed as they believed that the Canadians would never chance a crossing of the Canal du Nord. Even though the canal was not filled with water, the attack would be funnelled into a narrow kill ground, and if it was blunted, the infantry caught in the cauldron would be slaughtered. Currie understood the danger, but he unleashed his forces nonetheless and they leapt forward at 5:20 A.M. behind the creeping barrage fired by 785 artillery pieces. The Canadians' advance was too much for the Germans, who were thrashed in the initial assault and were thereafter left reacting to the rapidly shifting attacks. Strongpoints fell to Currie's soldiers, and the lead units crashed through a number of trench systems before being replaced by leap-frogging forces. Even as the enemy was awakened to the threat and responded by flooding the front with reinforcements that flowed out of Cambrai, the Canadians kept driving forward.

After nearly two weeks of battle, and with the Canadians utterly spent on October 9, the German defences buckled under the relentless advance. The prize of Cambrai fell to the Canadians, but Currie was correct to write that this battle, in which they defeated elements of twelve German divisions, was "the bitterest fighting we have ever experienced."[50] The Allied forces, with the

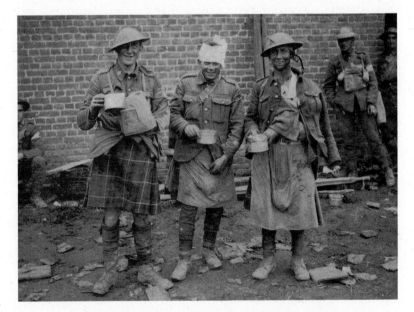

Wounded Canadians on their way to medical care.

Canadians in a spearhead role in several crucial campaigns, out-fought the Germans from August 8 to October 9. While other battles would be fought during October and early November, the German army's spine had been broken and its morale crushed in combat.

———

A 1919 official report from General Currie counted 42,628 Canadians killed, missing, or wounded in these three titanic campaigns.[51] However, the evolving tactics at the front led to a shift in the types of Canadian casualties recorded during the cataclysmic victories from August 8 to October 9, offensives that formed the core of what has become known as the Hundred Days campaign. Canadian soldiers in these battles suffered far more wounds from bullets than from shrapnel, high explosives, and shell splinters, and the medical services saw a steady increase in casualties from poison gas, which also tended to wound rather than kill.[52] At Amiens, Currie's report counted 11,362 casualties from August 8 to 22 (a slightly lower number than the 11,822 that was recalculated later). Of the 11,362 casualties, 2,259 Canadians were listed as killed and missing in action versus 9,103 wounded. This was a 1 to 4 ratio of killed and missing to wounded. During the Battle of Arras and the drive on Cambrai, in which 30,806 total casualties were counted from August 22 to October 11, 6,297 Canadians were killed and missing in action, for a ratio of 1 to 5 killed to wounded.[53] While the casualty numbers were horrendous during these sixty days of carnage, the ratio of killed and missing (8,556) to wounded (33,612) in the Canadian Corps was 1 to 3.93, a significantly less lethal ratio than at the Somme, Vimy, or Passchendaele.

This ratio of high wounding to death in the Hundred Days period has never been analyzed in any history book, but the data reveals four important elements of the fighting. First, the Canadian artillery dominated the German batteries, and the enemy relied heavily on machine guns in their defence. Though these elite German soldiers fought bravely, the Canadians captured an astonishing total of 2,745 machine guns during the Hundred Days campaign, and destroyed even more. And yet while these machine guns were mass killers, bullet wounds were less lethal than shrapnel and shell splinters.[54] Second, the successful Canadian drive in all three battles ensured that the wounded could be cleared in a timely manner, saving many men from dying of shock in No Man's Land. The operations were never perfect—with, for example, the first day at Amiens revealing the failure of placing the casualty clearing stations too far to the rear—but lives were saved when the Canadians were able to advance forward instead of being hurled backwards. Third, the warmer weather was a factor that kept soldiers from slipping into shock and hypothermia, providing far better conditions than those who suffered in the cold at the Somme, at Vimy, and especially at Passchendaele. Finally, the increase in survival can also be attributed to the evolution of care in the medical services, which ensured that those who had previously died from wounds to the abdomen and head, or had succumbed to blood loss, shock, and infection, now had a better chance of surviving. Connecting the medical services to the combat forces and to the higher survival rate of wounded soldiers in this intense period provides a major new insight into the Canadian fighting experience during the Hundred Days campaign and its most frenzied period of battle, the sixty days from August 8 to October 9. It also reveals how doctors and nurses, after more than three years of refinement and revolutionary treatment, found new ways to pull the wounded back from the abyss in the ongoing medical war for survival on the Western Front.

CHAPTER 17

A PANDEMIC OF MASS DEATH AND AN EPIDEMIC OF SEXUAL DISEASES

"We have the Hun absolutely where we want him on the Western Front," wrote Major Arnott Grier Mordy, while acknowledging that "the Canadian Corps has suffered very heavy casualties in the accomplishment of this."[1] With the capture of Cambrai on October 9, 1918, Mordy—who was writing from a hospital bed after receiving a gunshot wound to his left shoulder—and his comrades had inflicted another momentous defeat on the enemy. While the Canucks bled for that victory, the three battles of the first sixty days of this final campaign broke a series of crucial enemy defensive positions, with the fall of Cambrai fatal to the German war effort. Along the front, the Allies were pressing back the Kaiser's forces, and the Canadians continued to be in the vanguard. General Arthur Currie's Corps pursued a fleeing German army, hoping to finally end the war that only two months earlier most felt would not be concluded until at least 1919. The Canadians were not alone along the Western Front, but they fought in sustained battles longer than any other corps, and over the next four weeks they would continue to defeat the enemy in multiple skirmishes and small-scale battles.

This was also a period of liberation, with more than 70,000 French citizens given back their freedom.[2] Behind the main battle zone of the Western Front, the French had suffered through four years of cruel occupation. Their houses and properties had been pillaged of goods by the occupying force, and now, as the German army retreated eastward, the enemy laid waste to the countryside, poisoning wells and demolishing structures.[3] This was the hard hand of war. And yet amid this destruction, the Canadians liberated dozens upon dozens of villages and towns. Out of cellars and hiding places emerged French civilians, tentatively at first, and then with open delight. "They were so glad to see us," recounted Private J. Arthur Maguire of the 2nd Battalion. "They wept with joy."[4] In the words of the war diarist of the 4th Brigade, Canadian Field Artillery, "The people could not do enough for us. Every time the column halted, cups of steaming hot coffee and biscuits were handed to the men, and our horses were garlanded with flowers."[5] Homemade flags were waved, the French sang "Vive la Canadienne," and banners were unfurled welcoming the "liberators."[6] Infantryman Wilfred H.S. Macklin of the 19th Battalion recounted that "these people came out and greeted us with the greatest possible enthusiasm and this in itself was a great raiser of morale. The soldier felt that, after all, they've been telling us that we're fighting for freedom, and there are the people that we are liberating and the very reception that the soldier got was enough to convince him that this was, in fact, true."[7] Tired, worn out, and sometimes disillusioned by the terrible cost of victory, the battle-hardened warriors saw in these multiple acts of liberation a reminder of why they had fought so hard.

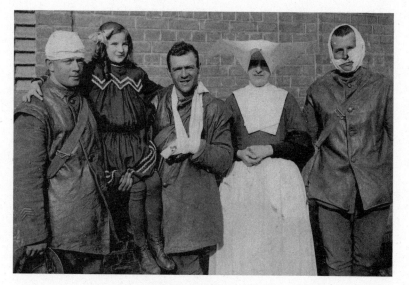

Injured Canadians with French civilians whom
they liberated in ferocious battle.

The mass liberation also thrust a new humanitarian crisis onto the Canadian Army Medical Corps. Despite the logistics-related famine the Canadians suffered as they outdistanced their supply lines in their steady pursuit of the retreating enemy, leading to shortages of food and other supplies, many of the soldiers freely shared their rations with the liberated French who were suffering from malnutrition and disease. Medical officer Charles Willoughby articulated the medical services' challenge of aiding the sick and wounded, but also their responsibility for the "sanitation of each new camp."[8] Using scorched-earth tactics, the Germans fouled water sources with dead animals to hinder the Canadians. Sanitation units and medical officers were ordered to test all wells and deploy chlorine to purify the water.

Lieutenant-Colonel John Alexander Gunn described the French, noting that they were given back their freedom after "living in daily terror" but also that "many of the people in the area were in very poor physical condition, and by far the greater part of the work of the ambulance was in attending to these poor people."[9] To aid civilians along the front, the CAMC established medical clinics that, according to one Canadian report, "countless inhabitants used for care."[10] "Many of them are ill with influenza," wrote Major T. Edgar MacNutt. "I remember one poor woman with her baby only two or three days old in her arms. The mother was ill and the baby was dying."[11] The emaciated and sick French were highly susceptible to the deadly pandemic that was moving through soldiers and civilians with its killing touch, and that would unleash a plague upon the world.

———

Sapper Harold Edward Cook, a grocery clerk from Woodstock, Ontario, who enlisted in May 1918, was ordered to a hospital in Seaford, England, on October 5, 1918, after falling gravely ill. A doctor observed he had been coughing heavily and that he had muscle aches and "pain in the stomach and vomiting." On the 11th, after struggling to breathe for several days and then seeming to recover, Cook endured a fever spike, leaving him convulsing periodically and in need of oxygen to breathe through congested lungs. The next day the sapper was "quite cyanosed" and "markedly worse," according to one physician.[12] The twenty-year-old died at 1:45 P.M. that day, his death given as pneumonia, although his medical case sheet said he had been admitted with influenza.

Thousands of Canadian soldiers had been laid low with influenza in June 1918, but save for those with gas-corrupted lungs or some unlucky few, most had recovered. However, a new killer virus swept through the armies of the Western Front in September 1918. Though it was known as the Spanish flu, it did not originate in Spain and was only identified first by medical practitioners in that neutral country because they were not subject to the same press censorship as the combatant nations.[13] Present-day scientists and medical detectives believe that the H1N1 virus mutated in the late summer of 1918 and that the lethal strain originated either in the army camps of southern England, in the U.S. Midwest, or in China.[14] The new variant of the virus, transmitted via particles in the air expelled through coughing, was highly contagious and far more deadly than the original form.

The flu virus first presented as a fever and cough, then deepened to bronchitis, and often ended as pneumonia, resulting in death. Canadians well understood the lethality of disease, with tuberculosis—the "white death"—having long been the greatest reaper of Canadians under the age of forty-five, but the mutated virus's terrifying speed of spread, its virility, and the fact that it killed the healthy as much as it did the very young and old sowed a new terror. The body's immune system often went into overdrive in fighting the virus, and increasingly sodden lungs filled with water, pus, and blood. Doctors now describe this as a cytokine storm, with the immune system overreacting to the virus and releasing inflammatory mediators that lead to organ failure.[15] That this happened most frequently in those with healthy immune systems was another sick twist of the knife after four years of war during which the old buried the young.

Some propagandists and rumour-mongers in the West believed that the Germans had concocted the virus in a laboratory in a desperate turn to biological warfare as they had done in their use of chemical weapons. After years of their countrymen being

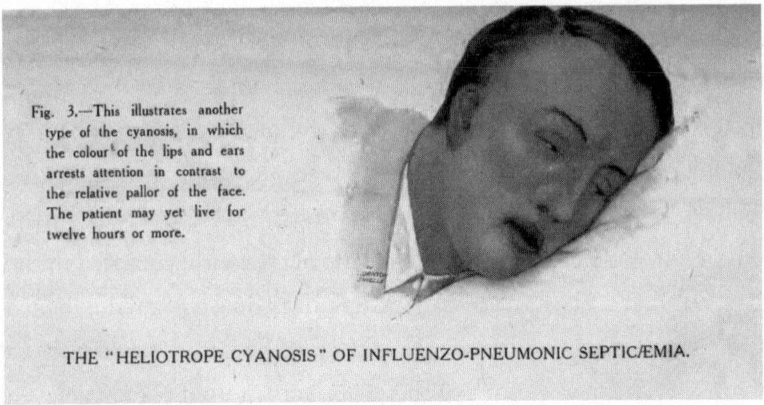

Fig. 3.—This illustrates another type of the cyanosis, in which the colour of the lips and ears arrests attention in contrast to the relative pallor of the face. The patient may yet live for twelve hours or more.

THE "HELIOTROPE CYANOSIS" OF INFLUENZO-PNEUMONIC SEPTICÆMIA.

A sketch from a contemporary British medical history that sought to document the slow death of an influenza victim. This late-stage patient is close to the end, with darkened lips and ears and pale skin because of lack of oxygen.

slaughtered in the trenches, journalists and politicians found the connection between "germs" and "Germans" easy to make within the hypercritical war environment. Others believed that the millions of rotting dead in Europe had created a sickening miasma that infected the living. This was not biological warfare, however, or even a bacteria as medical professionals believed, and it was not until 1933 that the influenza A virus was identified.[16] Far from creating and inflicting the virus, the German army was among those most vulnerable to its effects on the Western Front. The Kaiser's soldiers, already physically weakened by the Royal Navy blockade starving Germany of food supplies, were especially susceptible.[17] The flu did not end the war, although it contributed to the declining fighting efficiency of the German forces when the Allied onslaught rolled over them during the Hundred Days campaign.

The first mutated lethal flu strain victim was reported in Canada in mid-September 1918, and while the contours of the disease pathway are not easy to track with specificity, in broad terms the flu was carried across Canada, from east to west, via the rapid transmission of the virus among the population, particularly in the overcrowded cities.[18] The spread of the virus was intensified by the wounded soldiers from the Hundred Days campaign who, judged too badly injured to ever return to the front, were sent to Canada on hospital ships, their mangled bodies becoming transport vessels that carried the virus back home. Troop ships also steamed in the opposite direction, from Canada to England, bringing supplies, reinforcements, and the virus. With expediency trumping public health, visibly sick soldiers were stuffed into poorly ventilated and crowded hulls. The troopship *City of Cairo*, for example, which left Quebec on September 28 and arrived in Devonport on the October 11, was a veritable plague ship, with 32 deaths taking place at sea and the remaining 1,000 soldiers nearly all sick with the flu.[19]

Canadian papers began to track the virus in late September as it seeped across the country, first in the Maritimes, then through Quebec and Ontario, and eventually to the West. The bodies started to pile up, and the large cities, which had the greatest number of deaths, faced shortages of coffins and so many funerals that more grave diggers were hired. Public health officials were overwhelmed, with provinces having insufficient staff and relying on federal employees whose primary tactic was imposing a quarantine at ports, a policy aimed at immigrants. The strategy failed since returned soldiers were waved through, thereby imperilling health and leading to much condemnation of the federal response. In Montreal, at the time Canada's largest city, 16,266 cases of flu were reported in October and November, with 2,713 deaths. In a similar time frame, Toronto reported 1,259 deaths, Ottawa 570, and Halifax 153.[20] Given this mass death, all medical services were swamped, and accurate counting of the victims was not top of mind in most municipalities. The tabulation of the virus's impact has, as one scholar noted, "under-represented the extent of mortality."[21]

Back at the front, the flu was afflicting all the armed forces. Even with the war grinding to an end as Germany's allies surrendered—Turkey on October 30 and Austria-Hungary on November 3—the virus spread rapidly from early November onwards. "There are a great many cases of influenza over here," wrote Gunner Clarence McCann on November 7, "and so many deaths that the undertakers are unable to do their work properly."[22] Around the same time, Nursing Sister Mabel Clint was nearly overwhelmed by the flu patients who "almost filled every hut."[23] As nurses and caregivers sought to reduce the soldiers' agony, both overseas and at home, they too succumbed to the virus. Voluntary Aid Detachment worker Jeannette Bridges from Saint John, New Brunswick, penned a letter to her mother on October 30, 1918, from isolation in the "sick hut" of No. 1 Hospital at Reading as she was recovering from the virus. "When I tell you that one third of the staff on night duty & a great many on day duty are down with it," she wrote, "you would probably have been more surprised if I had escaped. . . . The pain in my head legs and back was something desperate. . . . The Influenza epidemic has been dreadful all over England."[24] Bridges survived, but many did not, and it was the medical practitioners, especially nurses and VADs, who bravely went into the wards and houses marked with illness to

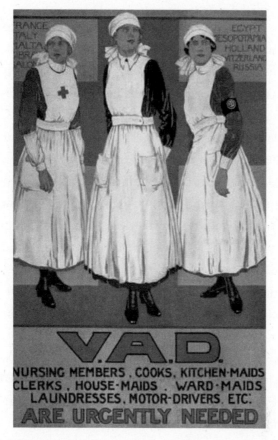

A VAD recruitment poster. Both overseas and in Canada,
VADs and nurses cared for influenza patients.

care for the needy. They often paid for their sense of duty and compassion with their lives.

Within the Canadian forces overseas, 45,960 flu cases were reported, of which 776 ended in death.[25] But in Canada, another 61,063 were in uniform in late 1918. Of these, 11,496 were tracked flu cases, of which 2,208 developed pneumonia and 716 died.[26] These two sets of statistics show a minimum of 1,492

Canadians in uniform listed as having died of the virus or compli-
cations, but that aggregate number must be considered low.
During this period many soldiers who were listed as dying from
pneumonia were also almost certainly victims of the pandemic.
From 1918 to 1920, across the Dominion some 55,000 Canadians
were killed by the virus, most of them in the seven-month period
from September 1918 to March 1919.[27] In the large cities and
rural areas, the flu laid waste to human life, and it was most deadly
in working-class neighbourhoods and especially in Indigenous
communities, where the mortality rate was five times that of the
national average.[28] The virus would eventually kill at least fifty
million people around the world.[29]

Despite the virus's virulence, effective public health measures
reduced the flu's impact in some communities, with theatres,
places of worship, schools, and businesses shuttered for extended
periods. Cloth and cotton masks were issued to many who cared
for the sick, but the rules for wearing them were applied haphaz-
ardly and with little enforcement. Within this heightened period
of uncertainty, charlatans emerged to peddle their fake medicine
to the sick and scared, including enemas and powders, chloroform, and other alcohol-based remedies. After a brief respite at the
beginning of 1919, when the number of deaths dipped, a second
deadly wave of the virus passed through the country. It too claimed
victims, although it was less devastating than the first wave. A new
round of closures was enacted to slow the spread, and even the
Stanley Cup finals in early April 1919, between the Seattle
Metropolitans and the Montreal Canadiens, were cancelled when
many of the players were stricken with the virus. The pandemic
began to burn itself out in the spring, aided by Canada's still being
a rural nation, which ensured much distance between neighbours.

The virus had cut through many communities: mothers and fathers buried children, while children mourned for parents taken before their time. And yet Canadians on the home front soldiered through the flu like they had the war.

The medical response to the pandemic in Canada was episodic, regional, uncoordinated, and often run through local charities, churches, voluntary nursing associations, and the limited number of hospitals. Dr. T.H. Whitelaw, Edmonton's medical officer of health, bemoaned the impotency of physicians in the face of the cataclysm, stating, "Never before has the medical profession been confronted with a more baffling problem presented by the influenza epidemic, both as to its possible prevention or treatment."[30] Though a vaccine was desperately sought, and several were in fact created and administered to a limited number of Canadians, they had no effect since the flu was thought to be a bacteria.[31] Scared and angry Canadians demanded a better public

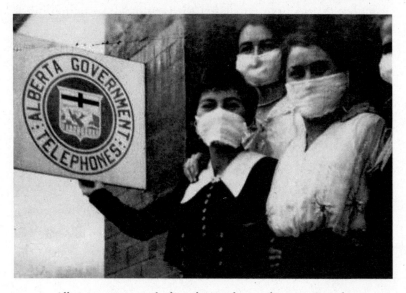

Alberta women masked up during the pandemic in Canada.

health plan, and, as we shall see, the pandemic was crucial in the formation of the Department of Health in 1919, a potent legacy of the war.

In the face of this pestilence, it is perhaps surprising that Canadians came together in huge crowds when word reached them of the armistice of November 11, 1918. Across Canada, celebrations included marching bands, raucous parties, and public burnings of the Kaiser's effigy, with photographic evidence showing very few people wearing masks. The shuddering end to the long crusade for victory trumped quarantine measures. Vincent Massey, a wealthy patron of the arts who would become governor general, was in Ottawa in the last year of the war as associate secretary of the War Committee of the Cabinet. Offering insight into the emotional climate in Canada at the time of the armistice, and the calamitous effects of the virus, he observed, "We would have been more shocked by the number of fatalities had it not been that this scourge came after the long list of casualties in the war years."[32]

———

"The nightmare of four and a half years is gone," wrote Arnold G.A. Vidler of Victoria, B.C., who had enlisted at Valcartier in September 1914, survived a gunshot wound to the head, and been discharged from the CEF by the armistice.[33] The cascading emotions of relief and grief were not easily captured in letters home, but Canadians along the Western Front were almost all surprised by the sudden end of the war on November 11, 1918. The Canadian Corps remained at the spearhead of the First British Army, having captured the ancient Belgian city of Mons on the last day of the war. It was the capstone to Canada's Hundred Days campaign, although the cost had been witheringly high at 45,835 casualties.[34] The four Canadian divisions met and defeated elements of forty-seven German divisions, albeit all of them understrength.[35] General Currie crowed of his Corps, "No force of equal size ever accomplished so much in a similar space of time during the war."[36]

While the armistice ended the firing on the Western Front, the occupation of Germany and the slow demobilization of the million-man armies would take place over a long period. After more than four years in service, Percy Kingsley of the 5th Battalion pondered his fate: "What would I do on return to life as a civilian

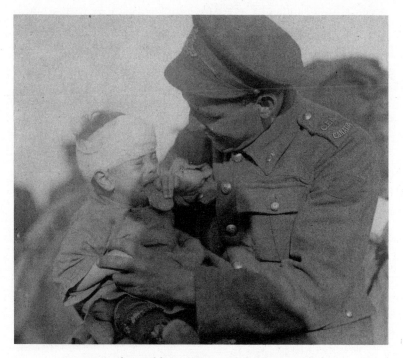

A Canadian soldier in Mons comforts a wounded
Belgian baby whose mother was killed in the fighting.

and why was I spared to see the end? It seemed incredible that I had survived."[37] This uncertainty at the front was shared by many citizen-soldiers, including the tens of thousands of Canadians in the medical system. Sergeant George Biddle of the 31st Battalion, a prewar theology student from Lethbridge, Alberta, who was in a hospital back home recovering from severe gassing when news of the armistice arrived, remembered, "I went into my room and wept when I thought of all the fellows I left behind over there."[38]

It would be months before large groups of Canadians could begin to travel across the Atlantic, with shipping shortages, postwar strikes in England, and iced-up ports in Canada preventing such movement, along with the challenge of documenting hundreds of thousands of Canadians—especially those with wounds and injuries—for future pension claims. However, more leave time was available for soldiers, who explored Britain and reconnected with family members. The YMCA and Salvation Army in

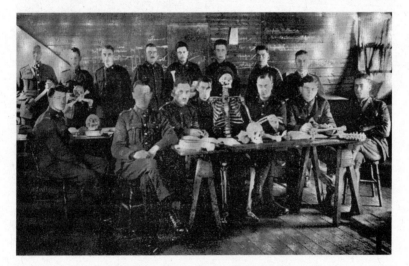

A class of Canadians in the Khaki University
studying osteology alongside a dressed-up skeleton.

Canada had done tremendous work during the war to raise money for the soldiers, and they continued to send sporting equipment and libraries overseas and to fund cinemas behind the lines, in the name of keeping service personnel active and staving off boredom.

These distractions were welcomed, but soldiers also turned to vice, using their stored-up pay to purchase drink and the services of women. Almost immediately after the armistice, medical officers warned that the incidence of venereal disease among Canadians had begun to rise.[39] The high command took note and the chaplains, doctors, and fighting officers were, as stipulated in one order, told to reinvigorate their lectures "on the dangers and evils of Venereal Disease."[40] Some soldiers walked away from the talks and lantern-slide presentations with the belief that if they sought out prostitutes their penises would rot off and they would be on the fast road to an insane asylum, but many were not deterred and medical officers made it clear in reports that they were losing the battle against sexually transmitted diseases.[41]

Stringent measures were put in place to monitor women and prostitutes, although these did not curb the rising venereal disease rates among Canadian soldiers in both December and January.[42] It would get worse, cautioned senior Canadian medical officers, who argued that only the removal of French and Belgian civilian women from their communities would reduce the incidence of sexual infections. The civilian authorities refused, aware that this would rapidly lead to the liberators being viewed as occupiers, and they told the Canadians to control their own soldiers.[43] The stern lectures and threats directed at the enlisted men continued, even as the numbers of sexually infected soldiers rose steadily, with 842 new cases recorded from February to March.[44]

While dealing with this epidemic of sexually transmitted diseases, the CEF also suffered through the second wave of the killer virus in early 1919. Nursing Sister Mabel Clint lamented that so many sick soldiers needed care that the patients had to lie on the floor of her hospital, and added that, in an awful irony, the medical staff "buried men at Mons who had enlisted in 1914 and escaped fatal wounds."[45] The virus spread widely as tens of thousands of Canadians were being pulled back from the Western Front and moved to England for eventual return home. The message in the long demobilization process was always "hurry up and wait," as men were gathered in holding camps for processing and forced to stew in enclosed spaces.[46] In early February, flu outbreaks erupted at Witley and then at Kinmel Park in Wales. These were already dismal camps, with few opportunities for entertainment and sports, inexperienced officers who leaned on discipline, and limited canteens for treats. A month later, frustrated Canadians rioted over the course of two days at Kinmel, ransacking the camp. In the widespread destruction on March 4 and 5, several dozen soldiers were wounded, five were killed, and much damage done.[47] Jack Hudgins, who had received the Distinguished Conduct Medal during the war, wrote after the riots about his shock upon finding that one of his chums was among the killed, a sad end to his service after having survived trench and open warfare along the Western Front. He also remarked in a letter, "Most everyone I know has the flu."[48]

British authorities responded to the riot with outrage and reproached the Canadians for their lawless ways. The senior Dominion command objected to the broad condemnation, but the Imperials, fearful of the mad colonials sowing death and destruction in nearby English or Welsh towns, fast-tracked their return to

Canada. Though the citizen-soldiers were happy to be on their way home, those with a venereal disease were not allowed on the troopships.[49] The condemned soldiers were funnelled into special hospitals where they underwent painful treatment and carried deep grievances as they were robbed of the opportunity to return with their comrades to be celebrated together as the heroes of the overseas war, and were perhaps also fated to face uncomfortable questions upon their delayed return.

The harsh treatment was demanded because venereal disease was considered a threat to the prevailing notions of the family and monogamous love, and was feared for its potential to weaken the next generation of Canadians, contributing to what was known at the time as "race degeneration." The swirling constellation of worry over the high rate of sexual diseases held more sway with the Canadian public than the concern over the plight of blinded soldiers, amputees, mental wounds, or, seemingly, the effects of the virus that was killing thousands. Moral reform groups mobilized and warned that soldiers' diseased bodies would infect the helpless collective of women back home, and that the disease would even be passed to babies, who would be born with mental and physical defects. This, it was argued, was nothing short of the path to moral and physical decline of Canadians.

Medical officers were involved in the battle against both the virus pandemic and the venereal disease epidemic, although they came to understand that little would help in the struggle against the flu other than isolation and basic medical acts of rehydration and pain relief. Furthermore, unlike the advances achieved in treating conventional wounds, not much headway would be made in the losing clash against venereal disease. In the face of the failed policy of threats and pleading, the doctors argued that a reduction

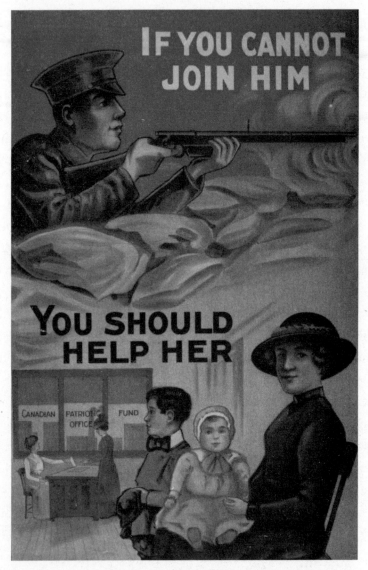

Distance and loneliness affected wartime relationships.
This Canadian Patriotic Fund poster was meant to elicit donations
from Canadians to support soldiers' dependants. It is a reminder, too,
of the challenge that separation for several years posed for families and
the stress that was put on marriages.

in these diseases would best be achieved through prevention rather than treatment, a lesson that medical officers and nurses would take back to Canada. This required open and honest discussion and the use of prophylactics, rather than threats and punishments. At the same time, some medical officers asked why such an effort was being made with the afflicted soldiers when about 10 to 15 percent of the male population in Canada carried venereal diseases and nothing was being done about them. It was Colonel George Adami who provocatively argued, "It is not the civil population that has to fear the soldier, but the soldier the civil population."[50] The soldiers had been surveilled and studied; they had been taught and warned about the danger associated with unprotected sex: the threat, Adami insisted, was from the rest of Canadians, as many had sexually transmitted diseases that ran unchecked and much of the population had a deplorably poor understanding of the issue.

———

It was a country ravaged by the flu that welcomed back the returned soldiers. After years of absence, agonizing reunions took place as daughters, sons, uncles, and fathers returned to a house or a farm only to find that a kid sister, a parent, or even a baby they had never met was now buried because of the virus. What a cruel fate to bear after surviving a devastating war. Economic ruin also stalked the land. Inflation was running wild and munitions jobs disappeared overnight with the war at an end. The misery deepened and rising labour unrest culminated in the Winnipeg General Strike in May 1919, which those in power saw only as a harbinger of the destabilizing effects of Bolshevism that had reordered Russia and that would usher in communism there. Canada roiled with unrest.

Upon hearing of the armistice, Gunner Bob Gillespie of the 23rd Battery, Canadian Field Artillery, responded with much feeling and no little eloquence, writing, "Now our great task is done. With what price we do not yet realize. Of our bravest, many now sleep on European soil; many more will bear henceforth on their persons the mark of war; still more will remember the war as a donor of weakened health and constitution. But we all—maimed, weakened, and untouched alike, united in a common sorrow as well as a common pride in those who sacrificed their all—but not in vain."[51] The Canadian liberators returned home to a new country, one that had passed through the trial of war and was stumbling forward into an uncertain future. On the medical front, learned battlefield lessons would be applied to aid a recovering society, bolstered by the prevalent feeling that medicine had been crucial in supporting the military crusade against Germany and that now it must be redeployed in a public health campaign to save Canadians.

CHAPTER 18

LESSONS AND LEGACIES

J ust as no battlefield victories would be won without a cost in
blood, no medical victories would be earned without a terrible
price in lives. And yet victory had been achieved, in the field and
on the operating table, and especially in preventative medicine,
surgical advances, and the art of healing and rehabilitation. The
seemingly forever war finally came to an end and Canadian medical staff returned to their communities throughout 1919. About
two dozen Canadian medical units—mostly hospitals, convalescent homes, and administrative sections—remained open in
England through the summer of 1919, which was frustrating for
the wounded who were recovering there and for the nurses and
physicians who were eager to be reunited with loved ones.

Despite these delays, most of the 15,580 doctors, nurses, surgeons, X-ray specialists, physiotherapists, and other medical caregivers who were overseas at the time of the armistice returned to
Canada with new knowledge and refined medical techniques that
had been learned on or near the killing fields.[1] They were desperate to return home even though the demobilization of the CAMC

in 1919 destroyed the best and most effective medical system ever created up to that point in Canadian history. Collectively, Canada's overseas medical units dealt with 539,690 patients admitted both during and immediately after the war. Of that total, 144,606 were battle casualties and 395,084 were those resulting from disease or serious illness.[2] These statistics come from the 1925 Canadian medical official history and have been slightly adjusted over the past 100 years as new information has come to light, but along with others they reveal that over 90 percent of the wounded who arrived at a medical unit survived because of the lifesavers' interventions.

All medical personnel at the front had saved countless lives and contributed to the victory by ensuring that the fighting forces were not ravaged by disease. Dr. G.A. Anderson, the president of the Alberta Medical Association, observed during a September 1919 Calgary address to welcome back the overseas medical veterans that they had engaged in "the prevention of disease and the alleviation of suffering," while "establishing new traditions and setting up for the profession a standard of unselfish devotion to the service of humanity such as will be difficult to emulate, but I trust, in civil life, we will make it our ambition to attain."[3] In short, the war had led to a monumental advancement of medical expertise in Canada, and it was felt by many physicians and members of the public that the devotion to soldiers overseas must now be turned towards Canadians across the Dominion. Colonel Alexander Primross, a wartime surgeon whose son was killed in action, noted in his 1919 presidential address to the Academy of Medicine in Toronto that "the men who have had the good fortune to have seen service at the Front have been profoundly influenced by their experiences."[4] Not all medical veterans would see it as good fortune, given the traumatizing sights they had witnessed, the agony of triage, the rush of patients, and the lack of time to devote to all of them, not to mention the fear of their own death or maiming in the war zone, but all of them learned through providing care and adapting treatment under such difficult circumstances. "We may assert the fact, universally recognized, that the experience of this war has had revolutionary effects upon the practice of medicine and surgery," said Primross, noting further that this experience would "produce a profound effect upon the theories and practices of our profession."[5]

———

The large-scale demobilization of hundreds of thousands of citizen soldiers over the spring and summer of 1919 led to the rapid disbandment of the Canadian Expeditionary Force and to a rush of veterans returning to their homes flush with payments from the state for their service. They found their communities changed, ravaged by the pandemic and depleted of available jobs. Some veterans settled on land in the West, taking advantage of public programs directed towards them, though they found that the government had secured vast tracts of low-quality fields, sometimes by appropriating land from Indigenous reserves. Many struggled with the return to normalcy, often being unable to talk to their loved ones about their war experiences and finding it easier to simply bury their memories deep.

Though almost all of the professors of medicine and senior surgeons were welcomed back to their universities or civilian hospitals, the path forward was less clear for younger doctors who tried to restart their private practices that had been shuttered when

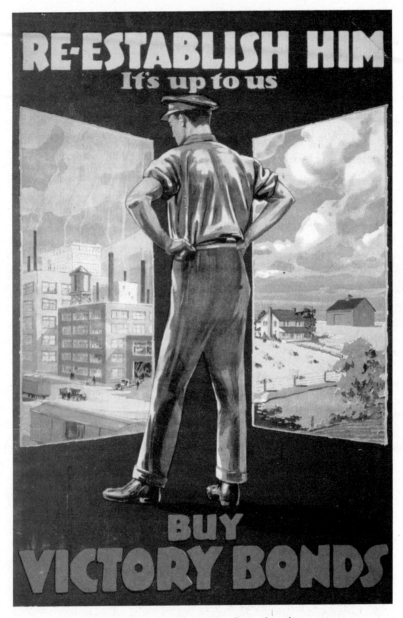

A wartime poster reminding Canadians that there was an ongoing obligation to help re-establish Canadian veterans.

they left to serve King and country. Some veterans of the medical services found that the civilian doctors who had stayed at home were not happy to share their expanded practices.[6] Many citizens in cities, towns, and villages would eventually return to the doctors who had served in uniform, but it would be a process that required patience and imposed no little financial hardship.

Those faced with the greatest challenge in carving out a practice upon their demobilization were young doctors, especially those who had hurried through their university years to enlist. Frederick Banting of Alliston, Ontario, was one of them. He had graduated from the University of Toronto in 1916, and then enlisted in the CEF, serving as a medical officer in England and at the front. A war hero who received the Military Cross for his bravery and devotion to wounded soldiers during the Battle of Arras in September 1918, he returned to Ontario quite unsure of what to do. Banting had enjoyed the comradery overseas and the rough life of soldiering, but he left these behind when he set up a practice in London, Ontario, in 1920. Patients were slow to arrive and he spent some of his free time thinking about better ways to treat the sick, especially those with the death sentence of diabetes. Rolling the dice in the summer of 1921, he left his practice and travelled to Toronto, where he pitched an idea about a possible cure for diabetes. He was given access to a graduate assistant, Charles Best, and a tiny laboratory, where the two men discovered insulin over the late summer. Their breakthrough came by blocking the pancreatic ducts in dogs so that they continued to produce insulin that would be extracted and then injected into sick patients to reduce their blood sugar. This insulin extract was refined through additional experimentation involving several researchers, and late in 1921, Banting began treatments on hopeless patients, including veterans, which proved remarkably successful.[7] Insulin was soon recognized as a miracle drug that would save tens of millions of lives over the century, and Banting was awarded the 1923 Nobel Prize in Physiology or Medicine, along with another scientist, J.J.R. Macleod. Though no other doctors returned to embark on such epic scientific discoveries, most took home the hard-earned lessons of the war to improve, prolong, and save Canadian lives.

———

In October 1914, the director-general of the Royal Army Medical Corps, Sir Alfred Keogh, had described the nightmare of infected war wounds at the start of the war, stating, "We have with this war gone straight back into all the septic infections of the Middle Ages."[8] And yet in this time before antibiotics, extraordinary success was achieved through innovation, especially in combatting infection through surgical work and irrigation of wounds. Reflecting on his service overseas, George Armstrong, an elderly professor of surgery at McGill and surgeon-in-chief at the Royal Victoria Hospital, noted that a doctor could acquire more knowledge about the body, disease, and treatment in a week of frenzied work on the Western Front than in a lifetime of civilian practice—even though "war surgery at the front is often carried on under distracting and terrorizing conditions."[9] The medical professionals in uniform learned to bring even the most badly wounded patients back from death, as operations were conducted closer to the front, the slain were mined for secrets to saving others, and new treatments to the body reduced mortality rates. In the words of John William

Hutchinson, a CAMC wartime surgeon who specialized in chest wounds, "The present war, by its magnitude and the diversity of its fighting machines, has afforded surgeons numerous opportunities of advancing their science along many lines, and of solving many problems in the diagnosis and the treatment of injuries of various parts of the body."[10]

John Alexander Gunn, who had commanded a field ambulance in the war and returned to Winnipeg to practise surgery, observed that blood transfusion was one of the critical wartime innovations, noting, "The vast scope for its application presented by the war has at least given an added impetus to the scientific study of its effect, and has proven beyond a doubt, in a practical way, that it is a life saving procedure of the greatest value."[11] Canada's most advanced practitioner in the field was Lawrence Bruce Robertson, who went by Bruce and who had served as a CAMC captain during the war, saving lives on the battlefield. After the war, Robertson continued to hone the application of transfusions in his treatment of burned children and cancer victims at Toronto's Hospital for Sick Children.[12] Many were saved. But in 1923 Robertson died at age thirty-seven of pneumonia, his lungs weakened by repeated cases of influenza and the strain of his wartime service. His early death truncated the impact of his revolutionary work on the Western Front, and it would be decades before the scientific world had a better understanding of the pioneering role played by the Toronto doctor.[13]

Aiding the surgeons were the new specialists in radiology. Captain Alexander Howard Pirie of McGill's No. 3 Canadian General Hospital took thousands of images of patients to determine the location of metal and fragments in bodies. Imaging the wounds of war proved the value of the X-ray in assisting surgeons, and Pirie shared his battlefield research, findings, and success with fellow doctors in lectures and publications.[14] Radiology would be used in Canada to assess many injuries and diseases, and especially in the fight against tuberculosis—the greatest killer of Canadians aged 15 to 45—a battle that was advanced by the wartime care of soldiers.[15]

The "fragments from France," as some disabled veterans sometimes darkly described themselves, required ongoing treatment and therapy. Medical services had saved many of the grievously wounded who would have died in past wars. Living with horrendous injuries, these survivors now faced an uncertain future, even as the state had a duty to care for them. This obligation was also new in the arena of medical treatment, an extension of the social contract between the state and the soldier and a powerful legacy of the war. Prosthetic limb factories were established across Canada to supply wooden or metal arms, feet, legs, and hands, and glass eyes, although this work fell to the civilian medical state agencies that emerged during the war.[16] Badly injured veterans faced a long journey to recovery or had to learn to live with their changed bodies, and some of the wartime doctors and nurses would aid them in newly created veterans' hospitals and facilities. Even with the state-of-the-art care, veterans had their lives cut short by the ghastly wounds, and the Canadian Legion, the largest group of organized veterans, estimated that 40,000 Canadian veterans died of wartime wounds in the decade following the armistice.[17] This was one of the hidden costs of the war, with some two thirds the number of the war's dead succumbing in the decade after the armistice from physical injuries, invisible wounds, suicide, and debilitating health conditions.

"The calamity of war has been necessary to startle the profession into a realization of the wide field that should be occupied

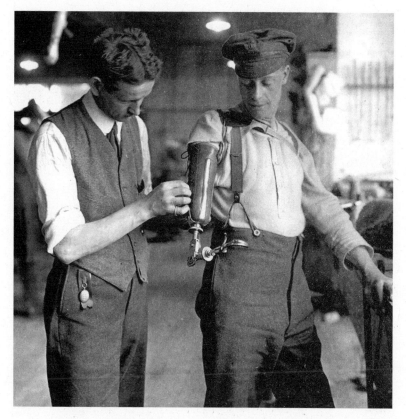

A Canadian soldier being fitted with a prosthetic arm.

by physical methods in the treatment of disease," wrote Canadian Robert Tait McKenzie, a celebrated sculptor and leader in the field of physical therapy. His skill had been honed overseas in the repair of soldiers, where he had witnessed how "torn and mangled bodies have to be patched and remade."[18] McKenzie was among the growing leaders in the field of physiotherapy. While the many wartime agencies in Canada that cared for veterans were slow to respond to the value of physiotherapy, undeniably successful results were recorded overseas as therapists worked with soldiers' scarred and broken bodies. As this cutting-edge therapy was taking shape in CAMC hospitals in Britain, in the spring of 1918 the Military School of Orthopaedic Surgery and Physiotherapy at Hart House at the University of Toronto began to train therapists and employ them in hospitals across Canada. One of them, Enid Finley, a twenty-four-year-old massage therapist, worked in the Dominion Orthopaedic Hospital for veterans on Christie Street in Toronto.[19] After treating veterans, she would become a leader in the field and advance the study of physiotherapy.

"Men who despaired of ever being happy or useful again, because of the horror of disfigurements" managed, in the words of one Canadian hospital wartime report, to find "healing and hope and courage, and the desire to live."[20] Facial reconstruction and skin burns were among the most complex of surgical reconstruction, with Harold Gillies and specialists like him furthering the art of remaking flesh and bone.[21] In Canada, at least 170 veterans had been transferred during or after the war to undergo facial reconstructive surgery in the state hospital system, which had started overseas and would continue in Canada for years to come.[22] "During the war there has been an opportunity such as never would occur in time of peace, for the study and development of plastic surgery," observed one doctor in the *Canadian Medical Association Journal*.[23] Some of these veterans returned to normal lives, while others rarely left hospitals or only worked in isolation and at night.

The advances in medical treatment during the war extended to haunted minds. Two Canadian doctors who dealt with the psychologically ravaged soldiers felt in 1919 that shell shock had become "the storm centre of military medicine."[24] Mental wartime injuries had a profound impact on psychiatry and they further legitimized this aspect of the medical profession. In 1923,

and the soldiers who refused, for the most part, to curb their behaviour. Much floundering between honest teaching and inexcusable shaming took place through a rolling barrage of lectures, sermons, pamphlets, films, and punishments. The war provoked some champions in the field, like Colonel George Adami, to demand that the profession address this crisis through the lens of treatment and not morals, leaving humiliation and outrage aside. Adami also publicly advocated for soldiers who had contracted debilitating venereal disease to receive a pension like other wounded soldiers, noting that a man's service had to be taken into account not only in acknowledging the source of exposure to the disease but also in recognizing how the strain of the war could lead to symptoms manifesting more rapidly. "It is unjust and immoral to deny that man a pension," Adami argued to authorities.[29] His voice held sway in many fields, but sadly not in this one, and sexually infected veterans faced stigma in the allocation of pensions, along with those suffering from shell shock and from chemical wounds that were difficult to attribute.[30] More often than not, these veterans were denied pensions or given a much-reduced rate that was impossible to survive on. The CAMC doctors—themselves veterans—returned to Canada, where they turned with vigour to addressing social diseases and the fight against the "secret plague."[31]

The medical services had triumphed in preserving the health of the soldiers within exceptionally trying conditions. The control of sanitation along the vast Western Front and in the rear areas was much lauded for having reduced the losses of soldiers to disease. A prewar 1911 Royal Army Medical Corps training manual had estimated that in a future war sick soldiers would outnumber the wounded by a factor of 25 to 1.[32] On the Western Front, the

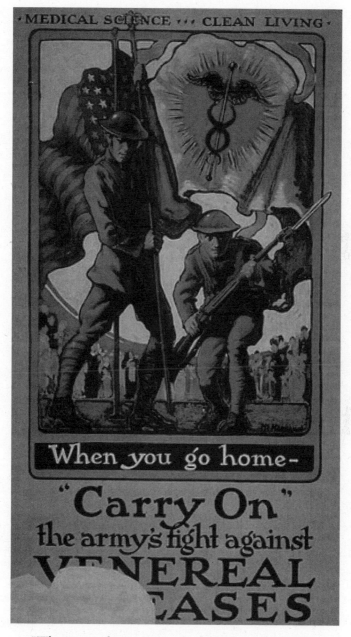

"When you go home—'Carry On' the army's fight against
Venereal Disease," reads this American poster.

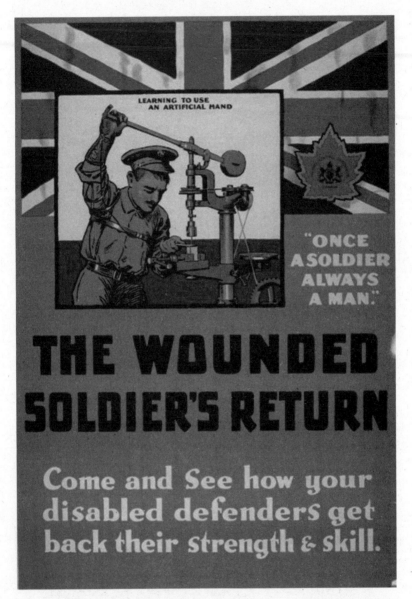

A poster encouraging the Canadian public to see wounded veterans as contributing members of society. "Once a soldier always a man," reads one message, shedding some light on issues of masculinity and disability.

figure was around 2.7 to 1, with a ratio of 1 disease death to every 10.4 from battle.[33] Vaccination, water purity, and the monitoring of early disease outbreaks protected the army from withering away in the cesspool of the trenches, although those figures also reveal the ferocity of modern weapons of war and their ability to kill in shocking numbers. As Canadian soldier Fred Bagnall of the 14th Battalion wrote in his memoir, "Thanks to the wonderful sanitary precautions and the use of serums, science overcame many of the diseases usual in war." He added ruefully, however, "We were maintained by science to be killed by shells."[34]

The sanitation victory overseas had been overshadowed by the catastrophic losses from the influenza pandemic, which had laid bare the failure of doctors to prevent mass death by a virus they did not understand. "Not within a century has medical science received a more staggering body blow than was inflicted by this elusive but fatal scourge," said Dr. G.A. Anderson in September 1919.[35] The high number of virus victims, added to the shuddering casualties of the war and the revelation of rampant venereal disease, led many to call for a renewed public health battle in 1919. "If the flu could not be defeated by medicine," said Anderson, "then the focus should be on preventative medicine." The same conclusion had been reached in combatting venereal disease. In the early 1920s another doctor suggested to his colleagues, "If it was possible among the millions of soldiers to reduce infectious disease to a vanishing point, should not a similar precaution be taken in civil life?"[36] The war led to a valorization of the medical profession, and now doctors talked of using their influence and skills to assist all Canadians. If before the war greater focus had been directed towards new ways of treating disease, the war showed that pre-emptive work in public health could win the battle without having to fight it. "Our soldiers have shown Canadians how to die," claimed the City of Ottawa's annual report on public health for 1918. "It is up to the health authorities to show the people how to live."[37]

In 1923, at the annual meeting of the Manitoba Medical Association, Dr. T. Glen Hamilton explained to his colleagues how the forced inoculation of soldiers had saved lives during the war. Now, he argued, "The public must be educated."[38] Another noted Canadian physician believed that vaccination of soldiers had proven so successful that it was "almost inconceivable that during the first year of the war, a determined effort was made by fanatical and ignorant civilians in Great Britain, chiefly members of anti-vaccination societies."[39] While some in Canada remained opposed to vaccination, a wartime editorial in the *CMAJ* observed that the person who opposed mass inoculation was a "misguided crea-ture" and "that the saner half of the public is losing patience."[40] The success of vaccines in protecting soldiers had proven the anti-vaccine advocates wrong, the medical profession declared, and "the precious liberty of the individual may justly be sacrificed to the manifest good of the state and, incidentally, to the individual's own good."[41] Battles over the efficacy of vaccination would continue, but the Great War proved an identifiable tipping point in the protection of soldiers and an undeniable moment of victory against disease and ignorance.

Also contributing to evangelical-style postwar public health debates were the wartime medical inspections that had exposed the shockingly poor health of tens of thousands of young recruits who had been turned away from enlistment because of tubercular lungs or malnourished bodies. This revelation during the war against Germany also stimulated the need to focus on Canadians' health generally. Some drew lessons that sent them down the darker path of eugenics, whereby pseudo-scientific theories, shaped by racial and cultural beliefs, sought to ferret out defects in intelligence, social hygiene, and morality. These dogmatic adherents to a false science classified people into superior and inferior groups, and addressed the public health issue through selective breeding, including sterilization of some of those deemed unfit in order to prevent "race degeneration."[42] A more positive legacy of wartime public health was a renewed focus on the care of mothers and babies, and a desire to raise their standard of living and well-being to ensure that the new generation would be hardier and more robust than the last.[43] "Our profession should do all in its power through properly organized clinics, supervised instruction and ethical propaganda to secure healthful prenatal conditions for the mothers of our land," believed Dr. G. Stewart Cameron, who linked his call to action to the evidence of wartime medical inspections that revealed tens of thousands of young men who had suffered through unhealthy upbringings and were unfit for service in a time of great need.[44] War imagery and language was often employed in this campaign to improve maternal care. Health-care professionals talked about "arming" mothers with education, training, and resources as they were the "first line of defence" for the helpless "infant soldier."[45]

These public health crusaders were aided by the creation in 1919 of the federal Department of Health, one of the significant legacies of care to emerge from the war.[46] "It has required a great war to arouse the people to a sense of the primary national need, the saving of its manpower," wrote Dr. Peter Henderson Bryce, chief medical officer of the federal Department of Immigration in

1920 and a leader in public health.[47] Having served in Canada during the war, while so many doctors were overseas, Bryce had also watched impotently as the state ignored his repeated warnings that the health of Indigenous children in residential schools was being neglected, leading to abnormally high death rates from disease. This "national crime," as Bryce called it in a report, was buried, and young Indigenous children continued to die in shocking numbers.[48] While the health of residential schools is beyond the scope of this book, Bryce had more success in instigating public health measures across Canada. "There is nothing like a war to discover the steps that should be taken for the protection of public health," mused the influential Senator James Lougheed, who also witnessed the enormous transformation wrought by the Great War.[49] The civil servants of public health would go forward into the 1920s with some success, but the department was not well funded and its officials were frequently caught between federal and provincial jurisdictional skirmishes.[50] The bane of disease, and the poverty that often exacerbated it, was not erased by the war or defeated by the doctors trained within it, although monumental medical advances were achieved in the war's aftermath.

———

While *Lifesavers and Body Snatchers* has examined the medical war, providing new ways to see the conflict and the care, its focus has been on the people: the soldiers in battle and the medical practitioners who battled to save them. And so it is fitting to end this chapter on the complex legacy of wartime care and its enduring impact with an exploration of five Canadians as a handful of representatives from the 620,000 who served in the Canadian Expeditionary Force.

Tens of thousands of Canadians suffered life-altering wartime wounds, and they returned to a complicated system of assigning pensions to wounded men that was based on the severity of their injuries and on whether those injuries could be firmly attributed to the war experience. The civilian agency responsible for veterans, the Department of Soldiers' Civil Re-establishment, assessed the scarred bodies of soldiers, and those with visible wounds—a missing hand or eye—usually received a generous pension (at least in comparison to British or German veterans). Attesting to the care of the CAMC in saving men who would have died in earlier wars, some 77,000 were collecting pensions by the early 1930s.[51] Among the worst of the wounded were the 2,780 Canadians who survived an amputation during the war.[52] While many more succumbed to the trauma or infection, these limbless warriors had refused to go under. The only surviving quadruple amputee was Ethelbert "Curley" Christianson, a Black American-born Canadian resident who enlisted at age thirty-three in Selkirk, Manitoba. At Vimy, he was working in logistical support when he was caught in an enemy shell bombardment. He lay unconscious for two days in the mud and his wounds were already infected when he was discovered. Not expected to live, he somehow survived multiple operations and the amputation of both hands and lower legs. The indomitable Christianson returned to Toronto in September 1917 and was fitted with prosthetics. During his recovery and rehabilitation at Euclid Hall on Jarvis Street, he fell in love with Cleopatra McPherson, a volunteer aide worker who had emigrated from Jamaica. They married and had a son, and Christianson became

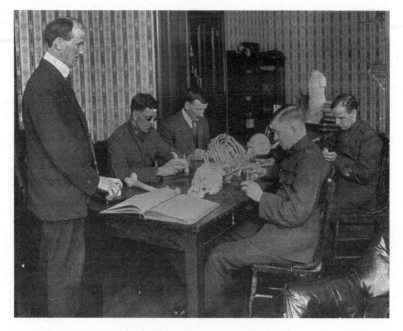

Blind soldiers learning to work on
human bones as part of a training course.

a prominent member of the Canadian Legion, remaining so until his death at age seventy in 1954.

With tens of thousands of Canadians having passed through hospital units with battlefield wounds, many of the survivors carried scars on their bodies from the steel and fire that lashed, severed, and gouged. Others had less visible wounds. The mental strain of the war, as revealed through shell shock, caused thousands of concealed injuries. Often the soldiers would be returned to the front after medical care, but many never fully recovered from the ordeal. One of those sufferers was Lieutenant-Colonel Samuel Sharpe, a prewar lawyer and militia officer from Uxbridge, Ontario, who raised the 116th Battalion and led it through the cauldron of battle at Vimy, Lens, Hill 70, and Passchendaele.

Undeniably brave, he was traumatized by seeing so many of his soldiers killed, and in December 1917 the lieutenant-colonel suffered a mental breakdown and was hospitalized for several months in England. It was during this period that he was awarded the Distinguished Service Order for his leadership at the front.[53] Major George F. Boyer, a CAMC doctor, described Sharpe and other patients like him who broke under the strain, observing, "He is driven by duty. The will is willing and impels, but the frame fails."[54] In early May 1918, Sharpe returned to Canada, although he could not escape the Western Front's long reach. He committed suicide that same month by throwing himself from the window of a second-floor room in a hospital where he had been receiving treatment. A casualty of the war, he was given a public funeral that attracted thousands, but many other veterans suffered with their wounds after the war in silence, often alone.

"To have come through this war alive will be to a great many like recovering from a terrible illness," wrote Nursing Sister Helen Fowlds in the aftermath of victory and having lost a brother to the maw of war.[55] Any doctor or nurse who had been at the front to witness the wreckage of combat, the shattered bodies, and the struggle to save men from infections, or those involved in trying to ease the pain, restore mobility, and allow the disabled a return to normalcy could never forget their experiences. Even though close to 3,000 nurses served on surgical teams, took over the anaesthetizing of patients, and engaged in important ward and rehabilitation work, they were not always rewarded in postwar Canada. With too few jobs available in the medical system, some of these war veterans left the profession, while others were hired in the United States. Those who remained in the nursing service continued to aid Canadians, raised the profile of nurses in the care system, and often became leaders in the field, having been propelled forward by their war experience.

War hero Francis Scrimger, VC, returned home to Montreal. He had lost a finger to infection during the war, and he was aware of the absence of so many McGill students and faculty when he joined the university as a lecturer in clinical surgery. He continued to practise and teach medicine for another two decades—acknowledged as a brilliant surgeon but a deadly boring lecturer—eventually rising to become chair of surgery at McGill and chief surgeon of the Royal Victoria Hospital.[56] Dr. Scrim, as his students called him, never flaunted his Victoria Cross, dying in 1937 after a fulfilling career. He did not have to live through the Second World War, in which his son, Captain Alexander Canon Scrimger, served and died in the Netherlands as he fought to liberate the Dutch. In 1986, a plaque bearing Scrimger's Victoria Cross citation was unveiled at the National Defence Medical Centre in Ottawa. He serves as a tangible reminder that heroism comes in many forms, and perhaps Scrimger best represents Canada's civilian-soldiers, ordinary men and women called to draw deep upon their courage, expertise, and care in the battle to save lives.

One of the many physicians who did not return from overseas was John McCrae. He had saved countless lives before the war and during the conflict, even as he suffered from a lingering gas wound, an invisible mental injury, and deteriorating health from overwork that left him susceptible to meningitis and pneumonia, which ended his life on January 28, 1918. How many more lives might McCrae have saved if he had survived the war and returned to Montreal to continue his healing work over the coming decades? While the war left an undeniable legacy of care and advancement, we will never be able to judge the unfulfilled advances and accomplishments of those caregivers whose lives ended in the war zone. That, too, is a dark legacy of the war. One admirer of McCrae, Captain Norman Guiou, recounted how the charismatic doctor, an expert on typhoid, had lectured to his field ambulance about the power of vaccination a few weeks before his death. McCrae testified to the importance of inoculations in saving lives, with the famous doctor concluding his address by stating to his fellow medical officers, "If I can go home to Canada and persuade the government to inoculate every man, woman and child against typhoid fever, I would consider my life well spent."[57] He never returned home, but others took up that battle.

McCrae was always a doctor first, even as he lives on in the Canadian consciousness mainly because of his poem. "In Flanders Fields" has become an icon of remembrance. Many of the nurses and doctors who had served and sacrificed had memorized the poem and were proud of its resonance across the English-speaking world. For them, the war would not be forgotten; and for many, the torch that was passed to them was not only about the need to remember but about the legacy of medical advances that emerged from the war, a guide handed by fallen medical personnel like McCrae to the living to light the way in saving lives in postwar Canada.

———

"Out of the welter of this terrible war, with all its misery and suffering, will emerge as some small measure of compensation a fuller knowledge of the prevention of disease, the treatment and cure of sickness and wounds and general surgical conditions, which knowledge will be used by the medical profession to the great benefit of living humanity and generations yet unborn," wrote one Canadian physician.[58] The Great War battlefields were a test of nations, an industrial charnel house, a place of tremendous suffering and heroics; they were also an uncontrolled, unstable, and charged laboratory of medical treatment. While mistakes were made at the front, with soldier-patients dying from experimental care or being left to expire because of the mass of wounded, many other lives were saved that would have been lost without medical intervention in the dismal sepulchre of the many fighting fronts. Doctors and nurses enlisted in the CEF, bringing their skills and expertise from civilian life, but the trials of war demanded constant change and evolution. Their mettle was tested and they were not found wanting. In fact, the period from 1914 and 1918, as well as the next world war's span, from 1939 to 1945, was the only time in Canadian history when a massive change to civilian care across multiple medical disciplines was driven by practitioners in military uniform. There was, in fact, no divide between military and civilian medicine, since almost all of the physicians and nurses in uniform were drawn from civilian society, and would return to it. However, these wartime lessons and legacies have never been fully acknowledged in the historical medical literature, even though irrefutable evidence of this progress can be seen in the widespread changes to care and its codification in scientific literature, technology, and practice for decades to follow. Not a single doctor or nurse would endorse war as a positive means to advance their profession; but not a single one could have avoided the conclusion that this brutal classroom taught them important lessons that forged a legacy of care for future generations of Canadians.

CHAPTER 19

MEMORIALIZING THE MEDICAL WAR

S helling and sniper fire, mortar bombs, chemical agents, and all the other weapons of war, together with accidents, disease, and infection, claimed over 68,411 Canadian and Newfoundland soldiers during and immediately after the war. Whirling metal or unseen bacteria did not discriminate between combatants and non-combatants. Lawrence Rogers was one medical man who spent much of the war caring for the wounded and sick. He had left behind his wife and two children in Quebec to enlist at the ancient age of thirty-seven. As he hugged his family goodbye, his daughter Aileen gave him a little teddy bear to keep him safe and to remind him of home. Rogers was a good soldier—smart, effective, and a leader in the ranks. Soon he was the senior medical orderly attached to the regimental medical officer of the 5th Canadian Mounted Rifles. He wrote of the wounded as they hobbled in to the regimental aid post, "helping each other, one propping the other up," and noted, "We don't allow ourselves to look on the blue side of things or the hardships [,] if we did we would all go to pieces."[1] At Mount Sorrel and on the Somme in 1916, he had seen men broken by shell shock and cut down by enemy fire, and he was awarded the Military Medal for his gallantry in treating his fellow comrades. Commissioned the next year, he served at Passchendaele in a forward medical unit on October 30, 1917. As he struggled to save the mangled soldiers who writhed in the blood-saturated mud, a shell burst above him, sending shrapnel balls and shell fragments tearing into his body. Lieutenant Rogers died while caring for others. His personal possessions, including his wedding ring, letters, and the teddy bear, were sent back to his family, and his body was buried, although it was later lost as shellfire destroyed the grave.[2] His name was inscribed on the Menin Gate at Ypres, forever enshrined in that massive memorial

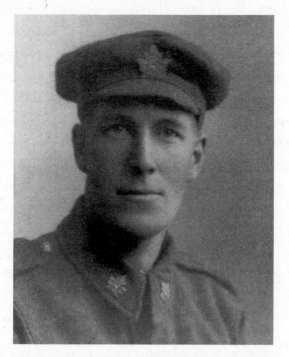

Lawrence Rogers was one of tens of thousands of Canadians and Newfoundlanders who never came home to their loved ones.

to the Empire's dead with no known graves on Belgian soil. The teddy bear—a smaller and more intimate memorial—was cherished by his family for decades, handed through the generations as an object representing a husband, father, and later grandfather who marched away, never to return. It is now on display at the Canadian War Museum as a poignant reminder of the cost of war. Every single one of the war's deaths was a man or woman taken from their loved ones, extended families, and communities, with their absence hollowing out the nation.

About two thirds of Canada's wartime dead lie buried in the Commonwealth War Graves Commission cemeteries that were erected after the war as the last resting place of hundreds of thousands of British, dominion, and other Empire soldiers. A wartime report by Field Marshal Sir Douglas Haig had noted that a proper grave for soldiers "has a symbolical value to the men that it would be difficult to exaggerate."[3] Some of these sites had previously been occupied by medical units and hospitals that were forced to create cemeteries for those who could not be saved. From the early 1920s, Canadian headstones were marked with a maple leaf and the name of the soldier, where known, but some 6,846 unidentified soldiers were interred in graves with headstones that read *"A Canadian Soldier of the Great War—Known Unto God."* Almost 7,000 Canadians are marked on the Menin Gate, while the Vimy Memorial is inscribed with the names of 11,285 Canadians who were killed without graves in France. Members of the Canadian Army Medical Corps have their names inscribed on both memorials, while the nurses and other medical practitioners who were killed in the *Llandovery Castle* attack are commemorated on the Halifax Memorial, which marks those who were lost at sea in wartime.[4] These commemorative sites make real the desire on the part of loved ones and survivors to ensure that the names of the fallen were forever memorialized, even as the bodies were consumed in fire, mud, and water.

At least 9.4 million soldiers were killed during the war, and another 21 million injured.[5] The figures for wounded must be treated with caution since they include soldiers with multiple wounds who were counted each time they passed through a hospital.[6] For instance, decorated German officer Ernst Junger was wounded at least fourteen times, and suffered from other less significant injuries, although it is unclear if all wounds were officially recorded. In other cases, certain minor wounds were not tracked, as was often the case in the German army. At all times, record-keeping was not a priority for the vanquished. What can be said with certainty is that the wounds from modern weapons in industrial warfare maimed and killed with frightening violence.

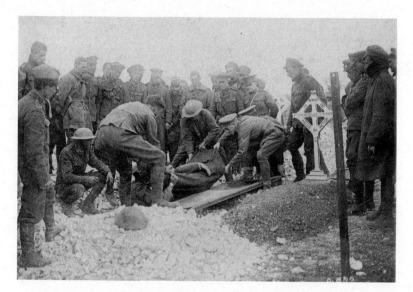

Canadians buried on the Western Front. After the war,
most bodies were reinterred in war cemeteries that remain to this day.

By the summer of 1919, most Canadians in uniform had returned home, where they continued to die from their wounds, from infection, from accidents, and from the flu virus. While the official Canadian cut-off date to mark Canada's total war dead was April 30, 1922, veterans still died afterwards from their wounds or from permanently damaged health. This date appears to have been arbitrarily chosen, but it acknowledges that the war continued to claim thousands of Canadians and Newfoundlanders into the 1920s and beyond. I have calculated that 3,792 Canadian soldiers and veterans died between 1919 and the end of 1921.[10] This is not a surprising figure if one considers the 172,950 instances where CEF soldiers and nurses were wounded (along with another 1,130 airmen), of which 138,166 were classified as battlefield casualties (with this figure slightly reduced from Macphail's calculation in 1925 of 144,606). The remaining thousands of wounded were attributed to injuries and accidents not occurring in battle but not including illness and disease.[11] About half of the wounds were severe, and tens of thousands of veterans lived with life-debilitating injuries.[12] The Imperial War Graves Commission's cut-off date for compiling the numbers of war dead was different from that of the Canadian state, which was set at August 31, 1921, but Canada's Book of Remembrance, as noted above, includes those who died up to April 30, 1922. Canada's book lists 66,755, while Newfoundland's book has 1,656 names, and both sacred memorial documents have occasionally been updated when new information is revealed through research. This jumble of numbers has often been shorn of its nuances, and in the twenty-first century the Canadian state usually presents the figure of 66,000 killed during the war, which doesn't align with any of the figures above. This number represents about one in nine of the total who enlisted and about one in six and a half of the roughly 425,000 who served overseas. The final figure of 68,411 includes Canadian deaths after the war, as well as Newfoundland's losses. This total gets us closer to a fuller understanding of the lethal cost of the war to Canadians and Newfoundlanders.

These were catastrophic losses for Canada and Newfoundland no matter how the statistics are tallied or presented. However, the deaths would have been significantly higher had it not been for the men and women of the CAMC. Tens of thousands of service personnel were saved by surgery and medical interventions, and even more avoided hospital treatment because of the medical service's preventative program in combatting disease. Of the 539,690 admissions of the sick and wounded to medical units, 21,455 died in care—a rate of slightly less than 4 percent.[13]

The CAMC also suffered losses as a result of enemy action and disease. Of over 20,000 medical officers, nurses, and other ranks who wore the CAMC badge, 30 medical officers were killed in battle or died of wounds, 31 more died of disease, and 99 were wounded. At least 61 nurses were killed or died of wounds.[14] In the other ranks of the CAMC, 453 were killed or died of wounds, 79 died of disease, and 589 were wounded.[15] The ratio of killed to wounded in other ranks was extremely high, testifying to the dangerousness of the stretcher-bearer's work on the Western Front, crucial labour that involved exposing oneself to enemy fire to care for and carry the wounded out of the kill zone.[16] Speaking shortly after the war about the service of doctors, nurses, and enlisted men, Lieutenant-Colonel John W.S. McCullough eulogized his comrades in the CAMC, promising "to keep their memories enshrined forever in our hearts, and to remember the valour and glory of their deeds rather than the tragedy of our loss," and declaring, "It is for us to keep the faith for which they yielded their lives."[17] These words were not unlike the sentiments expressed by politicians and pastors across the country, or intoned by parents and other loved ones. And yet how indeed would this memory of service and loss be enshrined?

———

With tens of thousands of loved ones buried overseas, a shroud of grief was cast over the country. Nearly every city and town had lost men to the maw of war. Adding to this carnage from battle, the flu pandemic burned through Canada from September 1918 to March 1919, with additional flareups in late 1919 and, in some parts of the country, into 1920, ultimately killing 55,000 people.[18] In the war's aftermath, however, the focus was on the war dead and not on those killed by the virus. While the pandemic's scythe cut across the country, wiping out thousands in a short period, Canadians did not build the same number of memorials to the flu victims—or almost any for that matter. Why? First, the flu slowly dissipated in 1919, claiming fewer and fewer lives, but no Armistice Day–style celebrations were held to mark a victory. It came and went with astonishing speed, virility, and impact, but it also faded with no climatic battle. More importantly, Canadians knew death by disease. Flu and sickness had always snatched Canadians—primarily, the youngest and elderly. Even though this virus also killed the healthy, the lack of memorials suggests that the flu was seen as a natural disaster, one separate from human agency and akin to disease deaths of the past, if extraordinary in its lethality. The virus came from the natural world, while in contrast the war was a man-made disaster with deliberate political goals that led to legions of dead. Was it the guilt aroused by sending the young to die in foreign fields that demanded memorials? Perhaps, although there is evidence that the pride in sacrificing for a just cause (which was how it was widely portrayed during the war and afterwards for at least a decade), the desire to mark service for a community, the need to create a space to honour absent bodies, and the fervent belief in standing by British and Canadian ideals were also powerful motivating factors for communities across the country to create memorials to the war dead. The thousands of memorials erected for Canada's wartime fallen were not just about loss and death; instead, they revealed a desire to forge meaning from the war within its dark shadow. The fallen soldiers—drawn from every class, language group, and race—would not be forgotten, even as the virus victims were laid to rest individually and without collective memorials.

Canadians turned to honouring the dead by constructing war memorials throughout the 1920s. Geographical features were named after those who died, while stained glass windows were installed in churches. Businesses and schools mounted plaques to name those who had served and who forever lay overseas. Community organizers raised funds to build cenotaphs—empty graves—to mark the service and loss, and these were placed in prominent spots where citizens could gather around and pay their respects. Armistice Day (renamed Remembrance Day in 1931), its two minutes of silence, and the poppy were other symbolic anchors in this new memorial landscape.

The CAMC was severely cut back after the war, with only 144 officers, nursing sisters, and other ranks remaining to meet the needs of the radically reduced army, but the fallen from the medical services were also marked in many ways.[19] Like other Canadians in

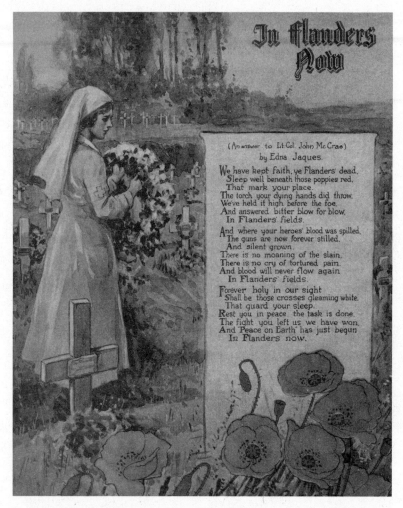

"In Flanders Fields" lived on as a literary legacy and a commemorative icon of remembrance. This is one of the many response poems to McCrae's work that was inspired by the original. Like this image, these illustrated versions were often adorned with red poppies.

uniform who never came home, medical service members also had their names inscribed on the local memorials, as well as in schools, churches, and other sites of memory. Most of the hospitals were commemorated at the universities where they had been raised, with plaques denoting service. While no separate monument to members of the CAMC was erected until 1984, when the Canadian Military Medical Service Memorial was unveiled at CFB Borden, other Canadian Forces' bases, units, and centres made note of the Great War contributions through the naming of buildings or the erection of plaques.

In Canada's Parliament, the service of nurses was commemorated with a bas-relief memorial that was unveiled in August 1926. It was to mark the 61 nurses who had died in service. Matron Margaret Macdonald, who had led them during the war, asked her "warrior sisters" to attend the event in Ottawa.[20] Paid for by the nurses through personal subscriptions, the ceremony saw some 250 veterans come together wearing their uniforms and medals to honour absent comrades. They were feted at the seat of democracy, with Governor General Lord Byng—the former Canadian Corps commander—in attendance along with senior cabinet ministers, politicians, and veterans. The marble sculpture near the Library of Parliament depicts military sisters aiding a wounded soldier. It links nurses' wartime service to Canada's earlier history of nursing care through a series of other sculptures providing aid through the country's history, while also drawing attention to the interplay of civilian and military care.[21] One of the allegorical female figures, noted a contemporary newspaper account, represents "History" and she "holds the Book of Records and draws aside the veil between past and present."[22]

Published unit histories were another means of marking service. Many of the hospital units turned to a learned doctor to compile a narrative. The results were often dense books tracking the officers, nurses, and other ranks who served, the organizational

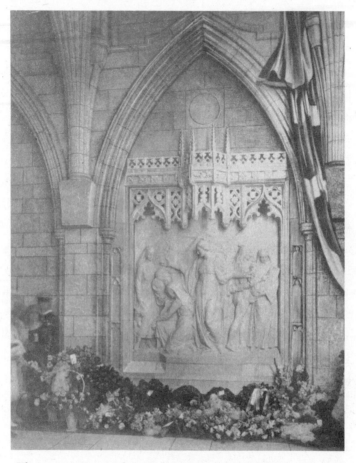

The nurses' memorial in Ottawa, unveiled in 1926, is a constant reminder to elected officials and visitors to Parliament of the service of women in uniform during the Great War.

changes of the hospital, and the evolving system of care.[23] Although they were primarily literary memorials, these hospital histories also sought, as one author noted, to capture in print "the administrative and scientific work of a general hospital as performed in war time."[24] No histories of the four Canadian casualty clearing stations were published, as these wartime necessities that emerged as the epicentre of forward surgical care disappeared after the war, with no place available for them in the much-reduced CAMC. Most of the field ambulances demobilized too, although a few histories were written to keep the memory of these units alive. One of the first, published in 1920, was a descriptive account by Lieutenant-Colonel John Nisbet Gunn and Staff Sergeant E.E. Dutton, laying forth the experiences of No. 8 Canadian Field Ambulance. Basing the narrative on the ambulance's war diary and medical records, the authors included a dedication: "To the memory of those who went out with us Never to return, but who rest 'over there.'" The book was also for survivors and casual readers, with Gunn and Dutton believing that the history "will help you to realize the greatness of the humane and necessary work of the field ambulance, with men ever ready at hand, in every dangerous experience, to minister to the men as they fought and fell."[25]

These print memorials were augmented by published accounts from a limited number of those who served in the CAMC. William Boyd, a professor of pathology at the University of Manitoba who was in uniform overseas as a surgeon, had returned to Winnipeg during the war to become a public health officer, and he published his diary. Characterized by Boyd as a "record of facts, experiences, and emotions," *With a Field Ambulance at Ypres* (1916) provides unique insight into the early struggle to save lives.[26] Other written accounts emerged, although one of the finest memoirs, masquerading as a regimental history, was written by Frederick W. Noyes, a literate sergeant whose *Stretcher Bearers at the Double* (1937) is a no-holds-barred account of the brutality of war and the stupidity of some of the decisions made by officers.[27]

Many nurses kept diaries and autograph books during the war. Georgianna Beach McCullough, who received the Royal

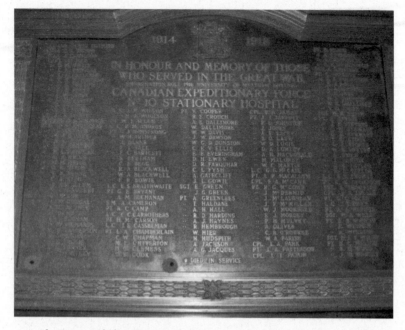

A plaque unveiled at Western University, in London, Ontario, to those who served with No. 10 Stationary Hospital during the Great War.

Red Cross Medal, Second Class, and served as a nursing sister in Salonika and France, added clippings and poems to her book throughout the 1920s, making it a complex object of service and memory.[28] McCullough's scrapbook was unpublished, like so many, and only four of the 3,000 Canadian nurses published memoirs in the twentieth century. Perhaps too many of these women would have agreed with their comrade, Nursing Sister Pearl Babbit, who wrote, "No one but those at the front and we who see the mangled bodies brought in still breathing, can have any idea of what is going on. . . . It is too awful to write about."[29]

One of the few published accounts, Mabel Clint's *Our Bit: Memoirs of War Service by a Canadian Nursing Sister* (1934), recounted Clint's pride in serving the Empire in a time of great need and in standing with her fellow nurses, although she believed that "of the conditions prevailing on the Islands of Imbros and Lemnos, and indeed in hospitals and camps in Egypt, the public knows nothing."[30] *Our Bit* was much admired by Matron Margaret Macdonald, who described it as a "red-letter day for the members of the nursing profession" when it was published during the Depression, and all the more so since Macdonald had failed to write a history of the nursing service.[31] With no place in Ottawa for Macdonald in the reduced postwar military service, despite her acknowledged skills as a tough if fair commander and as the first woman in the British Empire to achieve the rank of major, she had been ordered in 1920 to write a history of the nursing sisters before she was pushed into retirement. Macdonald understood the value of documenting the nurses' service, but she had trouble steadying herself after the long war. Furthermore, when she called out to the nursing veterans to supply stories and anecdotes, she received little response as most had moved on to a new phase in their lives. Most importantly, as Macdonald was not a trained historian, she had little idea of how to draw together the many threads of history into a tapestry representing the whole.[32] In one postwar speech, Macdonald had expressed her hope that "generations yet unborn will bless the memory of these heroic women" and declared that "the lofty ideals, aspirations and attainments of the Army Nurses . . . have given us traditions that will survive till time is at an end."[33] Alas, during two years of work, she produced little and the nurses' valued contributions faded from public memory for decades. It would be left to historians three generations later to begin the task of more fully writing this history.[34]

Without a historical work documenting deeds, service, and sacrifice, lived experience and fading memories are always in danger of being cast into oblivion.

———

After the American Civil War in the 1860s, chroniclers in the U.S. spent nearly three decades writing six volumes of medical history, and while these were of value to future generations, one lesson learned was the importance of beginning the historical work as events were unfolding.[35] Following in this vein, Sir William Grant Macpherson and a number of British historians and doctors would write and edit a thirteen-volume Great War series for the Royal Army Medical Corps—based on over 38,000 official war diaries, each of several hundred pages or more—which one of the assigned historians described as "an almost insuperable task."[36] The British-born Canadian nationalist Colonel George Adami also planned a multi-volume history, aware that Canada would have to tell its own story separate from that of the British, and throughout the war he urged medical units to create records and write historical narratives.[37] As historical medical recorder from 1915, Adami gathered, arranged, and studied war records, interviewed fellow medical officers to document their experiences, and wrote amid his many duties. In late 1918, Adami's *The War Story of the C.A.M.C., 1914–1915* was published; it was a "contemporary history," as he called it, but it was a very fine offering that explored the medical services in the early part of the war.[38] However, after his wife, Mary Stuart Cantilie, died in 1916, he handed off the subsequent volumes to future writers.

One of these was Colonel Arthur Evans Snell, who was five

times mentioned in despatches for his distinguished work and who served the Corps in 1918 as deputy director of the medical services. Serving along the Western Front, Snell gathered and arranged archival documents, including official records, diaries, and maps that underpinned a 300-page narrative during the war.[39] That document formed the basis for *The C.A.M.C. with the Canadian Corps during the Last Hundred Days of the Great War* (1924), a very technical book that straddled the line between a narrative and a doctrinal manual. The colonel explored the training for open warfare before the Hundred Days campaign and then the role of the medical services in aiding the wounded in those costly battles that broke the German army.[40]

Colonel Snell was assisted in this work by Colonel A.F. Duguid, a decorated artillery officer who was appointed Canada's official historian in 1921 and was tasked with writing a multi-volume series of Canada's entire war effort. The planned eight-volume history, with additional specialized books related to nurses, engineers, and the medical services, would be an epic account of the Canadian war effort overseas. Energetic, experienced, and informed, the decorated gunner had many strong qualities as a staff officer, but he was not a professionally trained historian. Confronting millions of pages of documentation and often pulled in many directions to assist regimental historians, defend Canada's reputation from the British official historians who slighted or downplayed the Canadian role in the war, and oversee heritage military projects, Duguid made little headway on his ambitious project.[41] As the years wore on, Canadian veterans complained loudly through their organizations and members of Parliament that their unwritten history had silenced their achievements on the battlefield and, far worse, had allowed the Americans most also recognized his untempered views. Attesting to his influence as a public intellectual, he was knighted for his service to Canada and the Empire in 1918.[45]

Macphail returned to Montreal after the war and continued to write despite living with poor health exacerbated by the strain of the war. The inexhaustible author and professor penned a long biographical essay in 1919 about his friend, John McCrae, giving voice to the poet-soldier-physician whose life had been cut short. A best-seller, the essay furthered the enduring reach of "In Flanders Fields."[46] That year also saw the emergence of another round in the war of reputations between Colonel Herbert Bruce and the CAMC, with the Toronto surgeon unleashing a new barrage by publishing a polemic about his controversial wartime report. Fired by a desire to redeem himself, Bruce's *Politics and the C.A.M.C.* (1919) incited another minor eruption. The book was not wholly ignored, with one paper calling it "a strange tale of sensational allegations," but most reviewers dismissed it as old news.[47]

The senior officers of the CAMC were not panicked by Bruce's book, but they felt that the service's significant wartime accomplishments deserved a wartime history and that the Toronto surgeon might be formally rebuked there. The CAMC high command turned to Macphail, the country's most distinguished medical writer next to William Osler, who passed away in 1919, still heartbroken over the wartime death of his son. Macphail set out to tell the medical story to the Canadian public, to refute Bruce's accusations, and to codify the war's lessons for future generations of medical service personnel. Commissioned in October 1921, he tackled his project at a feverish pace, even as he suffered from lingering pain after surviving an assassination attempt that same year by a deranged man who shot him in the right arm.

In almost every country—both the victors and the vanquished—official historians were writing multi-volume war series, although almost all would be staid, clinical accounts. The authors, who were often serving and senior officers, treaded softly through the minefield of reputations, while influential generals and politicians exerted pressure to curtail criticism, advance agendas, and shape the interpretation of history. Governments in Paris, London, Washington, and Ottawa had little inclination to open up the war archives for intense scrutiny, although public demand to know the story and officers' need to better understand the war's lessons were evident. And so it fell to the official historians to write these histories that, once completed, were sometimes described as official but rarely as history.

As a professor and essayist, Macphail refused to obscure the war effort with guarded language or safe platitudes. Having characterized the act of historical writing as "something more than record and something less than praise," he noted further that "it demands selection and judgement, judging events as if they were far in the past, and men as if they were already dead."[48] The prolific historian had a draft of some 500 pages ready by February 1922. His focus drifted from service history to medical minutia, although he wrote with flare, and insights peppered with eyewitness accounts for medical officers invigorated the narrative. Only decades later did historians discover that he had cloaked his own personal observations in ambiguous references to unnamed Canadian officers, quoting from his own diary.[49] While these remarks were disguised, his opinions, including his hatred for Sir Sam Hughes, were not.

In the opening section, Macphail laid bare the clash and challenge of bringing together "the civil and the military." Minister

Sam Hughes, said Macphail, "in time lost the confidence of his colleagues; he never had the confidence of the army after it became an Army. . . . When he resigned there was a sense of deliverance."[50] Macphail was not wrong, but some felt that this was not the forum in which to flay the minister. "War being polemical," responded an unrepentant Macphail, "writing about war must be polemical too. It is not intended to please."[51]

When the McGill doctor delivered his manuscript to senior CAMC officers in early 1922, the authorities read it with growing worry. Duguid prevailed upon Macphail to rewrite sections and to tone down his attacks on Hughes. The professor refused. To the senior officers' discomfort, the contract with Macphail revealed that the McGill professor owned the intellectual rights and that he could publish the work even if the authorities refused to support it.[52] A compromise of sorts was reached, with Macphail rewriting select parts and the Department of National Defence dragging its heels and only publishing the history in 1925.

The Medical Services attracted much attention and many readers, especially since Duguid's series had been delayed and the public remained interested in the war. "Under the cloak of the title of historian," the *Ottawa Journal* complained, "Sir Andrew Macphail has washed a lot of unclean linen, trifled with the memory of gallant if mistaken men and given a grossly misleading slant to the character of Canada's war effort."[53] While Macphail's attacks on Sam Hughes were sharp and well deserved, the discredited minister, who had made a career of outlandish verbal assaults, frightening rants, and full-blown lies, still had many champions after his death in August 1921. The *Canada Lancet* accused the book of being "neither impartial nor authentic." Other commentators applauded the work of history, with one describing *The*

Medical Services as "a valuable and courageously independent study" because it went beyond the medical services to lay forth the history of the larger Canadian war effort.[54] The official history could not be ignored, and *Maclean's* magazine applauded Macphail's monumental achievement while also highlighting the resulting "lively literary scuffle." It observed, too, that "the Canadian press never before gave so much space to the consideration of any book."[55]

Macphail also laid into Herbert Bruce, highlighting the failures of his 1916 report, especially easy-to-refute errors like the accusation that many medical officers were alcoholics, that operations were performed badly, and that the recovering wounded were cast adrift in British hospitals.[56] Some saw this rebuke of Bruce in the state-sponsored history as an official censure, and Bruce's 1919 book justifying his contentious report was soon lost to history, although, as lieutenant-governor of Ontario from 1932 to 1937, he had a long and notable career. He also had more than a few defenders in 1925, including the *Charlottetown Guardian*, which saw Macphail's assault on Bruce as revealing the writer to be a "ridiculous and venomous individual."[57] Macphail was used to literary controversies, and, shrugging off the attacks by lesser-known writers, he continued to produce in multiple fields of history, medicine, fiction, and literary criticism, remaining a public intellectual of the highest order until his death in 1938.

The Medical Services is episodic in nature and oddly structured, although it includes a multitude of facts, statistics, and fascinating contemporary medical observations.[58] While some of the statistics have since been revised and its judgments have not always stood the test of time, Macphail's book remained the foundational document of the CAMC for decades, informing all subsequent scholarship. In writing *Lifesavers and Body Snatchers*, one of my goals was to update the official history, while remaining indebted to the statistical breakdown if not the doctor's interpretations.

———

With or without the memorials and histories, the doctors and nurses went on with their lives, aiding fellow Canadians, advancing the art of medicine, and furthering health care. "Lest we forget," Canadians murmured on Remembrance Day in November at their local cenotaphs or at the national memorial after it was unveiled in Ottawa in 1939. But perhaps some medical professionals in Canada also occasionally reflected back on the pathological samples that were to have been the anchor around which a war museum would be established to present the struggle to save lives in the lands of death on the Western Front. What indeed had happened to the body parts, organs, and bone specimens of the Canadian soldiers that had been removed, labelled, and then placed on display in London? Where had the pathological samples gone that had been taken from those soldiers who died in service to the country, harvested after their deaths to be employed in new battles for the advancement of medical treatment?

CHAPTER 20

THE USE AND MISUSE OF HARVESTED SOLDIERS' ORGANS

"I Lie Here, Mother, But Victory Is Ours."

T his was the epitaph chosen by the parents of Private Thomas Mack, who was killed at age twenty-four, dying from wounds suffered in battle on April 29, 1917. The creation of the overseas cemeteries was comforting to some grieving Canadians who took solace in knowing that their sons and daughters, uncles, aunts, and fathers would be buried forever with their comrades, having given their lives in what most believed was a just and necessary war.[1] Frequently described as the "glorious dead," this silent army would forever be a reminder of the cost of the war: to Canada and its allies, to communities across the Dominion, and to individuals forever diminished by absence and sorrow.

And yet some Canadians were deliberately buried with their bodies missing organs. Medical officers had cut up the soldiers, extracting organs and bones as teaching specimens and museological oddities. "These specimens, in the years to come, must be of great value to the future Canadian war surgeon and more particularly will be of great value in the teaching of clinical surgery and pathology."[2] So wrote CAMC Captain Morton Hall, who in early 1919 was organizing and sorting the remaining Canadian body parts at the Royal College of Surgeons into sixty-three reinforced boxes. This final collection sent to McGill University followed the transfer a year earlier and consisted of bone machinations, brains, lungs, and other organs that totalled 618 specimens.[3] In Hall's words, the collection was "a very complete, valuable and instructive one, illustrating all varieties of gunshot injuries and more particularly the associated processes of repair and infection."[4] The pathological samples were supported by illustrated drawings, X-ray slides, watercolour sketches of pathological samples, and oil paintings by serving personnel.[5]

By the end of the war, over 4,000 pathological samples had been delivered to the curators at the Royal College, with some 1,200 objects on display in their galleries at the time of the armistice.[6] The collection documented almost every type of injury to the body. To enrich its value as a research tool, a typeset catalogue was created describing each object.[7] Ten medical papers were also published over a five-year span, which allowed for the collection's dissemination in specialized clinical circles. Some of this work also fed into the multi-volume British medical official history series, which described the pathological samples as holding a "value to the nation at large" that "cannot well be over-estimated."[8]

As curators continued to stabilize and arrange the pathological objects in the Royal College collection, with many additional years of organizing and cataloguing to follow, in August 1919 the last of the total of 799 body parts and bone samples were sent to McGill.[9] They primarily came from Canadian soldiers, with Captain Lloyd Philips MacHaffie having aggressively gathered

446

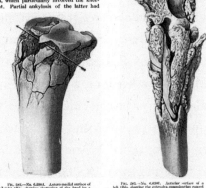

INFECTION AND REPAIR OF LONG BONES   309

through the head of the tibia, shattering it. Fissures extend down the shaft and across the articular surface. The soldier was wounded on Nov. 27, 1917, and lay out three days before evacuation. He was admitted to base hospital on Dec. 3, and an amputation was performed on account of severe infection of the knee-joint. It will be noted that erosion of the cortex along the fissures had already begun although the period of infection had been brief. The articular surfaces of the tibia had, however, escaped.

In specimen No. 6.6301 (*Fig.* 283) there has been an extensive comminution of the whole upper third of a left tibia by a missile, probably a shell fragment, which perforated the leg from side to side. The soldier was wounded on April 15, 1917, and extension was applied till June 2, when an amputation was performed because of the severe infection, which particularly involved the knee-joint. Partial ankylosis of the latter had

FIG. 282.—No. 6.6084. Antero-medial surface of a right tibia, showing shattering of the head by a bullet. Note the erosion of the cortex on the surface of the fragments along the fissures.

FIG. 283.—No. 6.6301. Anterior surface of a left tibia, showing the extensive comminution caused by a through-and-through shell-wound. Note the areas of smooth dead bone (sequestra), and the abundant callus on the surface of some of the fragments.

occurred, and the soft structures of the joint had degenerated. It will be seen that the entire upper third of the tibia, including the head, has been shattered into numerous fragments, some of which have been lost. Of those remaining, several died at the time of injury, and remain as smooth sequestra, while others survived, and on their surfaces new bone has been thrown out. In some of these, the margins were destroyed and have become entirely separated as sequestra. There has been complete destruction of the articular surface of the head of the tibia.

An illustration of a pathological bone sample published in an academic medical journal after the war. It was removed from a British or dominion soldier and became part of the Royal College of Surgeons collection.

together 978 bone and tissue samples since August 1918. His appointment as a medical officer dedicated to pathological samples had come after several years of Colonel Adami requesting an officer to focus solely on the task, and MacHaffie's collection was joined by the many other body parts sent by Canadian officers to London for ultimate transfer to Montreal.[10] The collection of specimens had arrived to Canada in installments, with 181 specimens sent first and another 618 in this final transfer, but not all of MacHaffie's specimens went to Canada because some were from

British soldiers.[11] Others were likely divided among the dominions, as British records show that 700 pathological samples went to Australia, and Canadian hospitals autopsied and selected body parts from both Australian and New Zealand soldiers who died on the operating table.[12]

One representative box of material sent to Canada in the 1919 transfer yielded almost twenty specimens, including a portion of a spinal cord, a brain, two hearts, two spleens, a kidney, a jugular vein and carotid artery, a left foot, a lung and liver set, another brain and spinal cord from an individual soldier, two lungs from different men, and a larynx, liver, and left kidney from the same man. These were accompanied by some of the bullets and fragments extracted from the lethal wounds represented among the specimens.[13] The spinal cord had been removed at No. 1 Canadian General Hospital from Private W. Asser of the 1st Battalion, London Regiment, after he had suffered multiple gunshot wounds on May 11, 1917. Asser survived long enough to be cared for in a field ambulance and a clearing station, but he died eleven days later from the bullet that passed through his clavicle, lungs, and finally lodged in his spine. Major John James Ower had removed the spinal cord with the bullet still embedded, before Private Asser was buried. Each of the body parts in the box was described and linked to the soldier from whom it was extracted, and this particular collection largely came from British soldiers because No. 1 Canadian General Hospital, where Major Ower served, took in Imperial and dominion soldiers. One of the extracted lungs came from Peter MacRae, a twenty-eight-year-old Canadian infantryman in the 2nd Battalion who died from his injuries on June 26, 1917, months after suffering from multiple gunshot wounds.

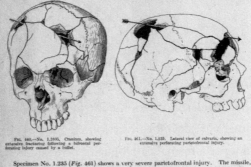

Illustration of a bullet wound to the cranium. The skull was harvested from the slain soldier and put on display, as well as being used to illustrate a medical article on gunshot injuries to bones.

His spleen, lungs, and liver were harvested and sent to Montreal because they all revealed noteworthy damage from tuberculosis.[14]

The 799 body parts and skeletal remains were drawn from individual Canadian and British soldiers, although some 28 Canadian specimens were left behind in the Royal College of Surgeons' national collection. Initiating a macabre horse trade of sorts, the Imperials substituted the body parts with an equal number from their collection.[15] Having served, fought, and sacrificed together, Canadian, British, and other dominion soldiers were buried together in the Imperial War Graves Commission cemeteries, and now they would be arranged, presented, and studied alongside each other as well.[16]

———

Dr. Maude Abbott, who had been excluded from overseas service because of her gender, now took control of the soldiers' pathological specimens at McGill University. Her goal was to conserve, arrange, and write a formal catalogue that would better allow the collection to be used as a teaching device when it was put on display at the future medical museum in Ottawa. A few months after the last of the pathological samples arrived from overseas, Abbott hosted a remarkable evening on November 7, 1919, four days before the Empire-wide observance of the first Armistice Day. She invited many of the professors who had served in the war with No. 3 Canadian General Hospital to give lectures, and the pathological samples were made available to illustrate their presentations.

The symposium attended by students and faculty was kicked off by Professor C.S. Peters, who had served in a field ambulance and hospital, and who spoke to the effects of gas on lungs, using two of the organs that showed spongy damage from chemical warfare. He also recounted his horror at seeing gassed victims, observing that "the pallid anxious face, the awful air hunger, the rapid shallow breathing, the restlessness, the coughing and vomiting, and groaning, together with the acute consciousness and the anxious appealing eyes, made one feel that the deepest hell is not deep enough for the men who first used gas." Peters was joined by Alfred Turner Bazin, a CAMC lieutenant-colonel and respected surgeon who lectured on damage to knee and elbow joints using two bone samples drawn from soldiers who died of infections. "In examining these specimens," Bazin said, "one is at once impressed by the serious complicating injury to bone." Gunshot wounds to the brain were the focus of Edward Archibald's talk, which drew attention to several preserved brains showing lacerations from bullets funnelling through the skull and into the grey matter, while the Victoria Cross recipient Francis Scrimger demonstrated the effects of surgical care on "penetrating wounds of the abdomen." The trauma to the specimen he used led Scrimger to "hazard a guess that this man had died within ten hours of his wounding, probably from a combination of shock and haemorrhage." Other speakers took the floor, including Laurence Joseph Rhea, who as the pathologist for No. 3 General had collected many of the bone and wet tissue samples that were on display in this symposium. Using reconstructed bone specimens, he spoke to the "great amount of injury to bone" as revealed by bullets and shell fragments. The evening ended with Major George Alexander Campbell, who had recently been appointed curator of the national medical museum in Ottawa, thanking Abbott for her work on the collection. Major Campbell urged her to continue to showcase the pathological samples and to give further "demonstrations at Medical Societies." He also hoped that this work would form the core of the planned "Museum of which the Canadian Army Medical Corps might justly be proud."[17]

Senior medical officers, both veterans of the war and those continuing in uniform with the much smaller CAMC, still desired that these body parts would eventually be put on display in the

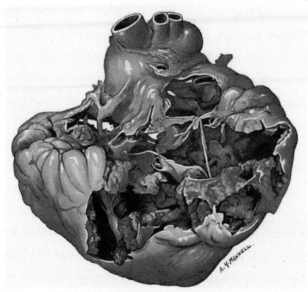

FIG. 67.—Extreme laceration of the heart caused by a fragment of high-explosive shell.

Drawing of a soldier's heart that was removed from his body and put on display. The caption reads, "Extreme laceration of the heart caused by a fragment of high explosive shell."

Ottawa medical military museum, which existed only in name at the time. Alexander Primross, in a 1919 address to the medical profession, made mention of the revolutionary changes to medicine that he witnessed as a CAMC lieutenant-colonel, but also emphasized the need to enshrine such legacies in a museum of "national importance." The collection of artifacts and pathological samples, along with wax models, X-ray images, and scientific drawings, would be of "great educational value" and would "constitute a permanent record in Canada of the part played by the Canadian Army Medical Corps."[18]

Lord Beaverbrook also envisioned a national war museum to house the relics, works of art, trophies, and historical records that had been created or collected to document the Canadian war effort that had so profoundly put the country on a new trajectory towards full nationhood. Two sets of plans were drawn up for a museum in Ottawa, but the country was mired in debt and successive governments found excuses to delay the museum's creation throughout the 1920s.[19] Beaverbrook became frustrated with the inertia and moved on to new projects, exploits, and scandals. During the wait for the war museum to be established, the stunning war art collection of over 800 works was housed at the National Gallery. However, after a number of successful tours and exhibitions, it was little displayed and became destined for the vaults.[20] Copies of the official photographs of the Canadian war effort, numbering over 5,000, were on sale for public purchase in the 1920s, when a significant demand for reproductions was expressed by businesses, patriotic women's associations, veterans' groups, and individuals. By the late 1920s, the original photographs were transferred to the Public Archives of Canada in Ottawa and became more difficult for Canadians to access. Even worse, most of the priceless film footage that was shot by combat cameramen during the war was misplaced for a decade and only re-emerged in the early 1930s, after which it was used to create an official film, *Lest We Forget* (1935).[21] The afterlife of these historical records is filled with tales of neglect and apathy, and many of the relics and artifacts were lost or left to disintegrate. Canadians seemed content to build thousands of local, provincial, national, and overseas memorials to the fallen, but to then allow the history of Canada's war effort to remain untold and unpreserved. The war would therefore increasingly be seen through the lens of the sacred and the sacrificial, a view that was further cemented by symbolic acts like Remembrance Day, the

Maude Abbott curated another exhibition for the surgeons, who were treated to a show of "Pathological Specimens from France."[24] The soldiers' lungs, brains, and other organs were displayed alongside bone structures, wax models, and artwork. Abbott's work had advanced since the Hamilton display in May 1918, and now the catalogue of this 1920 exhibition listed eighty-eight bone specimens, many shattered by bullets and shell fragments, which had been reconstructed and displayed dynamically to reveal the damage. Also exhibited were ninety-four organs—described as "wet specimens"—including fourteen respiratory tracts and lungs that had been removed from soldiers who died from poison gas inhalation.[25]

Presented professionally in long glass table cases, the body parts were divided into three groupings: bone specimens, pathological specimens, and medical prostheses. A series of plaster casts was also included, exposing damage to hands and, quite horrifyingly, facial wounds. The plasters had come from the Ontario Military Hospital at Orpington, and the exhibition presented over 40 of these, revealing shattered jaws, broken chins, and missing eyes.[26] Accompanying them were a number of photographs of facially disfigured soldiers that documented the progression of recovery through multiple operations in a series of images over time. At least seven plaster hand models were mounted on bases, most of them illustrating scarring wounds. Arranged on a table, the disembodied hands appeared to be reaching out, almost like the limbs of buried men. The bone samples were housed in a series of glass cases and several artworks were presented on the wall, along with the "wet" pathological samples that were on tables with caption labels.

In Abbott's personal archives, a letter from the chair of the program committee thanking her for curating the display reads,

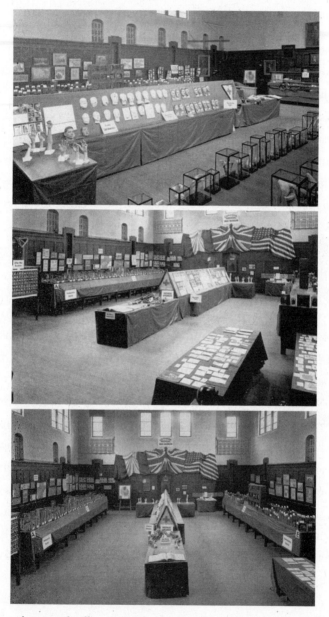

Three photographs illustrating the display of bone and organ samples in Montreal in October 1920, along with works of art, models, and artifacts. A sign above the flag reads, "Canadian Medical War Museum."

"No one who ever attended a meeting of the American College of Surgeons has ever before seen anything like it, and the catalogue you issued of all of the exhibits was a perfect marvel to everybody. How you ever managed to get this catalogue out of the Government none of us have the slightest idea; but it just made complete an exhibition which was really wonderful."[27] Though the admiring letter writer was amazed by Abbott's ability to wrangle money from the government during the debt-laden postwar years, the surgeon may also have been curious about how Abbott had been able to display the human remains of soldiers during a period of memorial-making across the Dominion.

Indeed, how could the fallen be revered as Christlike soldiers who gave their lives in a war against German aggression while the body parts of some of the same soldiers were being put on display for medical examination or for the diversion of curious gawkers?[28] This apparent contradiction may conjure images of sinister conspiracy or of plotting mad scientists. But Abbott made no secret of the body parts that had been collected, and nor did the curators at the Royal College of Surgeons. In fact, in the early 1920s, Abbott wrote several articles in the *CMAJ* to keep the Canadian medical profession apprised of the collection's development and of how it was being prepared for presentation and education. The pathological samples were also mentioned in Sir Andrew Macphail's 1925 medical history, which provided an account of the medical museum and the plans for Abbott's descriptive catalogue.[29] And although *The Medical Services* elicited much commentary and criticism, no journalist was disturbed by Macphail's fulsome section on the medical museum and the soldiers' body parts.

The medical museum consultant board met throughout 1921, and it periodically reported to Canadian director general of medical services John Taylor Fotheringham. None of this was a secret, and the collection was better known after June 15, 1921, when the Department of National Defence submitted a brief to Parliament describing the value of the collection and the Privy Council authorized $10,000 for the continued preparation of pathological samples. Prime Minister Borden had left office at this point, exhausted and close to death (though he rallied and lived until 1937), but the government led by Arthur Meighen bolstered the body parts collection through this act of financial support that would today amount to around $145,000.[30] This was quite remarkable in an age of debt and cutbacks to the military forces, and all the more so as it was set against the backdrop of the high-profile interring and burying of tens of thousands of Canada's fallen overseas as they were moved to permanent cemeteries. Again, the collection of body parts was not a secret conspiracy dreamed up by Frankensteinian doctors, although it is nearly impossible to reconcile with Canadians' perception of the fallen soldiers at the time and ever since.

The answer to how this collection could be funded and supported by the state is to be found in the long tradition of using medical autopsies to discover the secrets to life in the bodies of the dead. Furthermore, the powerful legacy of medical learning energized by the Great War was part of the equally long-established tradition of sharing knowledge through the use of pathological specimens as teaching tools. To codify the lessons revealed through the pathological samples, it was agreed at an April 1921 meeting between Abbott and medical authorities in Ottawa that the state would fund a comprehensive catalogue, which Abbott speculated, given the extent of the "Bones and Moist specimens," would "occupy approximately 800 pages."[31] The catalogue was also to be illustrated with photographs of the pathological samples, X-ray slides, and artifacts. This agreement having been secured, work continued on mounting and preserving the organs and bones, with Abbott and other medical colleagues driven by the desire to take the evil of the war and transform it into a public good in times of peace, even if that action was diametrically opposed to the broader societal urge that was ennobling the fallen through commemorative acts, symbols, and new structures of remembrance.

———

As George Adami had fought so hard for the Canadian pathological samples to go to Canada, he would have been an influential champion for the medical museum, but in 1919 he was appointed vice-chancellor of the University of Liverpool. Invigorated by his new post and having remarried in 1922, he continued to investigate diseases and publish widely in Canadian and Imperial journals until his death in 1926 at the age of sixty-four.[32] Had Adami returned to McGill, he would surely have used his considerable influence to carve out the military medical museum and a permanent place for the pathological samples.

The idea of a military museum stagnated in Ottawa in the early 1920s, with sporadic debates over the creation of a memorial museum inciting fierce pledges to remember the service and sacrifice of Canadians, and this was followed by foot-dragging and delay on the part of the Liberal government of William Lyon Mackenzie King, prime minister from December 1921. And so, although Britain had created its Imperial War Museum and almost every other belligerent nation was building a war museum, Canada dithered. It was not until 1942, in the middle of the Second World

War, that a small, ugly building in downtown Ottawa was finally opened to the public. Though it was stuffed with war trophies, posters, and artifacts, the body parts remained at McGill. Before this, however, Abbott had continued to dedicate her time to the military pathology collection, serving as its only remaining guardian. And yet she was frustrated by Ottawa's lack of support and by the refusal by senior CAMC officers to allow the publication of the catalogue, which she completed in 1922. Why, she wondered, had there been such a loss of interest on the part of the CAMC senior military leadership, which had previously been so supportive of a museum and the pathological collection? The lack of committed action from several governments towards establishing a national military museum must have troubled the senior medical leadership, and it certainly made no sense to have a separate medical museum without a national war museum. But why not publish the catalogue to which significant public funds had already been allocated? It is clear that the fierce reaction to and fallout from Macphail's official history made the CAMC senior leadership gunshy about future controversies. If the condemnation of Hughes had excited a verbal and printed barrage, what would be the reaction of the grieving next of kin to a catalogue itemizing harvested slain soldiers' body parts? But the reaction to Macphail's book had been in 1925, and the catalogue was delayed even before that.

It appears that, in the period between the summer of 1921, when the government allocated $10,000 in funding for the catalogue, and the next year, a radical change of heart took place in Ottawa. Where once enthusiasm was clear, now there was resistance as the military medical authorities pulled back in late 1922, unwilling to be associated with the harvested soldiers' organs and bones. The next year, at a meeting in Ottawa on March 14, 1923, with McGill represented by Abbott and Sir Arthur Currie—the former corps commander now university principal—the university came to an agreement with the director general of medical services in Ottawa, Colonel A.E. Snell. Even though Snell was a champion of the cause, the political environment was too toxic for the medical services to hold on to the pathological collection, and Snell formally placed it under Abbott's care, even agreeing to pay her a yearly $300 honorarium, as one McGill report noted, to "defray the upkeep of the museum."[33]

The display of citizen-soldiers would remain hidden to the Canadian public, although it would continue to serve as teaching material for medical students. In a country haunted by the spectres of the fathers, sons, daughters, brothers, and sisters who never came home, the wartime fervour of collecting body parts for study was progressively weakened. Though the Department of National Defence continued to send annual payments to Abbott to care for the collection, all talk of a museum to display them in the capital ceased and the catalogue was denied publication. Military medical authorities saw the collection as a dark legacy of the war that was at odds with the commemorative impulse of grieving Canadians who were memorializing the fallen.

While the body parts were shrouded from sight at McGill, they were not destroyed. Museums, archives, and collections need guardians, however, and as Ottawa felt it necessary to pull back and Adami was in Liverpool and then buried, that left only Abbott. Though capable and motivated, she was perplexed as to why Ottawa was not allowing the publication of the catalogue, and was clearly never told the reason why it could not be made available for a wider audience. The collection was put aside in 1923 when Abbott set off on new professional endeavours, accepting a two-year appointment as acting head of the Department of Pathology at Women's Medical College of Pennsylvania in Philadelphia. This move provided a welcome respite for Abbott; having long faced discrimination at McGill because of her gender, she was feted in the United States. During and after Abbott's sabbatical, no more formal exhibitions of the collection took place, but Department of National Defence records indicate that the military continued to pay Abbott $300 per year to care for the pathological samples, and that she made at least one trip to Ottawa in 1927 to discuss the collection.[34] She did so as an assistant professor at McGill and while continuing to hone her reputation as a world leader on congenital heart disease.

The body parts were still stored at McGill in "glass bottles," noted Abbott, and she observed in the *McGill Medical Journal* in 1928 that she continued to hope that the wartime pathological collection would be displayed in a purpose-built museum with an interpretative catalogue to better understand its value.[35] The catalogue would never be made available (and the information has now been lost), and the political will for a museum had long since withered away. The conscientious Abbott even offered to use the surplus defence department payments to print it. She received no positive response and Ottawa clearly wished to have no association with these relics.[36] The optics of a catalogue showcasing former Canadian soldiers' body parts would be, at the very least, a public relations disaster. Even worse, it would perhaps strike at the core of the cherished memory of service and sacrifice, and could dim the torch held aloft in memory of the sacred fallen.

———

In England, the First World War medical samples remained on display at the Royal College of Surgeons for over two decades. They became more important to a new generation of physicians who would serve in uniform when Britain, Canada, and the Commonwealth stood with France against Nazi Germany in September 1939. The collapse of France in June 1940 was a shocking blow to the Allies. The British, battered but defiant, kept fighting, even after Nazi dictator Adolf Hitler unleashed an aerial bombardment on London and other cities in the hope of bludgeoning the British people into submission. "We can take it!" went out the cry, but this was at a fearful cost of more than 40,000 citizens killed in 1940–1941. On the night of May 11, 1941, the Royal College of Surgeons was hit with bombs, and flames consumed medical specimens and artifacts collected over two centuries. Almost the entire Great War pathological collection was destroyed, with only fourteen specimens surviving. As Arthur Keith, the collection's former curator, remarked sadly in his diary from his retirement home in Kent, "Bombs of one war blotted out the treasured scar of its predecessor."[37]

A few months before this, Abbott, the only remaining guardian of the Canadian pathological collection, had died on September 2, 1940. The vulnerable collection survived at McGill through the Second World War, although it was little used in the training of medical officers, and a new dean of medicine in 1947 signalled his lack of interest in the "unused and ancient medical material."[38] After some negotiations, and then a shuffling of the collection from depot to base, the body parts finally found their way to the Royal Canadian Army Medical Corps School at CFB Borden, some 100 kilometres north of Toronto. Starting in February 1952, two part-time curators—Professors John Hamilton and H.J. Barrie of the University of Toronto—developed the Army Medical Pathological Museum at the RCAMC School, to which the Great War collection was added.[39] It is not clear if the soldiers' organs were ever put on display, but the two professors were paid to mount and catalogue the collection for the "purpose of instruction," according to one official document, because the "rare specimens" had "historical value."[40] As Hamilton and Barrie processed and conserved the Great War collection, they also added several dozen new pathological specimens, including a "prepyloric ulcer," a "squamous cancer hand," and "early carcinoma of kidney."[41] Interestingly, one of the additional bone samples was labelled as "traumatic damage to cartilage of talus in air crash," suggesting that it came from an airman, likely in uniform, who was in a fatal air accident or one that resulted in the amputation of his foot.[42] The archival records make no mention of where these pathological and bone samples came from to fill the museum's display cases, and few base records have survived from this time period. However, in 1955 the funding was cut and work on the Pathological Museum, as an official memo called it, was halted.[43] The official Department of National Defence file on the subject was closed on June 21, 1961, and the Great War collection was likely destroyed sometime around then. No further surviving records documenting its fate have been found.

———

Adami's program of collecting body parts, begun in the summer of 1915, became more sustained and sophisticated during the course of the war, with some 799 pathological and bone samples transferred to Montreal in 1918 and 1919. The post-mortem work was not simply about chopping up and jarring organs of every slain soldier who died in the many medical units; no, the selected body parts and bone fragments were preserved because they revealed interesting and unique wounds. And so the 799 samples that were in the care of McGill from 1919 onwards were drawn from almost as many individuals. The idea that the pathological collection of 799 body fragments may have represented almost that many individual soldiers is a staggering revelation that draws into question how Canada dealt with its dead. For over 100 years, Canadians have been told that their Great War soldiers lie in foreign fields under the Commonwealth War Graves Commission headstones, that those with no known graves had their names inscribed on monuments at Vimy or the Menin Gate, and that they were buried in Canada, having died as veterans.[44] The fact that some 799 soldiers—most of them Canadians—were brought home in the form of harvested body parts is a revelation that shakes the core concept of the sacred honouring of the fallen.

The best hope is that, at Camp Borden, the pathological samples were buried when they were abandoned in the mid-1950s; more likely, however, they were thrown out in the garbage or incinerated. The men to whom these body parts and bones once belonged had all long been buried in their graves in Western Europe. The removal of these fragments without the soldiers' or their families' consent, to be used for medical teaching purposes, was supported by the ethos before, during, and after the war of the medical community that had done so much to save lives. But two or three generations later, in the mid-1950s, some members of the Canadian armed forces must have viewed these specimens taken from distant comrades as more than simply tissue and bone. They were once men; they were once soldiers. They had lived, felt dawn, saw sunset glow, as McCrae had written, loved and were loved, and parts of them lay far from Flanders fields.

As this book has revealed, the lifesavers were also body snatchers, selecting pieces of slain soldiers to be removed by surgical knife, harvested for knowledge, stored in formaldehyde, and sent back to London and then to Montreal, all without loved ones' knowledge and with no record of this action being included in the soldiers' personnel files. When Canadians turned to commemorating the fallen, the idea of a museum of body parts was unpalatable, and these strange objects remained as oddities under glass at McGill until they were unceremoniously destroyed.

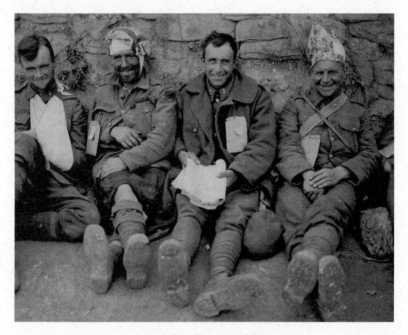

Remember them as soldiers;
remember them as men who served and sacrificed.

This story has been buried in the archives for more than 100 years. Now it has been told. These Canadian soldiers deserved a better fate after death.

———

Blood. Tissue. Viscera. Bone fragments. The Canadian medical soldiers, doctors, and nurses of the Great War were eyewitnesses to every type of horror amid the screams and moans of maimed and dying men. Even the unimagined trauma of chemical gas wounds, shell fragments through the brain, and looping intenstines severed by steel were encountered daily. But the shredded and mutilated were cared for and often brought back from nearly certain death, especially as the war progressed and lessons were learned in the cauldron of the medical care centres. It was a war of contractions, and the situation was no different within the many medical battles along and behind the Western Front. The caregivers bore a heavy emotional weight, giving freely of their expertise and empathy, and yet many were hardened by the process, sometimes in order to save their sanity. Often willing to sacrifice themselves to save the wounded, the doctors and nurses were also the high command's gatekeepers, tasked with holding genuinely ill or fought-out soldiers in the line as well as returning them there before they were fully healed. "Jekyll and Hyde," muttered the soldiers. The front-line doctors understood this contradiction and tried to navigate through the awful moral conundrums they confronted, but it was never easy to know where to draw the line between refusing to let soldiers leave the battle front and finding ways to bolster their morale to keep them in the line. This issue and many others reveal that the medical services were deeply integrated into the industrial war, and without a doubt the fighting effectiveness among the combat arms would have been much reduced if not for the support of the doctors and nurses. In this war of contradictions, it is not surprising that body parts were collected as part of the long process of teaching and learning from the dead. And yet these were not simply the bodies of the old and sick, or the destitute and unlucky. They were the citizen-soldiers of Canada who stepped up and left their loved ones to fight overseas, giving their all. It was in the Canadian body parts collection, drawn from almost 800 soldiers, that some of the grimmest contradictions of war were revealed, where healers became gears in the war machine and soldiers were expected to keep up the fight after death, employed as medical and teaching tools against their will. This was indeed a war of lifesaving and body snatching.

ENDNOTES

INTRODUCTION

1 J.G. Adami, *War Story of the Canadian Army Medical Corps* (London: Canadian War Records Office, 1918) 120.

2 W.D. Mathieson, *My Grandfather's War: Canadians Remember the First World War, 1914–1918* (Toronto: Macmillan, 1981) 136.

3 John W.S. McCullough, "Sanitation in War," *Canadian Medical Association Journal* [hereafter *CMAJ*] 9.9 (September 1919) 783; and J.A. Grant, "The Medical Profession and the Militia," *CMAJ* 4.9 (September 1914) 758.

4 Richard A. Gabriel and Karen S. Mietz, *A History of Military Medicine, Volume II* (New York: Greenwood Press, 1992) 187.

5 See Tom Scotland and Steven Heys, *Wars, Pestilence and the Surgeon's Blade: The Evolution of British Military Medicine and Surgery During the 19th Century* (Solihull: Helion, 2013).

6 R.A.L., *Letters of a Canadian Stretcher Bearer* (Toronto: Thomas Allen, 1918) 40.

7 There is a deep literature on this subject. For Canada, start with Bill Rawling, *Surviving Trench Warfare: Technology and the Canadian Corps, 1914–1918* (Toronto: University of Toronto Press, 1992).

8 Katherine McCuaig, *The Weariness, the Fever, and the Fret: The Campaign against Tuberculosis in Canada, 1900–1950* (Montreal: McGill-Queen's University Press, 1999) 37.

9 Cynthia Toman, *Sister Soldiers of the Great War: The Nurses of the Canadian Army Medical Corps* (Vancouver: UBC Press, 2016) 39.

10 Report of the Overseas Ministry, *Overseas Military Forces of Canada, 1918* (London: OMFC, 1919) 394; "Canadian Army Medical Corps: Re-Organization," *CMAJ* 11.12 (1921) 964; G.W.L. Nicholson, *Seventy Years of Service: A History of the Royal Canadian Army Medical Corps* (Ottawa: Borealis, 1977) 112.

11 Tim Cook, *Shock Troops: Canadians Fighting the Great War, 1917–1918* (Toronto: Viking, 2008) 613.

12 Report of the Overseas Ministry, *Overseas Military Forces of Canada, 1918*, 387.

13 Sir Andrew Macphail, *The Medical Services* (Ottawa: F.A. Acland, 1925).

14 George Armstrong, "The Influence of War on Surgery, Civil or Military,"
    CMAJ 9 (1919) 399.

CHAPTER 1

1 There are hundreds of books on the start of the war; I have benefited from
   Michael Neiberg, *Dance of the Furies: Europe and the Outbreak of World War*
   I (Cambridge: Belknap Press, 2011).

2 James Wood, *Militia Myths: Ideas of the Canadian Citizen Soldier, 1896–1921*
   (Vancouver: UBC Press, 2010).

3 Tim Cook, *At the Sharp End: Canadians Fighting the Great War 1914 to 1916,*
   Volume One (Toronto: Viking Canada, 2007) 26; Colonel Guy Carleton Jones,
   "The Importance of the Balkan Wars to the Medical Profession of Canada,"
   CMAJ 4 (1914) 779.

4 See Andrew Holman, *A Sense of Their Duty: Middle-Class Formation in*
   Victorian Ontario Towns (Montreal: McGill-Queen's University Press, 2000);
   Robert D. Gidney and W.P.J. Millar, *Professional Gentlemen: The Professions*
   in Nineteenth-Century Ontario (Toronto: University of Toronto Press, 1994);
   S.E.D. Shortt, "Physicians and Psychics: The Anglo-American Medical
   Response to Spiritualism, 1870–1890," *Journal of the History of Medicine and*
   Allied Sciences 39.3 (1984) 339–55.

5 Ian Ross Robertson, *Sir Andrew Macphail: The Life and Legacy of a Canadian*
   Man of Letters (Montreal: McGill-Queen's University Press, 2008) 183; and
   Royce MacGillivray, "Body Snatching in Ontario," *Canadian Bulletin of*
   Medical History 5 (1988) 51–60.

6 H.L. Burris, *Medical Sage: The Burris Clinic and Early Pioneers* (Vancouver,
   1967) 81–82. Also see, N. Tait McPhedran, *Canadian Medical Schools: Two*
   Centuries of Medical History, 1822–1992 (Montreal: Harvest House, 1993).

7 S.E.D. Shortt, "'Before the Age of Miracles': The Rise, Fall, and Rebirth of
   General Practice in Canada, 1890–1940," in Charles Roland (ed.), *Health,*
   Disease and Medicine: Essays in Canadian History (Toronto: T.H. Best Printing
   Company, 1984) 129–30.

8 Cynthia R. Comacchio, *"Nations Are Built of Babies," Saving Ontario's Mothers*
   and Children, 1900–1940 (Montreal: McGill-Queen's University Press, 1993) 3.

9 David Naylor, *Private Practice, Public Payment: Canadian Medicine and the*
   Politics of Health Insurance (Montreal: McGill-Queen's University Press,
   1986).

10 Charles M. Godfrey, *Bruce: Surgeon, Soldier, Statesman, Sonofa* (Madoc:
    Codam, 2001) 9.

ENDNOTES

11 Robert Manion, *Life Is an Adventure* (Toronto: The Ryerson Press, 1936) 89; Shortt, "'Before the Age of Miracles,'" 136.

12 Richard Holmes, *Tommy: The British Soldier on the Western Front, 1914–1918* (London: HarperCollins, 2004) 483.

13 Carman Miller, *Painting the Map Red: Canada and the South African War, 1899–1902* (Montreal and Kingston: McGill-Queen's University Press, 1993) 110–22; Frank W. Schofield, "Anti-Typhoid Inoculation," *CMAJ* 5.12 (December 1915) 1070–75; Mitchell and Smith, *Medical Services. Casualties and Medical Statistics*, 270.

14 John W.S. McCullough, "Sanitation in War," *CMAJ* 9.9 (September 1919) 785.

15 W.H.B. Aikins, "The Medical Profession and the War," *CMAJ* 5 (1915).

16 Desmond Morton, *When Your Number's Up: The Canadian Soldier in the First World War* (Toronto: Random House of Canada Ltd., 1993) 71.

17 Herbert Rae, *Maple Leaves in Flanders Fields* (Toronto: William Briggs, 1916) 7.

18 Timothy Winegard, *For King and Kanata: Canadian Indians and the First World War* (Winnipeg: University of Manitoba Press, 2012).

19 Nic Clarke, *Unwanted Warriors: Rejected Volunteers of the Canadian Expeditionary Force* (Vancouver: UBC Press, 2015) 3. Also see David Silbey, "Bodies and Cultures Collide: Enlistment, the Medical Exam, and the British Working Class, 1914–1916," *Social History of Medicine* 17.1 (2004) 61–76.

20 James Marsh, "The 1885 Montreal Smallpox Epidemic," *The Canadian Encyclopedia*, online; and Michael Bliss, *Plague: A Story of Smallpox in Montreal* (Toronto: HarperCollins, 1991); and Katherine Arnup, "'Victims of Vaccination?' Opposition to Compulsory Immunization in Ontario, 1900–90," *Canadian Bulletin of Medical History* 9 (1992) 159–76.

21 Simon Walker, "The Greater Good: Agency and Inoculation in the British Army, 1914–18," *Canadian Bulletin of Medical History*, 36.1 (2019) 131–57.

22 Mark Harrison, *The Medical War: British Military Medicine in the First World War* (Oxford: Oxford University Press, 2010) 142–52; Ian R. Whitehead, *Doctors in the Great War* (Barnsley: Pen and Sword Military, 2013) 221–22.

23 J.G. Adami, *War Story of the Canadian Army Medical Corps* (London: Canadian War Records Office, 1918) 43.

24 Colonel George Adami, "Medicine and the War," *CMAJ* 10.10 (1920) 884.

25 Rae, *Maple Leaves in Flanders Fields*, 23–24.

26 "Compulsory Inoculation," *CMAJ* 5.3 (March 1915) 220.

27 For a discussion, see S.W. Hewetson, "National Defence and the Medical Profession," *CMAJ* 4.10 (October 1915) 886–89.

28 Quoted in Bill Rawling, *Death Thine Enemy: Canadian Medical Practitioners and War* (self-published, 2001) 51–52.

29 Kenneth Cameron, *No. 1 Canadian General Hospital, 1914–1919* (Sackville: The Tribune Press, 1938) 5.

30 Macphail, *The Medical Services*, 17.

31 Susan Mann, *Margaret Macdonald: Imperial Daughter* (Montreal: McGill-Queen's University Press, 2005) 74.

32 Cynthia Toman, *Sister Soldiers of the Great War: The Nurses of the Canadian Army Medical Corps* (Vancouver: UBC Press, 2016) 47–51.

33 Report of the Overseas Ministry, *Overseas Military Forces of Canada, 1918*, 403.

34 R.C. Fetherstonhaugh, *No. 3 Canadian General Hospital (McGill), 1914–1919* (Montreal: Gazette Printing, 1928) 6–7, 9.

35 Robin Glen Keirstead, "The Canadian Military Medical Experience during the Great War, 1914–1918," (Master's thesis: Queen's University, 1982) 31; *A History of No. 7 (Queen's) Canadian General Hospital* (London: C.W. Faulkner, n.d.) 4.

36 A.M. Jack Hyatt and Nancy Geddes Poole, *Battle for Life: The History of No. 10 Canadian Stationary Hospital and No. 10 Canadian General Hospital in Two World Wars* (Waterloo: Laurier Centre for Military Strategic and Disarmament Studies, 2004) 15.

37 Adami, *War Story of the C.A.M.C.*, 93.

38 George Nasmith, *On the Fringe of the Great Fight* (Toronto: McClelland, Goodchild & Stewart, 1917) 6.

39 Jeff Keshen, "The Great War Soldier as Nation Builder in Canada and Australia," in Briton C. Busch (ed.), *Canada and the Great War: Western Front Association Papers* (Montreal: McGill-Queen's University Press, 2003) 3–26; Tim Cook, "Documenting War & Forging Reputations: Sir Max Aitken and the Canadian War Records Office in the First World War," *War in History* 10.3 (2003) 265–95.

40 A.F. Duguid, *Official History of the Canadian Forces in the Great War 1914–1919, Volume 1* (Ottawa: J.O. Patenaude, 1938) 135–36.

41 W.D. Mathieson, *My Grandfather's War: Canadians Remember the First World War, 1914–1918* (Toronto: Macmillan, 1981) 34.

42 Harold Baldwin, *Holding the Line* (Chicago: A.C. McClurg, 1918) 36.

43 On training, see Andrew Iarocci, *Shoestring Soldiers: The 1st Canadian Division at War, 1914–1915* (Toronto: University of Toronto Press, 2008).

44 J. Clinton Morrison, Jr., *Hell upon Earth: A Personal Account of Prince Edward Island Soldiers in the Great War, 1914–1918* (P.E.I.: J. Clinton Morrison Jr., 1995) 28.

45 Daniel G. Dancocks, *Welcome to Flanders Fields* (Toronto: McClelland & Stewart, 1988) 63.

46 "A Letter from No. 1 General Hospital, CEF," *CMAJ* 5.6 (June 1915) 550–51.

47 LAC, RG 9, III-C-10, v. 4563, folder 3, file 3, Synopsis of Work Done by No. 1 General Hospital, CEF, n.d. [ca. February 1915].

48 Cameron, *History of No. 1 Canadian General Hospital*, 122; G.W.L. Nicholson, *Seventy Years of Service: A History of the Royal Canadian Army Medical Corps* (Ottawa : Borealis Press, 1977) 77; Duguid, *Official History*, 141.

49 Report of the Overseas Ministry, *Overseas Military Forces of Canada, 1918*, 382.

50 Arthur Hunt Chute, *The Real Front* (New York: Harper and Brothers Publishers, 1918).

51 Anonymous, "Meningitis in Camps," *CMAJ* 5 (1915) 225–27; Macphail, *The Medical Services*, 252–53.

52 Nasmith, *On the Fringe*, 20.

53 The casualty figures are unsettled, but see Ian Beckett, *Ypres: The First Battle, 1914* (London: Longmans, 2006) 466–68.

54 On casualties, Leo van Bergen, *Before My Helpless Sight: Suffering, Dying and Military Medicine on the Western Front, 1914–1918* (Surrey: Ashgate, 2009) 65.

55 Derek Linton, "Was Typhoid Inoculation Safe and Effective during World War I? Debates within German Military Medicine," *Journal of the History of Medicine and Allied Sciences* 55.2 (April 2000) 107–10; and Robert Engen, "Force Preservation: Medical Services," in Douglas Delaney and Serge Durflinger (eds.), *Capturing Hill 70: Canada's Forgotten Battle of the First World War* (Vancouver: UBC Press, 2016) 168.

56 van Bergen, *Before My Helpless Sight*, 23.

57 LAC, MG 30 E53, John Fotheringham papers, v. 4, folder 22, Foster to Kemp, 12 January 1918.

58 Anonymous, "Meningitis in Camps," *CMAJ* 5.3 (March 1915) 224.

CHAPTER 2

1 Canadian Bank of Commerce, *Letters from the Front: being a partial record of the part played by officers of the Bank in the Great European War, 1914–1919* (Toronto: Canadian Bank of Commerce, 1920) 9.

2 Ian R. Whitehead, *Doctors in the Great War* (Barnsley: Pen and Sword Military, 2013) 219.

3 Benoît Majerus, "War Losses (Belgium)," in *1914–1918-online. International Encyclopedia of the First World War*, issued by Freie Universität Berlin, Berlin 2016-01-25. DOI: 10.15463/ie1418.10812.

4 Diane Graves, *A Crown of Life: The World of John McCrae* (St. Catharines: Vanwell, 1997) 180.

5 Cook, *At the Sharp End,* 101.

6 LAC, RG 9, II-B-2, v. 3751, Diary of William M. Hart, 14 April 1915.

7 D.J. Goodspeed, *The Road Past Vimy: The Canadian Corps 1914–1918* (Toronto: General Paperbacks, 1969, 1987) 19.

8 John Swettenham, *McNaughton* (Toronto: Ryerson Press, 1968) 44–45.

9 Leo van Bergen, *Before My Helpless Sight: Suffering, Dying and Military Medicine on the Western Front, 1914–1918* (Surrey: Ashgate, 2009) 191.

10 LAC, RG 9, v. 4823, Report of Operations.

11 *Letters from the Front,* 10–11.

12 *Letters from the Front,* 15–16.

13 Harold Peat, *Private Peat* (New York: Grosset and Dunlap Publishers, 1917) 159.

14 Herbert Rae, *Maple Leaves in Flanders Fields* (Toronto: William Briggs, 1916) 164.

15 Andrew Macphail, *In Flanders Fields: and Other Poems* (Toronto: W. Briggs, 1919) 61.

16 Macphail, *In Flanders Fields: and Other Poems,* 73.

17 It was also called Shell Trap Farm. William F. Stewart, *The Embattled General: Sir Richard Turner and the First World War* (Montreal: McGill-Queen's University Press, 2015) 48.

18 Sir Andrew Macphail, *The Medical Services* (Ottawa: F.A. Acland, 1925) 193.

19 LAC, RG 9, III, v. 3751, Private War Diary of Captain P.G. Bell, 25 April 1915.

20 LAC, RG 9, v. 5027, War Diary of No. 3 Canadian Field Ambulance, 22 April 1915.

21 William Boyd, *With a Field Ambulance at Ypres* (Toronto: The Musson Book Company, 1916) 64.

22 F.G. Scott, *The Great War as I Saw It* (Ottawa: CEF Books, 2000) 38.

23 LAC, MG 30 E113, George Bell Papers, memoir, 27; see also Armine Norris, *Mainly for Mother* (Toronto: The Ryerson Press, 1919) 164.

24 The rifle became the object of a grim political battle and most Canadian units did not get rid of it until early 1916, when it was replaced with the British Lee-Enfield.

25 LAC, RG 9, II-B-2, v. 3751, F.A.C. Scrimger diary, 22 April 1915.

26 LAC, RG 9, II-B-2, v. 3751, F.A.C. Scrimger diary, 25 April 1915; Anonymous, "Captain F. A. C. Scrimger," *CMAJ* 6.4 (1916) 334–36.

27 Citation, *The London Gazette,* 22 June 1915.

28 LAC, RG 9, III, v.3751, Lt. Col. J.G. Adami's personal war diary, Appendix, "Notes of conversation with Major Gordon McLellan, late of 2nd Battalion, 20 August 1918."

29 LAC, MG 30 E321, William Johnson Papers, letter home, 3 May 1915.

30 Daniel Dancocks, *Welcome to Flanders Fields* (Toronto: McClelland & Stewart, 1988) 154.

31 G.W.L. Nicholson, *Canadian Expeditionary Force, 1914–1919* (Ottawa: Queen's Printer, 1964) 92. The most accurate breakdown of casualties is in Andrew Iarocci, *Shoestring Soldiers: The 1st Canadian Division at War, 1914–1915* (Toronto: University of Toronto Press, 2008) 180–85.

32 Major T.J. Mitchell and G.M. Smith, *Medical Services: Casualties and Medical Statistics of the Great War* (London: The Imperial War Museum, 1997 (original, 1931) 108. The percentage of total battle casualties: 14.17 were killed; 5.63 died of wounds; 5.39 were missing (and presumed killed); 6.5 were prisoners of war; and 68.31 were wounded.

33 Fiona Reid, *Medicine in First World War Europe: Soldiers, Medics, Pacifists* (London: Bloomsbury, 2017) 72–73.

34 Morrison, *Hell upon Earth*, 71–72.

35 LAC, RG 9, v. 3618, file 25-13-6, J.H. Elliot and Harold Murchinson Tovell, *The Effects of Poisonous Gases as Observed in Returning Soldiers* (December 1916).

36 A.F. Duguid, *Official History of the Canadian Forces in the Great War 1914–1919, Volume 1* (Ottawa: J.O. Patenaude, 1938) 851; LAC, RG 24, v. 1874, file 22(3), Second Ypres 1915 Casualties; Sir W.G. Macpherson et al., *Official History of the War: Medical Services Diseases of the War, Volume II* (London: 1923) 274; Tim Cook, *No Place to Run: The Canadian Corps and Gas Warfare in the First World War* (Vancouver: UBC Press, 1999) 32–34.

37 Tim Cook, "Forged in Fire," in Amanda Betts (ed.), *In Flanders Fields: 100 Years: Writing on War, Loss and Remembrance* (Toronto: Alfred A. Knopf, 2015) 43–50.

38 For the poem's legacy, see several articles in Amanda Betts (ed.), *In Flanders Fields: 100 Years.*

CHAPTER 3

1 CWM, MHRC, *The Listening Post* 1 (10 August 1915), n.p.

2 LAC, RG 24, v. 1820, file GAQ 5-11, Casualties, Canadian Division, Festubert.

3 Marjorie Barron Norris (ed.), *Medicine and Duty: The World War I Memoir of Captain Harold W. McGill, Medical Officer, 31st Battalion, C.E.F.* (University of Calgary Press, 2007) xvii.

4 Andrew Macphail, *The Medical Services: Official History of the Canadian Forces in the Great War 1914–19* (Ottawa: F.A. Acland; 1925) 127–28.

5 A. Mackenzie Forbes, "Number One Canadian General Hospital as a Part of the Canadian Medical Organization in France," *Canadian Medical Association Journal* 6.4 (April 1916) 295.

6 R.A.L., *Letters of a Canadian Stretcher Bearer* (Boston: Little, Brown, and Co., 1918) 55.

7 LAC, RG 9, III, v. 3751, personal diary of Major G.S. Strathy, 5 October 1917.

8 Macphail, *The Medical Services*, 131.

9 Norris (ed.), *Medicine and Duty*, 119. Also see Mark Harrison, *The Medical War: British Military Medicine in the First World War* (Oxford: Oxford University Press, 2010) 72.

10 LAC, RG 9, III, v. 3751, personal diary of P.G. Bell, 23 December 1914.

11 Macphail, *The Medical Services*, 247.

12 LAC, RG 9, III, v. 3751, file 2-1-1-2, Duties of officer in Medical Charge of a Unit [n.d.]; Great Britain, War Office, *Manual of Elementary Military Hygiene, 1912* (London: HMSO, 1912 [reprinted 1914]).

13 LAC, RG9, III-B-2, v. 3752, Measures for Prevention of Sickness, Canadian Troops, 8 December 1915.

14 See Cook, *At the Sharp End*, 231.

15 RG 9, v. 4542, 4/15, Conservancy in Trenches and Billets, 13 April 1916; Lawrence Burpee, "The Canadian Army Medical Corps," *Canada in the Great World War*, volume 6 (Toronto: United Publishers, 1921) 110–12.

16 CLIP, Charles Henry Savage, untitled memoir, n.p. [written in 1936].

17 E.G. Black, *I Want One Volunteer* (Toronto: Ryerson Press, 1965) 145.

18 *Letters from the Front*, 50.

19 Lance-Sergeant A.D. Peacock, *The Louse Problem at the Western Front* (1916) 16–17.

20 LAC, RG 9, III, v. 3745, Adami Papers, "Measures for the Prevention of Sickness Canadian Troops," December 1915, 1.

21 For a contemporary account, see Major W. Byam et al., *Trench Fever: A Louse-Borne Disease* (London: Henry Frowde, 1919); and for a modern exploration, R.L. Atenstaedt, "Trench Fever: The British Medical Response in the Great War," *Journal of the Royal Society of Medicine* 99.11 (November 2006) 564–68.

22 It is now known as *Bartonella quintana*. Kenneth Cameron, *No. 1 Canadian General Hospital, 1914–1919* (Sackville: The Tribune Press, 1938) 231.

23 Macphail, *The Medical Services*, 180.

24 Victor W. Wheeler, *The 50th Battalion in No Man's Land* (Ottawa: CEF Books, 2000) 216.

25 John S. Haller, Jr., "Trench Foot: A Study in Military–Medical Responsiveness in the Great War, 1914–1918," *Western Journal of Medicine* 152.6 (1990) 729–33.

26 F. McKelvey Bell, "Effects of Wet and Cold: Trench Feet," *CMAJ* 6.4 (1916) 289–94; "Trench Feet," *CMAJ* 6.4 (1916) 331–34.

27 LAC, RG 9, III, v. 3884, folder 30, file 8 [hereafter 30/8], G.155, from Corps Headquarters, 18 November 1915; and RG 9, III, v. 4551, Chilled Feet and Frostbite, 28 November 1915.

28 LAC, RG 9, III, v. 4040, file 2, 1st Canadian Division, AQ 23-1, [trench foot]; also see, RG 9, III, v. 4131, 10/1, 2nd Division to all units, A.1-17, 25 October 1916.

29 Macphail, *The Medical Services*, 265, 279.

30 Anonymous, "Venereal Prophylaxis among the Troops," *CMAJ* 15 (1915) 216.

31 Macphail, *The Medical Services*, 130.

32 LAC, MG 30 E113, George Bell papers, *Back to Blighty*, 113.

33 See Joanna Bourke, "'Swinging the Lead': Malingering, Australian Soldiers, and the Great War," *Journal of the Australian War Memorial* 26 (April 1995) 10–18.

34 LAC, RG 9, III-B-1, v. 2246, file A-5-30, pt. III, Report of Accident, Pte. G. Renaud, 1105202, 31 July 1918.

35 *The Listening Post* 29 (1 December 1917), no page numbers. Also see Tim Cook, "Anti-heroes of the Canadian Expeditionary Force," *Journal of the Canadian Historical Association* 19.1 (2008) 171–93.

36 *The Iodine Chronicle* 7 (10 May 1917) 7.

37 Norris (ed.), *Medicine and Duty*, 174. Also see Bruce Cane, *It Made You Think of Home: The Haunting Journal of Deward Barnes, Canadian Expeditionary Force, 1916–1919* (Toronto: The Dundurn Group, 2004) 140.

38 RG 9, v. 3751, personal diary of Major G.S. Strathy, Addendum, "Malingering or Scrimshanking, and Self-Inflicted Wounds."

39 For quote, see Robert Manion, *A Surgeon in Arms* (Toronto: McClelland, Goodchild, & Stewart, 1918) 107–8; also see Tim Cook, "'More as a Medicine Than a Beverage': 'Demon Rum' and the Canadian Trench Soldier in the First World War," *Canadian Military History* 9.1 (Winter 2000) 7–22.

40 Ian Whitehead, "Third Ypres—Casualties and British Medical Services: An Evaluation," in Peter H. Liddle (ed.), *Passchendaele in Perspective: The Third Battle of Ypres* (London: Pen & Sword, 1997) 179.

41 Manion, *Life Is an Adventure*, 107.

42 CLIP, James Fargey papers, letter to mother, 5 December 1915.

43 Macphail, *The Medical Services*, 250.

44 *The Listening Post* (October 1915) n.p.

45 Roger Cooter, "Malingering in Modernity: Psychological Scripts and Adversarial Encounters during the First World War," in Roger Cooter, Mark Harrison, and Steve Sturdy (eds.), *War, Medicine and Modernity* (Stroud, UK: Sutton, 1998) 130.

46 Manion, *A Surgeon in Arms*, 105.

CHAPTER 4

1 CLIP, Douglas George Buckley, letter, 1 November 1915.

2 D.J. Corrigall, *The History of the Twentieth Canadian Battalion* (Toronto: Stone and Cox, 1935) 131.

3 *Letters from the Front*, 155–56.

4 Tim Cook, *The Secret History of Soldiers: How Canadians Survived the Great War* (Toronto: Allen Lane, 2018) 10–20.

5 Lutz D.H. Sauerteig, "Sex, Medicine and Morality during the First World War," in Roger Cooter, Mark Harrison and Steve Sturdy (eds.), *War Medicine and Morality* (Stroud, UK: Sutton), 1998); Michelle K. Rhoades, "Renegotiating French Masculinity: Medicine and Venereal Disease during the Great War," *French Historical Studies* 29.2 (2006) 293–327.

6 J. George Adami, *The War Story of the Canadian Army Medical Corps, 1914–15* (Toronto: Canadian War Records Office, 1918) 63, 74–75.

7 Repeated in almost every Canadian history book, including by this author in previous works.

8 Michael Bliss, "'Pure Books on Avoided Subjects': Pre-Freudian Sexual Ideas in Canada," in S.E.D. Shortt (ed.), *Medicine in Canadian Society* (Montreal: McGill-Queen's University Press, 1981) 259.

9 Dianne Graves, *In the Company of Sisters: Canada's Women in the War Zone, 1914–1919* (Montreal: Robin Brass Studio, 2021) 215.

10 Lyndsay Rosenthal, "Venus in the Trenches: The Treatment of Venereal Disease in the Canadian Expeditionary Force, 1914–1919," (Ph.D. dissertation: Wilfrid Laurier University, 2018) 139.

11 "Venereal Prophylaxis among the Troops," *CMAJ* 5.3 (1915) 216–17.

12 For British policy, see David Simpson, "The Moral Battlefield: Venereal Disease and the British Army during the First World War" (Ph.D. dissertation: University of Iowa, 1998).

13 Jay Cassel, *The Secret Plague: Venereal Disease in Canada, 1838–1939* (Toronto: University of Toronto Press, 1987) 125–26.

14 LAC, RG 9, v. 5024, War Diary, DDMX, Canadian Corps, 17 January 1917; RG 9, III, v. 91, 10-12-22, Report on Venereal Diseases, 18 June 1917.

ENDNOTES

15 Desmond Morton, "A Canadian Soldier of the Great War: The Experiences of Frank Maheux," *Canadian Military History* 1.1 (1992) 82.

16 CWM, 19760148-061, "Facts for Fighters," 8, 11.

17 See Brent Brenyo, "Whatsoever a Man Soweth: Sex Education about Venereal Disease, Racial Health, and Social Hygiene during the First World War," *Canadian Military History* 27 (2018) 1–35.

18 LAC, RG 9, III, v. 4131, 10/1, Memorandum, Venereal Disease, 3 January 1918; RG 9, III, v. 3751, file 2-1-1-2, Duties of officer in Medical Charge of a Unit [n.d.].

19 RG 9, III, v. 91, 10-12-22, soldiers' conduct in England, Report on Venereal Diseases, 18 June 1917.

20 K. Craig Gibson, "'My Chief Source of Worry': An Assistant Provost Marshal's View of Relations between 2nd Canadian Division and Local Inhabitants on the Western Front, 1915–1917," *War in History* 7.4 (October 2000) 413–41.

21 "Venereal Prophylaxis among the Troops," *CMAJ* 5.3 (1915) 216–17.

22 LAC, RG 9, III, v. 4555, Memorandum, Venereal Disease, 27 January 1917; Colonel J.G. Adami, "The Policy of the Ostrich," *CMAJ* 4.4 (April 1919) 297.

23 K. Craig Gibson. "Sex and Soldiering in France and Flanders: The British Expeditionary Force Along the Western Front, 1914–1919," *The International History Review* 23.3 (September 2001) 543.

24 Macphail, *The Medical Services*, 274.

25 Joanna Bourke, *Dismembering the Male: Men's Bodies, Britain, and the Great War* (London: Reaktion, 1996) 85.

26 Kenneth Cameron, *No. 1 Canadian General Hospital, 1914–1919* (Sackville: The Tribune Press, 1938) 93; LAC, RG 9, III, v. 3740, History of the Canadian Special Hospital, Etchinghill [n.d.].

27 Adami, "The Policy of the Ostrich," 297; on nurses, see Toman, *Sister Soldiers of the Great War*, 115.

28 "Canadian Special Hospital, Etchinghill," *Bulletin of the Canadian Army Medical Corps* 1 (1918) 13; Cheryl Krasnick Warsh, *Moments of Unreason: The Practice of Canadian Psychiatry and the Homewood Retreat, 1883–1923* (Montreal: McGill-Queen's University Press, 1989) 60.

29 Rosenthal, "Venus in the Trenches," 16, 169. There were at least fifty British deaths linked to treatment. Also see Macpherson, *Diseases of the War*, 141–42.

30 Macphail, *The Medical Services*, 293; Cassell, *The Secret Plague*, 123; Alexia Moncrieff, *Expertise, Authority and Control: The Australian Army Medical Corps in the First World War* (Cambridge: Cambridge University Press, 2020) 141–42.

31 Martha Hanna, *Anxious Days and Tearful Nights: Canadian War Wives during the Great War* (Montreal: McGill-Queen's University Press, 2020).

32 Brenyo, "Whatsoever a Man Soweth," 9–10; also see *Canadian House of Commons Debates*, 1917, 4059–61.

33 Colonel George Adami, "Medicine and the War," *CMAJ* 10.10 (1920) 896.

34 LAC, RG 9, III, v. 3718, Report on Etchinghill, 20 December 1917; "The Venereal Disease Problem," *Canada Lancet* 52.1 (September 1918) 10–11. The Australians followed a similar trajectory, see Raden Dunbar, *The Secrets of the Anzacs: The Untold Story of Venereal Disease in the Australian Army, 1914–1919* (London: Scribe Publication, 2014).

35 "Venereal Prophylaxis among the Troops," *CMAJ* 5.3 (1915) 216–17.

36 CWM, 19801226-276, 58A 1 60.5, Assistant Director of Medical Services of 3rd Canadian Division, 10 February 1918; Clare Makepeace, "Male Heterosexuality and Prostitution during the Great War," *Cultural and Social History* 9.1 (2012) 65–83.

37 Victor N. Swanston, *Who Said War Is Hell!* (Self-published, 1983) 47.

38 Bill Freeman and Richard Nielsen, *Far from Home: Canadians in the First World War* (Toronto: McGraw-Hill, 1999) 134–35.

39 Morton, *When Your Number's Up*, 200; Harrison, *The Medical War*, 157; Cassel, *The Secret Plague*, 126.

40 Van Bergen, *Before My Helpless Sight*, 149.

41 LAC, RG 9, III, v. 91, 10-12-22, G.L. Foster, Report on Venereal Diseases, 18 June 1917.

42 Canada Commission of Conservation, *Report of the Tenth Annual Meeting: Held at Ottawa—February 17, 1919* (Ottawa: Canada Commission of Conservation, 1919) 201.

43 Cameron, *No. 1 Canadian General Hospital*, 135.

CHAPTER 5

1 LAC, RG 9, III, v. 5034, War Diary of Matron, 2 Canadian General Hospital, 2 July 1916.

2 Canadian Bank of Commerce, *Letters from the Front*, 142.

3 Canadian Bank of Commerce, *Letters from the Front*, 46.

4 CWM, 20090121-004, Charles Clarke, *One Man's Warfare* (n.d.) 61.

5 CLIP, letter, Charles Willoughby, letter, 29 June 1918.

6 LAC, RG 9, III, v. 4089, folder 19, file 3, Medical Arrangements, Defence Scheme, 1st Canadian Division, 5 November 1916.

7 Morrison, *Hell upon Earth*, 208.

8 For an overview of the Somme, see Robin Prior and Trevor Wilson, *The Somme* (New Haven: Yale University Press, 2005).

9 CLIP, Charles Henry Savage, memoir, n.d. [1936].

10 Morrison, *Hell upon Earth*, 94–95.

11 Louis Keene, *Crumps, The Plain Story of a Canadian Who Went* (Boston: Houghton, 1917) 95.

12 Lt-Colonel E.J. Williams, "Gunshot Wounds of the Present War," *CMAJ* 6.12 (1916) 1057.

13 R.A.L., *Letters of a Canadian Stretcher Bearer* (Boston: Little, and Brown, 1918) December 1916.

14 Morrison, *Hell upon Earth*, 207.

15 R.A.L., *Letters of a Canadian Stretcher Bearer*, 3 March 1917.

16 Scotland and Heys, *War Surgery 1914–18*, 64.

17 Mark Harrison, *The Medical War: British Military Medicine in the First World War* (Oxford: Oxford University Press, 2010) 71–72.

18 LAC, RG 150, Books of Soldiers Killed in the CEF, Henry Ruddock.

19 William D. Mathieson, *My Grandfather's War: Canadians Remember the First World War, 1914–1918* (Toronto: Macmillan, 1981) 137.

20 LAC, RG 9, III-B-2, v. 3751, Personal diary of Major G.S. Strathy, 16 June 1916.

21 Norman Miles Guiou, *Transfusion: A Canadian Surgeon's Story in War and in Peace* (Nova Scotia: Sentinel Printing Ltd, 1985) 47.

22 Tim Cook, "The Politics of Surrender: Canadian Soldiers and the Killing of Prisoners in the Great War," *Journal of Military History* 70.3 (July 2006) 637–65.

23 LAC, RG 9, III, v. 4715, folder 107, file 20, No. 10 Canadian Field Ambulance, Mobilization, 12 January 1916; and War Office, *Royal Army Medical Corps Training* (London: Hist Majesty's Stationery Office, 1911 [reproduced 1915]).

24 R.A.L., *Letters of a Canadian Stretcher Bearer*, 70.

25 Frederick Noyes, *Stretcher Bearer . . . at the Double!* (Toronto: Hunter-Rose, 1937) 124.

26 Percy G. Bell, "Notes on Special Work in a Field Ambulance," *CMAJ* 6.12 (1916) 1091; Manion, *A Surgeon in Arms*, 134–35.

27 LAC, War Diary, Number 4 Canadian Field Ambulance, 14–15 September 1916.

28 CLIP, Charles Henry Savage, memoir, n.p., [1936].

29 Macphail, *The Medical Services*, 87.

30 Mathieson, *My Grandfather's War*, 138.

31 CLIP, Harry Morris, letter, 5 April 1917.

32 CWM, MHRC, CBC *Flanders Fields*, episode 8, page 22.

33 William F. Stewart, *The Canadians on the Somme, 1916. Canada's Neglected Campaign* (Solihull: Helion, 2017) Table C.7 Death by Arm/Branch.

34 Morrison, *Hell upon Earth*, 102.

35 Deborah Cowley (ed.), *Georges Vanier: Soldier, The Wartime Letters and Diaries, 1915–1919* (Toronto: Dundurn Press, 2000) 112.

36 Stewart, *Canadians on the Somme*, 290.

37 See LAC, MG 30 E379, Hubert Morris papers, war diary, 16 September 1916; O.C.S. Wallace (ed.), *From Montreal to Vimy Ridge and Beyond: The Correspondence of Lieut. Clifford Almon Wells, B.A. of the 8th Battalion, Canadians, B.E.F. November, 1915–April 1917* (Toronto: McClelland, Goodchild and Stewart, 1917) 271.

CHAPTER 6

1 J.M. Elder, "Notes from the McGill General Hospital," *CMAJ* 6 (1916) 494.

2 George Armstrong, "Influence of War on Surgery," *CMAJ* 9 (1919) 399.

3 See Aaron Taylor Miedema, *Bayonets and Blobsticks: The Canadian Experience of Close Combat, 1915–1918* (Kingston: Legacy Books Press, 2011).

4 H.E. Munroe, "Remarks on the Character and Treatment of Wounds in War," *CMAJ* 5.11 (1915) 962; also see R.D. Rudolf, "Boulogne in War Time," *CMAJ* 5.3 (March 1915) 257.

5 T.J. Mitchell and G.M. Smith, *History of the Great War based on Official Documents. Medical Services. Casualties and Medical Statistics* (London: HMSO, 1931) 40.

6 Paul Cornish, "Unlawful Wounding: Codifying Interaction between Bullets and Bodies," in Paul Cornish and Nicholas J. Saunders (eds.), *Bodies in Conflict: Corporeality, Materiality and Transformation* (London: Routledge, 2013) 12–13.

7 Major Edward Archibald, "A Brief Survey of Some Experiences in the Surgery of the Present War," *CMAJ* 6 (1916) 781.

8 Archibald, "A Brief Survey of Some Experiences," 791.

9 Munroe, "Remarks on the Character and Treatment of Wounds," 963.

10 Black, *I Want One Volunteer*, 66.

11 Lt-Colonel E.J. Williams, "Gunshot Wounds of the Present War," *CMAJ* 6.12 (1916) 1056–57.

12 Canadian Bank of Commerce, *Letters from the Front*, 262.

13 Captain Donald Hingston, "Notes on War Surgery," *CMAJ* 7.4 (April 1917) 308.

14 Harvey Cushing, *From a Surgeon's Journal, 1915–1918* (Toronto: McClelland and Stewart, 1936) 176.

15 Tom Scotland, *A Time to Die and a Time to Live* (Warwick: Helion, 1919) 44.

16 J.A. Gunn, "Lessons from War Surgery," *CMAJ* 10.4 (1920) 354; Ian R. Whitehead, *Doctors in the Great War* (Barnsley: Leo Cooper, 1999) 205.

17 Wilmot Herrington, *A Physician in France* (London: Edward Arnold, 1919) 78–79.

18 H.H. Hepburn, "Notes on Tetanus," *CMAJ* 12.5 (May 1922) 312–15; Colonel A. Primross, "War Activities in Medicine and Surgery," *CMAJ* 9.9 (1919) 5.

19 Frederick A. Pottle, *Stretchers: The Story of a Hospital Unit on the Western Front* (New Haven: Yale University Press, 1929) 138–39.

20 Robin Glen Keirstead, "The Canadian Military Medical Experience during the Great War, 1914–1918" (Master's thesis: Queen's University, 1982) 118.

21 Sir W.G. Macpherson (ed.), *Medical Services Pathology* (London: His Majesty's Stationery Office, 1923) 35.

22 Toman, *Sister Soldiers of the Great War*, 121–22.

23 Anonymous, "War Wounds—The Prevalence of Infection—Treatment," *CMAJ* 5 (1915) 717.

24 Pottle, *Stretchers*, 109–10.

25 Boyd, *Field Ambulance at Ypres*, 26.

26 Archibald, "A Brief Survey," 775.

27 Archibald, "A Brief Survey," 778.

28 Archibald, "A Brief Survey," 778.

29 Bell, "Notes on Special Work in a Field Ambulance," 1094.

30 T.A. Malloch, "War Notes, II," *CMAJ* 5.4 (1915) 362; also see Major H.E. Clutterbuck, "The Causes of Death in Men Who Died from Gunshot Wounds of the Abdomen," *CMAJ* 10 (1920) 428.

31 CLIP, Alfred Andrews, diary, 10 April 1916.

32 Archibald, "A Brief Survey," 782.

33 Lieutenant Colonel N.B. Gwyn and Major H.E. MacDermot, "Wounds of the Chest," *CMAJ* 10 (1920) 62.

34 Harrison, *The Medical War*, 102.

35 Major Edward Archibald, "Abdominal Wounds as seen at a Casualty Clearing Station," *CMAJ* 7.4 (1917) 303.

36 William Hutchinson, "A Study of Four Hundred and Fifty Cases of Wounds of the Chest, with Special Reference to a New Method of Treatment for Infected Hæmothorax," *CMAJ* 8.11 (1918) 972–87; Robert Rudolf, "Boulogne in War Time," *CMAJ* 5 (1915) 257.

37 Hutchinson, "A Study of Four Hundred and Fifty Cases of Wounds of the Chest," 986–87.

38 CLIP, Cobourg World, Paul Skidmore to mother, 28 May 1915.

39 Harrison, *The Medical War*, 102.

40 Major T.J. Mitchell and G.M. Smith, *Medical Services: Casualties and Medical Statistics of the Great War* (London: The Imperial War Museum, 1997 (original, 1931) 17.

41 CLIP, Archibald MacKinnon, letter, 19 October 1916.

42 A.H. Pirie, "Shrapnel Balls. Their X-ray Characteristics, Compared with Bullets and Other Foreign Bodies," *CMAJ* 7.9 (1917) 780.

43 P.M. Robinson and M.J. O'Meara, "The Thomas Splint: Its Origins and Use in Trauma," *The Journal of Bone and Joint Surgery* 91 (April 2009) 540–44.

44 R.A.L., *Letters of a Canadian Stretcher Bearer*, 64.

45 Fetherstonaugh, *No. 3 Hospital (McGill)*, 36–37, 95.

46 Pirie, "Shrapnel Balls," 778.

47 Morton, *When Your Number's Up*, 193; Macphail, *The Medical Services*, 393–94.

48 Macphail, *The Medical Services*, 248. Across the BEF, the RAMC dealt with 1,989,060 casualties in France and Flanders, of which 151,356 died. This is a 7.6% death rate. Scotland and Heys (eds.), *War Surgery 1914–18*, 47.

49 Mitchell and Smith, *Medical Services: Casualties and Medical Statistics of the Great War*, preface.

50 Gunn, "Lessons from War Surgery," 355.

51 George Armstrong, "Influence of War on Surgery," *CMAJ* 9.9 (1919) 403.

CHAPTER 7

1 All information drawn from his personnel file, which is digitized on the Library Archives of Canada site, like most members of the CEF. Private George Gibson, 148282.

2 LAC, RG 9, III, v. 3604, file 24-4-0, pt. I, WOC. 2344, G. Gibson, Pte, No. 148282.

3 Silvia Cavicchioli and Luigi Provero, *Public Uses of Human Remains and Relics in History* (New York: Taylor Francis, 2020); and Tinnie Claes, *Corpses in Belgian Anatomy, 1860-1914: Nobody's Dead* (Cham: Palgrave, 2019).

4 S.J.M.M, *Morbid Curiosities: Medical Museums in Nineteenth-Century Britain* (Oxford: Oxford University Press, 2011); and Elizabeth Hallam, *Anatomy Museum: Death and the Body Displayed* (London: Reaktion, 2016).

5 See Michael Bliss, *William Osler: A Life in Medicine* (Toronto: University of Toronto Press, 1999); and Elizabeth T. Hurren, *Dying for Victorian Medicine: English Anatomy and Its Trade in the Dead Poor, c.1834-1929* (Houndsmill: Palgrave Macmillan, 2012).

6 Scott Belyea, "A Century of Grave-Robbing in Kingston, Ontario," *Ontario History* 108.1 (2016) 24–42; David Marshall, "'Death Abolished': Changing

Attitudes to Death and the Afterlife in Nineteenth Century Canadian Protestantism," in Norman Knowles (ed.), *Age of Transition: Readings in Canadian Social History, 1800–1900* (Toronto: Harcourt Brace Canada, 1998); and Suzie Lennox, *Bodysnatchers: Digging up the Untold Stories of Britain's Resurrection Men* (Barnsley: Pen and Sword History, 2016).

7 Maude E. Abbott, "The Pathological Collections of the Late Sir William Osler and His Relations with the Medical Museum of McGill University," *CMAJ* 10 (1920) 91–102.

8 "Maude Abbott," Maude Abbott Medical Museum, McGill: https://www .mcgill.ca/medicalmuseum/introduction/history/physicians/abbott; also see Douglas Waugh, *Maudie of McGill: Dr. Maude Abbott and the Foundations of Heart Surgery* (Oxford: Dundurn Press, 1992).

9 Humphry Rolleston, "John George Adami, C.B.E., M.D., F.R.S., F.R.C.P., F.R.C.S., Hon. D.Sc., LL.D," *British Medical Journal* (11 September 1926) 2 (3427) 507–10.

10 Editorial, "Lieutenant-Colonel John McCrae, B.A., M.B., M.R.C.P.," *CMAJ* 8.3 (March 1963) 246.

11 CEF personnel file, https://central.bac-lac.gc.ca/. item/?op=pdf&app=CEF&id=B0021-S023.

12 On Adami's role, see W.G. Macpherson, *Medical Services: General History*, volume 1 (London: H.M. Stationery, 1921) viii.

13 Thomas Scotland and Steven Heys (eds.), *War Surgery 1914–18* (Solihull: Helion, 2012) 47–48.

14 Scotland and Heys (eds.), *War Surgery 1914–18*, 64.

15 Macphail, *The Medical Services*, 311–15; and Sir W.G. Macpherson (ed.), *Medical Services Pathology* (London: His Majesty's Stationery Office, 1923) 574–75.

16 LAC, RG 9, III, v. 3604, file 24-4-0, pt. 1, Circular Memorandum, 121/Medical/329, 19 April 1915.

17 LAC, RG 9, III, v. 3604, file 24-4-0, pt. 1, J.G. Adami and E.L. Judah, The Preservation of War Material for Museum Purposes.

18 Arthur Keith, *An Autobiography* (London: Watts, 1950).

19 Royal College of Surgeons, History of John Hunter, https://www.rcseng.ac.uk /museums-and-archives/hunterian-museum/about-us/john-hunter.

20 Samuel J.M.M. Alberti, "The 'Regiment of Skeletons': A First World War Medical Collection," *Social History of Medicine* 28.1 (2015) 112–13.

21 Frederic Manning, *Her Privates We* (London, 1986, original 1929) 205.

22 Morrison, *Hell upon Earth*, 72.

23 LAC, RG 9, III, v. 3604, file 24-4-0, pt. 1, Memorandum re Pathological Specimens, 11 October 1915; Alberti, "The 'Regiment of Skeletons,'" 113.

24 RG 9, III, v. 3604, file 24-4-0, pt. 1, Lt. Col. ADMS to the Chief Paymaster, Canadian Contingents, 22 December 1915; LAC, RG 9, III, v. 3604, file 24-4-0, pt. 1, War Office, 121/Medical/329 (AMD 2) 13 December 1915; LAC, RG 9, III, v.3751, Lt. Col. J.G. Adami's personal war diary, 23 October 1915.

25 LAC, RG 9, III-C-10, v.4568, 12/1, Adami to No. 2 Canadian General Hospital, 23 December 1915; LAC, RG 9, III, v.3751, Lt. Col. J.G. Adami's personal war diary, 27 November 1915.

26 LAC, RG 9, III, v. 3604, file 24-4-0, pt. 1, Lt. Col. ADMS, Canadian Contingents, to Captain J.J. Ower, CAMC, No. 1 Canadian General Hospital, 23 November 1915.

27 Sean Dyde, "The Chief Seat of Mischief: Soldier's Heart in the First World War," *Journal of the History of Medicine and Allied Sciences* 66.2 (2011) 216–48; LAC, RG 9, III, v. 3604, file 24-4-0, pt. 1, Lt. Col ADMS to No. 1 Canadian Stationary Hospital, Mediterranean, 23 December 1915.

28 LAC, RG 9, III, v. 3604, file 24-4-0, pt. II, Adami to Auld, 8 December 1917; RG 9, III, v. 3604, file 24-4-0, pt. 1, Adami to J.J. Ower, 16 April 1917.

29 On Mount Sorrel, see Cook, *At the Sharp End*, 343–79; on the quote, LAC, RG 9, III, v. 3604, file 24-4-0, pt. 1, Adami to No. 5 Canadian Mobile Laboratory, 14 June 1916.

30 LAC, RG 9, III, v. 3604, file 24-4-0, pt. 1, Lt. Col. ADMS [Adami] to Elliot, 18 January 1916; and Elliot to Adami, 23 February 1916.

31 Kenneth Cameron, *No. 1 Canadian General Hospital, 1914–1919* (Sackville: The Tribune Press, 1938) 215; LAC, RG 9, III, v. 3604, file 24-4-0, pt. 1, War Office, 121/Medical/329 (AMD 2) 13 December 1915; LAC, RG 9, III-C-10, v.4571, 5/6, Medical Society, Minutes of Meetings, 3rd Can. Gen. Hosp.

32 "The Clinical Society at No. 1 Canadian General Hospital," in *Bulletin of the Canadian Army Medical Corps*, v. 1, (1918) 14–15.

33 Cameron, *No. 1 Canadian General Hospital*, 345.

34 Jean-Jaques Ferrandis, "Les collections anatomiques realises durant la guerre de 1914–1918 au muse du Service de santé des armées," *Histoire des Sciences Médicales* 38 (2004) 233–42; Amy Lyford, "The Aesthetics of Dismemberment: Surrealism and the Musée du Val-de-Grâce in 1917," *Cultural Critique* 46 (2000) 45–79. For a Canadian view of the French museum with its pathological collection, see LAC, RG 9, III-B-2, v.3604, file 24-3-4 to 24-3-12, Primross to A.M.D.D., Museum de Val de Grace, 27 November 1917.

35 Cay-Rudiger Prüll, "Pathology at War 1914–1918: Germany and Britain in Comparison," in Roger Cooter, Mark Harrison and Steve Sturdy (eds.), *Medicine and Modern Warfare* (Amsterdam: Rodopi, 1999) 131–61.

36 Tim Cook, "Black-hearted Traitors, Crucified Martyrs, and the Leaning Virgin: The Role of Rumor and the Great War Canadian Soldier," in Michael Neiberg and Jennifer Keene (ed.), *Finding Common Ground: New Directions in First World War Studies* (Leiden: Brill Academic Publishers, 2010) 21–42.

37 Arthur Keith and M.E. Hall, "Bones Showing the Effects of Gunshot Injuries, in the Army Medical Collection Now on Exhibition in the Museum of the Royal College of Surgeons of England," *British Journal of Surgery* 6 (1918) 537.

38 Keith and Hall, "Bones Showing the Effects of Gunshot Injuries," 537.

39 "The Army Medical Collection of War Specimens at the Royal College of Surgeons of England," *British Medical Journal* 2.2964 (1917) 532.

40 L.J. Rhea, "Method Used in the Army Zone for the Preparation of Bone Lesions Resulting from the Injuries of War," *Bulletin of the International Association of Medical Museums* 8 (1922) 4–48.

41 Fetherstonaugh, *No. 3 Hospital (McGill)*, 52, 163.

42 LAC, RG 9, III, v. 3604, file 24-4-0, pt. 1, Adami to Osler, 3 August 1918.

43 Macphail, *The Medical Services*, 313.

44 LAC, RG 9, III, v. 3604, file 24-4-0, pt. 1, Memorandum re disposal of pathological Specimens, n.d. [ca. December 1915].

45 See Shauna Devine, *Learning from the Wounded: The Civil War and the Rise of American Medical Science* (Chapel Hill: University of North Carolina Press, 2014).

46 LAC, RG 9, III, v. 3604, file 24-4-0, pt. 1, Surgeon-General, Director of Medical Services to Secretary, Militia Council, Department of Militia and Defence, 4 January 1916.

47 LAC, RG 9, III, v. 3604, file 24-4-0, pt. 1, Surgeon-General, Director of Medical Services to Secretary, Militia Council, Department of Militia and Defence, 15 January 1916.

48 LAC, Records of the Department of External Affairs (hereafter RG 25), v. 259, file P-3-19, Order-in-Council 3117, 6 January 1915.

49 See Tim Cook, "Immortalizing the Canadian Soldier: Lord Beaverbrook, the Canadian War Records Office in the First World War," in Briton Busch (ed.), *Canada and the Great War: Western Front Association papers* (Montreal and Kingston: McGill-Queen's University Press, 2003) 46–65.

50 LAC, RG 9, v. 4746, 175/1, CWRO, Report, 11 January 1917. Also see Peter Robertson, *Relentless Verity: Canadian Military Photographers since 1885* (University of Toronto Press, 1972); Robert McIntosh, "The Great War, Archives and Modern Memory," *Archivaria* 46 (Fall 1998) 1–31; Maria Tippett, *Art at the Service of War: Canada, Art and the Great War* (University of Toronto Press, 1984); Tim Cook, "Canada's Great War on Film: *Lest We Forget* (1935)," *Canadian Military History* 14.3 (Summer 2005) 5–20.

51 LAC, RG 9, III, v. 3604, file 24-4-0, pt. 1, W.E. Hodgins to the Adjutant-General and the Medical Services, 13 March 1916; LAC, RG 9, III, v. 3604, file 24-4-0, pt. 1, Surgeon General to Militia Council, 3 April 1916.

52 LAC, MG 30 E400, Claude Vivian Williams papers, letter, 18 November 1916.

CHAPTER 8

1 CWM, 20040015-005, letter, 20 June 1917.

2 Lord Moran, *Anatomy of Courage* (New York: Avery, 1987) 3.

3 Tracey Loughran, "A Crisis of Masculinity? Re-writing the History of Shell-Shock and Gender in First World War Britain," *History Compass* 11.9 (2013) 727–738; Mark Humphries, "War's Long Shadow: Masculinity, Medicine, and the Gendered Politics of Trauma, 1914–1939," *Canadian Historical Review* 91.3 (2010) 503–31.

4 Colin Russel, "A Study of Certain Psychogenetic Conditions among Soldiers," *CMAJ* 7 (1917) 712.

5 Victor Wheeler, *The 50th Battalion in No Man's Land* (Ottawa: CEF Books, 2000) 55.

6 Black, *I Want One Volunteer*, 82.

7 CLIP, Charles Henry Savage, memoir, n.p. [1936].

8 Coningsby Dawson, *The Glory of the Trenches* (New York: John Lane Company, 1918) 32.

9 CWM, 20000013-001, George Ormsby, letter, 4 October 1916.

10 War Office, Report of the War Office Committee of Enquiry into "Shell Shock," (London: HMSO, 1922) 123.

11 LAC, MG 30 E53, John T. Fotheringham collection, v. 4, file 21, diary, 16 February 1916.

12 Lieutenant-Colonel John McCombe and Captain A.F. Menzies, *Medical Service at the Front* (New York: Lea and Febiger, 1918) 29. Also see Colonel J. Edward Squire, *Medical Hints for the Use of Medical Officers Temporarily Employed with Troops* (London: Hodder and Stoughton, 1915) 10–11.

13 Patrick Brennan, "'Completely Worn Out by Service in France': Combat Stress and Breakdown among Senior Officers in the Canadian Corps," *Canadian Military History* 18.2 (Spring 2009) 5.

14 LAC, RG 24, v. 1844, file GAQ 11-11-E, Major J.P.S. Cathcart, "Group A21—Neurasthenia, Shell Shock and Hysteria Admissions Corresponded to Date of Admission by Months."

15 George Nasmith, *Canada's Sons in the World War* (Toronto: John C. Winston, 1919) 116.

16 See Diane Graves, *A Crown of Life: The World of John McCrae* (St. Catharines: Vanwell, 1997); and Cook, "Forged in Fire," 48.

17 LAC, RG 24, v. 1844, file GAQ 11-11-E, Epidemic Shell Shock: 1st Division, June 1916—Hill 60, Mount Sorrel.

18 Marjorie Barron Norris, ed., *Medicine and Duty: The World War I Memoir of Captain Harold W. McGill, Medical Officer, 31st Battalion C.E.F* (Calgary: University of Calgary Press, 2007) 172.

19 Gordon Reid, *Poor Bloody Murder* (Oakville: Mosaic Press, 1980) 172.

20 See Leonard Smith, *The Embattled Self: French Soldiers' Testimony of the Great War* (Ithaca: Cornell University Press, 2007) and Alexander Watson, *Enduring the Great War: Combat, Morale and Collapse in the German and British Armies, 1914–1918* (Cambridge: Cambridge University Press, 2008).

21 Rawling, *Death Thine Enemy*, 68.

22 Captain Edward Ryan, "A Case of Shell Shock," *CMAJ* 6.12 (December 1916) 1095–99.

23 See, for instance, Edward Shorter, *A History of Psychiatry: From the Era of the Asylum to the Age of Prozac* (New York: Wiley, 1997).

24 Mark Osborne Humphries and Kellen Kurchinski, "Rest, Relax and Get Well: A Reconceptualization of Great War Shell Shock Treatment," *War and Society* 27. 2 (October 2008) 89–90. Also see, Fiona Reid, *Broken Men: Shell Shock, Treatment and Recovery in Britain 1914– 1930* (London: Continuum, 2010).

25 Canadian Bank of Commerce, *Letters from the Front*, 223.

26 Morrison, *Hell upon Earth*, 204–5.

27 Macphail, *The Medical Services*, 274.

28 Mark Osborne Humphries, *A Weary Road: Shell Shock in the Canadian Expeditionary Force, 1914–1918* (Toronto: University of Toronto Press, 2018) 150.

29 Captain H.P. Wright, CAMC, "Suggestions for a Further Classification of Cases of So Called Shell Shock," *Canadian Medical Association Journal* 7.7 (July 1917) 629–35.

30 War Office, *Report of the War Office Committee of Enquiry into "Shell Shock,"* 17–18.

31 Caroline Alexander, "The Shock of War," *Smithsonian Magazine* (September 2010) online. Also see, Lewis Ralph Yealland, *Hysterical Disorders of Warfare* (London: MacMillan, 1918).

32 Tom Brown, "Shell Shock and the Canadian Expeditionary Force, 1914–18: Canadian Psychiatry in the Great War," in Charles Roland (ed.), *Health, Disease and Medicine: Essays in Canadian History* (Toronto: Hannah Institute, 1983) 319.

33 LAC, RG 9, III, v. 4162, 8/10, 1st Division to all units, A-25-91, 8 November 1916.

34 LAC, RG 9, III, v. 4162, 8/10, 1st Division to all units, A-25-91, 8 November 1916.

35 Humphries, *A Weary Road*, 184–96.

36 LAC, RG 9, III, v. 3752, file 3-1-4-2, Treatment of Shell Shock Cases at the Front. Also see Tracey Loughran, "Shell Shock, Trauma, and the First World War: The Making of a Diagnosis and Its Histories," *Social History of Medicine* 22. 1 (2009) 83–88.

37 LAC, RG 9, III, v. 916, 63-3, ADMS, circular, Shell Shock, 21 February 1917.

38 Tom Brown, "Shell Shock in the Canadian Expeditionary Force," 318–19; Rawling, *Death Thine Enemy*, 99. For other claimed success rates, see Ben Shephard, *War of Nerves: Soldiers and Psychiatrists, 1914–1994* (London: Pimlico, 2002) 60–62.

39 A.O. Hickson, *As It Was Then* (Wolfville: Acadia University, 1988) 70–71.

40 Manion, *A Surgeon in Arms*, 164.

41 Thaddeus Hoyt Ames, "The Prevention of War Neuroses," *CMAJ* 8 (1918) 1022.

42 For the evolution of treatment, see Humphries, *A Weary Road*.

43 Humphries, "In the Shadow," 513; van Bergen, *Before My Helpless Sight*, 241.

CHAPTER 9

1 Kate Wilson, *Lights Out!* (Ottawa: CEF Books, 2004) 77.

2 The best synthesis is Robin Prior, *Gallipoli: The End of the Myth* (New Haven: Yale University Press, 2010).

3 Richard Cramm, *The First Five Hundred of the Royal Newfoundland Regiment* (St. Philips, NFLD: Boulder Publishing, 2015) 36–37.

4 See Tim Cook and Mark Humphries, "The Forgotten Campaign: Newfoundland at Gallipoli," *Canadian Military History* 27.1 (2018) 1–39.

5 On disease, see Lieut.-Col. E.J. Williams, "Malaria in the Army," *CMAJ* 8.6 (June 1918) 523–29.

6 For a good introduction, see Loukianos Hassiotis, "Greece," in *1914–1918-online. International Encyclopedia of the First World War*; and David Dutton, *The Politics of Diplomacy: Britain and France in the Balkans in the First World War* (London: I.B. Tauris, 1998).

7 Alexia Moncrieff, *Expertise, Authority and Control: The Australian Army Medical Corps in the First World War* (Cambridge: Cambridge University Press, 2020) 19.

8 Constance Bruce, *Humour in Tragedy: Hospital Life Behind 3 Fronts* (London: Skeffington, 1919) 23.

9   Mabel Clint, *Our Bit: Memories of War Service by a Canadian Nursing Sister* (Montreal: The Royal Victoria Hospital, 1934) 62.

10 LAC, Laura Gamble collection, digitized diary, 17 November 1915.

11 Mackenzie, *No. 4 Canadian Hospital*, 68.

12 Clint, *Our Bit*, 59–60.

13 Michael Tyquin, *Gallipoli, The Medical War* (1993); Nicholson, *The Fighting Newfoundlander*, 181, 183.

14 Wilson-Simmie, *Lights Out*, 94.

15 Lester B. Pearson, *Mike: The Memoirs of the Right Honourable Lester B. Pearson*, volume 1 (Toronto, 1972) 25. On typhoid, see J.J. Mackenzie, *Number 4 Canadian Hospital*, 129.

16 Nicholson, *Canadian Expeditionary Force*, 498.

17 See Tim Cook, *The Madman and the Butcher: The Sensational Wars of Sam Hughes and General Arthur Currie* (Toronto: Allan Lane, 2010) 30–31.

18 William Boyd, *With a Field Ambulance at Ypres* (Toronto: The Musson Book, Company, 1916) 43; Duguid, *Official History*, 164.

19 For an overview, see Maj-Gen Jean-Robert Bernier and Lt-Col Vivian C. McAlister, "The Canadian Army Medical Corps Affair of 1916 and Surgeon General Guy Carleton Jones," *Canadian Journal of Surgery* 61.2 (2018) 85–87.

20 LAC, MG 30 E3, Babtie Papers, v. 1, *Report on the Canadian Army Medical Service by Colonel Herbert A. Bruce*

21 Morton, *When Your Number's Up*, 203.

22 Nic Clarke, *Unwanted Warriors: Rejected Volunteers of the Canadian Expeditionary Force* (Vancouver: UBC Press, 2015) 52.

23 Richard Holt, *Filling the Ranks: Manpower in the Canadian Expeditionary Force, 1914–1918* (Montreal: McGill-Queen's University Press, 2017); and Tim Cook, "'He Was Determined to Go:' Underage Soldiers in the Canadian Expeditionary Force," *Histoire sociale—Social History* 41.81 (May 2008) 41–74.

24 J.L. Biggar, "State Medicine and Rehabilitation," *CMAJ* 9.11 (November 1919) 1013.

25 Clarke, *Unwanted Warriors*, 70.

26 Militia Council, Army Medical Corps Instruction No. 165, 3 October 1916; Colonel J. Edward Squire, *Medical Hints for the Use of Medical Officers Temporarily Employed with Troops* (London: Hodder and Stoughton, 1915) 8. Also see David Silbey, "Bodies and Cultures Collide: Enlistment, the Medical Exam, and the British Working Class, 1914–1916," *Social History of Medicine* 17 (2004): 61–76.

27 Herbert A. Bruce, *Report on the Canadian Army Medical Service by Colonel Herbert A. Bruce* (Ottawa, 1916).

28   Sir W.G. Macpherson (ed.), *Medical Services Pathology* (London: His Majesty's Stationery Office, 1923) 477, 480; Morton, *When Your Number's Up*, 60.

29   Jay Cassel, *The Secret Plague: Venereal Disease in Canada, 1838-1939* (Toronto: University of Toronto Press, 1987) 133.

30   Mann, *Margaret Macdonald*, 85.

31   Macphail, *The Medical Services*, 196; Godfrey, *Bruce*, 65.

32   Ronald G. Haycock, "Sam Hughes," *Dictionary of Canadian Biography*, online.

33   Bliss, *William Osler*, 428–31.

34   See Donald M.A.R. Vince, "Development in the Legal Status of the Canadian Military Forces, 1914–1919, as Related to Dominion Status," *The Canadian Journal of Economics and Political Science* 20.3 (August 1954) 357–70.

35   Desmond Morton, *A Peculiar Kind of Politics: Canada's Overseas Ministry in the First World War* (University of Toronto Press, 1992).

36   Anonymous, "The Canadian Medical Profession and the War," *CMAJ* 7 (1917) 1009–10.

37   "The Need for Conscription of Canadian Doctors," *CMAJ* 8.10 (1918) 933–34; LAC, RG 9, III-B-2, v. 3749, file Adami, Extract from No. 1 Field Ambulance, War Diary, 27 November 1915; Editorial, "The Nursing Crisis," *CMAJ* 8.9 (September 1918) 842–43.

38   William F. Stewart, *The Embattled General: Sir Richard Turner and the First Word War* (Montreal: McGill-Queen's Press, 2015).

39   For a list of all hospitals, see OMFC Report, 395–99. Also see LAC, RG9, III-C-10, v. 4540, file 1, Disposition of Canadians of All Ranks in Hospital in the UK, 31 August 1917.

40   John Pateman, *The Ontario Military Hospital, Orpington, Kent* (Lincolnshire: The Pateran Press, 2012) 43.

41   See Hansard, 18 May 1917; J.L. Granatstein and J.M. Hitsman, *Broken Promises: A History of Conscription in Canada* (Toronto: Oxford University Press, 1977); R.C. Brown and D. Loveridge, "Unrequited Faith: Recruiting the CEF 1914–1918," *Revue Internationale d'Histoire Militaire* 51 (1982) 63.

CHAPTER 10

1   CLIP, David McLean, 799658, letter to Lettie, 12 November 1916.

2   Anthony Clayton, *Paths of Glory: The French Army, 1914–18* (London: Cassell, 2003) 70.

3   Susan C. McGrath (ed.), *The Long Sadness: World War I Diary of William Hannaford Ball* (Seanachie Press, 2014) 91.

4   CWM, 19730295-007, Sergeant W.M.L. Draycott, PPCLI, Intelligence Department, 9 April 1920.

5 Michael Boire, "The Underground War: Military Mining Operations in Support of the Attack on Vimy Ridge, 9 April 1917," *Canadian Military History* 1. 1–2 (1992).

6 Bank of Commerce, *Letters from the Front*, 181.

7 LAC, RG 9 III-C-10, v. 4546, folder 6/ file 2, Report on the medical service in the Somme fighting.

8 LAC, War Diary, No. 1 Casualty Clearing Station, 5 January 1917.

9 *The Listening Post* 29 (1 December 1917) 36. Also see, *Now and Then* 3 (15 June 1916) 7; Frank Walker and Mary F. Gaudet, *From a Stretcher Handle: The World War 1 Journals and Poems of Pte. Frank Walker* (Charlottetown: University of Prince Edward Island, 2000) 120, 122.

10 Walker, *From a Stretcher Handle*, 120.

11 CWM, 20040015-005, Lawrence Rogers, letter, 23 December 1916.

12 LAC, RG 9, III, v. 3846, 51/5, Report on Operations of Canadian Corps against Vimy Ridge, 9.

13 George S. Nasmith, *Canada's Sons in the World War* (Toronto: The John C. Winton Company, 1919) I: 133–34.

14 T.H. Whitelaw, "Presidential Address," *CMAJ* 6.11 (November 1916) 962.

15 LAC, RG 9, v. 4542, 4/15, reports from sanitation officer, HQ, Canadian Corps, 16 January 1917.

16 See, for example, LAC, RG 9, III-C-10, v.4568, 12/1, 17 and 18 August 1918.

17 LAC, RG 9, Series III, v. 3748, Adami Papers, No. 3 Sanitary Section, n.d., p. 2; LAC, RG 9, III, v. 4553, 5/3, The Incineration of Faeces, 12 September 1916; Scotland and Heys (eds.), *War Surgery 1914–18*, 40.

18 Macphail, *The Medical Services*, 250; LAC, RG 9, v.4542, 4/15, 1st Division HQ to all units, 13 October 1916.

19 Lieut. Col. H.B. Yates, "Prophylactic Inoculation against Typhoid Fever," *CMAJ* 5.6 (June 1915) 481–88.

20 CLIP, Charles Henry Savage, untitled memoir, n.p. [written in 1936].

21 Simon Walker, "The Greater Good: Agency and Inoculation in the British Army, 1914–18," *Canadian Bulletin of Medical History* 36.1 (2019) 134.

22 LAC, RG 9, III-A, v. 92, file 10-12-39, Routine Order 2966.

23 CLIP, Cobourg World, Watson to mother, 9 March 1915.

24 John W.S. McCullough, "Sanitation in War," *CMAJ* 9.9 (September 1919) 788–89.

25 LAC, MG 30 E400, Claude Williams papers, letter, 28 December 1916.

26 CLIP, Gordon Stuart Robertson, letter, 21 February 1917.

27 LAC, RG 9, III, v. 4555, 4/5, Comparative Statement by Divisions of Canadian Corps, 3 April 1917.

28 The British calculated 2,690,054 battle casualties versus 3,528,486 non-battle casualties. Major T.J. Mitchell and G.M. Smith, *Medical Services: Casualties and Medical Statistics of the Great War* (London: The Imperial War Museum, 1997 (original, 1931) 107.

29 Colonel George Adami, "Medicine and the War," *CMAJ* 10.10 (1920) 882.

30 CWM, 19920187-002, H.H. Burrell, diary, 28 March 1917.

31 Ibid., 9 April 1917.

32 Ibid., 9 April 1917.

33 Ibid., 9 April 1917.

34 R.G. Kentner, *Some Recollections of the Battles of World War I* (self-published, 1995) 36.

35 Jeffrey Booth (ed.), *Opened by Censor* (Aylmer Express, 2008) 145.

36 For the evacuation of the wounded, see Heather Moran, "The Canadian Army Medical Corps at Vimy Ridge," in Geoffrey Hayes et al. (eds.), *Vimy Ridge: A Canadian Reassessment* (Waterloo: Laurier Centre, 2007) 139–47.

37 CWM, 19800218-014, Joseph Harrison MacFarlane, diary, 9 April 1917.

38 For references to the splint, see WD, No. 1 Canadian Field Ambulance, 9 April 1917.

39 LAC, RG 9, III-B-2, v. 3750, Report on the Collection and Evacuation of Wounded in the Canadian Corps during the Operations of 9 April 1917; WD, No. 8 Canadian Field Ambulance, April 1917, appendix 1.

40 CWM, 20180639, Major Stanley Graham Ross, diary, 11 Vimy 1917.

41 CLIP, Sydney Winterbottom, letter, 28 April 1917.

42 LAC, RG 24, v. 1844, file GAD 11-11D, Total Casualties, All Units, Canadian Corps, April 1917.

43 CLIP, Cobourg World, letter from Blue to mother and father, 11 May 1917.

44 Tim Cook, *Vimy: The Battle and the Legend* (Toronto: Allen Lane, 2017).

45 This figure consists of the wounded on the 9th, but also some from the fighting on the 10th.

CHAPTER 11

1 LAC, MG 30 E 290, Sophie Hoerner papers, letter, 7 June 1918.

2 See Linda J. Quiney, *This Small Army of Women: Canadian Volunteer Nurses and the First World War* (Vancouver: UBC Press, 2017).

3 Canadian Bank of Commerce, *Letters from the Front*, 185.

4 Cook, *The Secret History of Soldiers*, 74–78.

5 See Peat, *Private Peat*, 201.

6 Macphail, *The Medical Services*, 247.

7 Rawling, *Death Thine Enemy*, 65; and see Michel Litalien, *Dans la Tourmente*:

Deux Hôpitaux Militaires Ccanadiens-français dans la France en Guerre (1915–1919) (Outremont, Qué.: Éditions Athéna, 2003).

8   G.W.L. Nicholson, *Seventy Years of Service: A History of the Royal Canadian Army Medical Corps* (Ottawa: Borealis Press, 1977) 90.

9   Major T.J. Mitchell and G.M. Smith, *Medical Services: Casualties and Medical Statistics of the Great War* (London: The Imperial War Museum, 1997 (original, 1931) 31.

10 Canadian Bank of Commerce, *Letters from the Front*, 161.

11 Rawling, *Death Thine Enemy*, 68.

12 CLIP, Charles Henry Savage, memoir, n.d. [1936].

13 T. A. Malloch, "Correspondence from the Seat of War," *CMAJ* 5.8 (1915) 735.

14 Fetherstonaugh, *No. 3 Hospital (McGill)*, 31.

15 J.A. Gunn, "Lessons from War Surgery," *CMAJ* 10.4 (1920) 355; also see Alexis Carrel, *The Treatment of Infected Wounds* (Toronto: Macmillan, 1917).

16 Pottle, *Stretchers*, 154–55.

17 L. Iris Newbold and K. Bruce Newbold (eds.), *Without Fear and with a Manley Heart: The Great War Letters and Diaries of Private James Herbert Gibson* (Waterloo: Wilfrid Laurier Press, 2019) 94.

18 Canadian Bank of Commerce, *Letters from the Front*, 90.

19 Macphail, *The Medical Services*, 215.

20 For soldiers' culture, see Cook, *The Secret History of Soldiers*.

21 LAC, MG 30 E31, T.B. Smith papers, memoir, 122. Also see Jeffrey S. Reznick, *Healing the Nation: Soldiers and the Culture of Caregiving in Britain During the Great War* (Manchester: Manchester University Press, 2004) 65–98.

22 CLIP, R.A. Todd, letter to mother, 5 December 1917.

23 Some papers include: *The Iodine Chronicle; N.Y.D.; The Iodine Chronicle; The Splint Record; Now & Then; The Ontario S-t-r-e-t-c-h-er.*

24 John Pateman, *The Ontario Military Hospital, Orpington, Kent* (Lincolnshire: The Pateran Press, 2012) 7.

25 Fetherstonaugh, *No. 3 Hospital (McGill)*, 22.

26 R.A.L., *Letters of a Canadian Stretcher Bearer*, 20–21.

27 Morrison, *Hell upon Earth*, 211–22.

28 Morrison, *Hell upon Earth*, 84.

29 Pte William Chisholm Millar, *From Thunder Bay through Ypres with the Fighting 52nd* (self-published, 1918; republished, 2010) 89.

30 Toman, *Sister Soldiers*, 173–74; Mann, *Margaret Macdonald*, 196.

31 CWM, MHRC, 19920088-005, Margaret Elliot Reilly, autograph book, 78.

32 CWM, MHRC, 19740213-009, Georgina Beach McCullough, autograph book, n.p.

33 CWM, MHRC, 20020161-002, Gertrude Mills, autograph book, 45; for ward culture, see Ana Carden-Coyne, *The Politics of Wounds: Military Patients and Medical Power in the First World War* (Oxford: Oxford University Press, 2014).

34 Katherine Wilson-Simmie, *Lights Out! The Memoir of Nursing Sister Kate Wilson, Canadian Army Medical Corps, 1915–1917* (Ottawa: CEF Books, 2004) 127.

35 Sandy Callister, "'Broken Gargoyles': The Photographic Representation of Severely Wounded New Zealand Soldiers," *Social History of Medicine* 20.1 (April 2007) 116–17.

36 Marjorie Gehrhardt, *The Men with Broken Faces: Gueules Cassées of the First World War* (Oxford: Peter Lang, 2015).

37 See Harold D. Gillies, *Plastic Surgery of the Face: Based on Selective Cases of War Injuries of the Face Including Burns* (London: H. Frowde, Hodder and Stoughton, 1920); and Kerry Neale, "Without the Faces of Men: Facially Disfigured Great War Soldiers of Britain and the Dominions" (Ph.D. thesis: UNSW Australia, 2015).

38 J.N. Roy, "War Surgery—Perforating Gunshot Wound of the Face with Extensive Destruction of the Superior Maxillæ," *CMAJ* 9.12 (1919) 1089.

39 Roy, "War Surgery," 1088–94.

40 Roy, "War Surgery," 1088.

41 Whitehead, *Doctors in the Great War*, 244.

42 Macphail, *The Medical Services*, 225–26.

43 Jason Bate, "Bonds of Kinship and Care: RAMC Photographic Albums and the Making of 'Other' Domestic Lives," *Social History of Medicine* 33.3 (2020) 772–97.

44 Pateman, *The Ontario Military Hospital*, 49.

45 Toman, *Sister Soldiers*, 99.

46 CLIP, Gordon MacKay papers, letter to mother, 2 September 1917.

47 Morton, *When Your Number's Up*, 194.

48 Wilson-Simmie, *Lights Out!*, 127–28. For an exploration of this emotional labour, see Margaret R. Higonnet, "Introduction," in Margaret R. Higonnet (ed.), *Nurses at the Front: Writing the Wounds of the Great War* (Boston: Northeastern University Press, 2001).

49 Canadian Bank of Commerce, *Letters from the Front*, 185.

50 CLIP, Harry Morris, Letter, 5 April 1917.

51 CLIP, Archie Polson papers, letter, Nursing Sister to Mrs. Polson, 10 April 1917.

52 Ibid., mother to Archie, 17 April 1917.

53 Ibid., Paine to mother, 25 April 1917.

54 Ibid., Tyler to Polson, undated, ca. September 1917.

ENDNOTES

55 A. Primrose, "Disabilities, Including Injuries, Caused by Bullets, Shrapnel, High Explosives," *CMAJ* 5.10 (1915) 853; Nick Bosanquet, "Loss and Devastation: The Costs of the Great War," in Peter Liddle (ed.), *Britain and Victory in the Great War* (Barnsley: Pen and Sword, 2018) 316.

56 A.M.J. Hyatt and Nancy Geddes Poole, *Battle for Life: The History of No. 10 Canadian Stationary Hospital* (Waterloo: Laurier Centre, 2004) 43.

57 It was established in the BEF in July 1916. Soldiers qualified for wounds but not self-inflicted ones, or accidents or sickness.

58 Canadian Bank of Commerce, *Letters from the Front*, 119.

59 Overseas Military Forces of Canada, *Report of the Ministry* (London: OMFC, 1919) 384.

60 Fetherstonaugh, *No. 3 Hospital (McGill)*, 249.

61 See Chapter 19 in this book.

62 G.E. Armstrong, "Letter from Lieutenant-Colonel G.E. Armstrong, C.A.M.C," *CMAJ* 7.8 (1917) 747.

CHAPTER 12

1 Captain R.J. Manion, MC, *A Surgeon in Arms* (Toronto: McClelland, Goodchild and Stewart, 1918) 79.

2 John William Lynch, *Princess Patricia's Canadian Light Infantry, 1917–1919* (New York: Exposition Press, 1976) 186.

3 Tim Cook, "Creating Faith: The Canadian Gas Services in the First World War," *Journal of Military History* 62 (October 1998) 755–86.

4 LAC, RG 9, v. 3619, file 25-13-6, Lecture by Captain C.A.R. Gordon, CAMC on the Medical Aspects of Chemical Warfare, 6.

5 CLIP, W.J. Stares, letter, 8 July 1917.

6 LAC, RG 9, v. 3931, folder 15 / file 8, Lessons from Recent Hostile Gas Attacks, August 1916.

7 Simon Jones, "Under a Green Sea, the British Response to Gas Warfare, Part II," *The Great War* 2.1 (1989) 18.

8 See LAC, RG 9, III, v. 3618, file 25-13-6, The Symptoms and Treatment of Late Effects of Gas Poisoning, 10 April 1918; Sir W.G. Macpherson, *Official History of the War: Medial Services Diseases of the War*, volume II (London: HMSO, 1923) 282.

9 R.C. Fetherstonhaugh, *No. 3 Canadian General Hospital (McGill), 1914–1919* (Montreal: The Gazette Printing Company, 1928) 105.

10 Keirstead, "The Canadian Military Medical Experience," 244.

11 LAC, RG 9, v. 3977, 7/2, "Suggestions Regarding the Treatment of Cases Suffering from the New Shell Gas Poisoning."

12 R.A.L., *Letters of a Canadian Stretcher Bearer*, 266.

13 LAC, RG 24, v. 1837, file G.A.Q. 9-37, "Attack Methods."

14 Robert Harris and Jeremy Paxman, *A Higher Form of Killing* (London: Windus, 1982) 27.

15 LAC, RG 9, III, v.3851, 63/2, Appreciation of the Enemy's Defences and Dispositions around Hill 70. For the battle, see Douglas E. Delaney and Serge Marc Durflinger (eds.), *Capturing Hill 70: Canada's Forgotten Battle of the First World War* (Vancouver: UBC Press, 2016).

16 London Gazette (Supplement) no. 30372, 6 November 1917, 11569; and Michael Kevin Dooley, "'Our Mickey': The Story of Private James O'Rourke, VC, MM (CEF), 1879–1957," *Labour/Le Travail* 47 (Spring 2001): 171–84.

17 LAC, RG 9, III, v. 3831, 14/8, Report by Divisional Gas Officer on the Gas Bombardment of the 1st Canadian Division Night of 17/18 August 1917.

18 LAC, RG 9, III, v. 3831, 14/8, Report on Gas Bombardment; and LAC, RG 9, III, v. 3831, 14/8, BM4-16.

19 LAC, RG 9, III-B-2, v. 3752, Report on Evacuation of Wounded in the Canadian Corps Operations for the Capture of Hill 70, 15–16 August 1917.

20 LAC, RG 9, III-B-2, v. 3752, War Diary, DDMS Canadian Corps, Report on Canadian Corps Operations for Hill 70, 17 August 1917.

21 CLIP, Clair Barrey, letter, 17 August 1917.

22 Wheeler, *The 50th Battalion in No Man's Land*, 142.

23 Norm Christie (ed.), *Letters of Agar Adamson, 1914 to 1919: Lieutenant Colonel, Princess Patricia's Canadian Light Infantry* (Nepean: CEF Books, 1997) 304.

24 Tim Cook, *No Place to Run: The Canadian Corps and Gas Warfare in the First World War* (Vancouver: UBC Press, 1999) 132; Tim Cook, *Shock Troops: Canadians Fighting the Great War, 1917–1918* (Toronto: Penguin, 2008) 306.

25 Tim Cook, "Warfare Most Foul," *Legion Magazine* (July–August 2020) 32–39.

26 Lyn MacDonald, *They Called It Passchendaele* (London: Penguin, 1978) 87. Also see LAC, MG 30 E31, T.B. Smith Papers, memoir, 197; LAC, RG 9, v. 4060, 5/1, No. 1403 (G).

27 LAC, RG 9, III-B-2, v. 3750, War Diary, DDMS Canadian Corps, Report on Canadian Corps Operations for Hill 70, August 1917.

28 LAC, RG 9, v. 4196, 1/16, "Report On Hostile Bombardment with Gas T.M. Bombs on the 9th Divisional Front on the Night of June 5th/6th, 1917."

29 Gunn and Dutton, *Historical Records of Number 8 Canadian Field Ambulance 1915–1919*, 63.

30 LAC, RG 9, v. 3751, War diary of Major G.S. Strathy, 22.

31 LAC, RG 9, v. 4547, 1/2, "Suggestions Regarding the Treatment of Cases

Suffering from the New Shell Gas Poisoning"; John Ellis, *Eye-Deep in Hell* (London: Croom Helm, 1976) 66.

32 Canon Frederick Scott, *The Great War as I Saw It* (Ottawa: CEF Books, 2000) 143.

33 All information in the paragraph is taken from G.B. Peat, "The Effects of Gassing as Seen at a Casualty Clearing Station," *CMAJ* 8.1 (January 1918) 17–24. On pain, see Ana Carden-Coyne, "Men in Pain: Silence, Stories and Soldiers' Bodies," in Paul Cornish and Nicholas J. Saunders (eds.), *Bodies in Conflict: Corporeality, Materiality and Transformation* (London: Routledge, 2013) 43–65.

34 Denis Winter, *Death's Men: Soldiers of the Great War* (London: Penguin, 1985) 123.

35 LAC, RG 9, v. 3618, file 25-13-6, John C. Meakins and T.W. Walker, *The After-Effects of Irritant Gas Poisoning, 1918*, 8.

36 LAC, RG 9, v. 3977, 7/2, "Notes for Treatment of Cases of Yellow Cross Gas Poisoning and Suspicious Cases in the Trenches"; LAC, RG 9, v. 945, file G-5-3 part 1, Report O.C., No. 58 Casualty Clearing Station; A.E. Snell, *The CAMC with the Canadian Corps during the Last Hundred Days of the Great War* (Ottawa: F.A. Cland, 1924) 211.

37 LAC, RG 9, v. 945, file G-5-3 part 1, New German Gas.

38 Macpherson, *Official History of the War: Medial Services Diseases of the War*, volume II, 394.

39 Fetherstonaugh, *No. 3 Canadian General Hospital (McGill)*, 106; LAC, RG 9, v. 4551, 1/9, D.G./E./280.87.

40 "No. 1 Canadian General Hospital Clinical Society," *CMAJ* 8.6 (June 1918) 576.

41 R.A.L., *Letters of a Canadian Stretcher Bearer*, 67.

42 Cook, *No Place to Run*, 168–211.

43 LAC, RG 9, v. 3751, War Diary of G.S. Strathy, 34.

44 LAC, RG 9, v. 3981, 1/2, Effects of Gas Shell Bombardments, 17/7/17; LAC, RG 9, v. 3975, 1/16, "Note on the Invaliding Factors amongst Casualties Caused by Dichlorethylsulphide."

45 LAC, MG 30 E 156, Robert N. Clements Papers, "Merry Hell. The Way I Saw It," 233.

CHAPTER 13

1 Patricia Jalland, *Death in the Victorian Family* (Oxford: Oxford University Press, 1996) 2–3. Also see Luc Capdevila and Daniele Voldman, *War Dead: Western Societies and the Casualties of War* (Edinburgh: Edinburgh University Press, 2006).

2 Ross Wilson, "The Burial of the Dead: The British Army on the Western Front, 1914–18," *War and Society* 31.1 (2012) 22–41; and Jeremy P. Garrett, Tribute to the Fallen; The Evolution of Canadian Battlefield Burials during the First World War, (Ph.D. thesis: Western University, 2018).

3 Tim Cook, "Grave Beliefs: Stories of the Supernatural and the Uncanny among Canada's Great War Trench Soldiers," *Journal of Military History* 77.2 (April 2013) 521–42.

4 LAC, RG 24, v. 1216, file HQ 512-19-1-A, Policy, Location of Graves, CEF, 8 March 1917.

5 LAC, RG 9, III, v. 4137, 1/18, letter by O.C., 28th Battalion, 24 October 1915.

6 "The Army Collection of War Specimens: The Opening of the Exhibition," *Lancet* 2.4912 (1917) 620–21; "The Great War Exhibit at the Royal College of Surgeons," *CMAJ* 8.1 (1918) 52–55. Also see Christine Quigley, *Dissection on Display: Cadavers, Anatomists, and Public Spectacle* (Jefferson, N.C.: McFarland & Co., 2012).

7 "The Army Collection of War Specimens: The Opening of the Exhibition," *Lancet* 2.4912 (1917) 621.

8 "The Great War Exhibit at the Royal College of Surgeons," *CMAJ* 8.1 (1918) 52.

9 "The Royal College of Surgeons and the CAMC," *Bulletin of the Canadian Army Medical Corps* 1.1 (March 1918) 16.

10 "The Great War Exhibit at the Royal College of Surgeons," *CMAJ* 8.1 (1918) 54.

11 Samuel J. M. M. Alberti, "The Regiment of Skeletons: A First World War Medical Collection," *Social History of Medicine* 28.1 (2015) 122.

12 Macphail, *The Medical Services*, 307.

13 "The Great War Exhibit at the Royal College of Surgeons," *CMAJ* 8.1 (1918) 52.

14 "The Need of an Army Medical Museum as Part of the Army Medical Service," *CMAJ* 8.1 (1918) 50.

15 LAC, RG 9, III, v. 3604, file 24-4-0, pt. 1, Adami to Surgeon-General, 7 August 1917.

16 On collecting and museums in the war, see Jennifer Wellington, *Exhibiting War: The Great War, Museums and Memory in Britain, Canada, and Australia* (Cambridge: Cambridge University Press, 2017).

17 LAC, RG 9, III, v. 3604, file 24-4-0, pt. I, Lt. Colonel, ADMS, Medical Historical Recorder to DMS, 8 October 1917: Memorandum re: Medical Section, National War Museum [ca. 8 October 1917].

18 Ibid.

19 LAC, RG 9, III, v. 3604, file 24-4-0, pt. I, Lt. Col. ADMS to Lt. Col. E. Seaborn, No. 10 Canadian Stationary, 21 March 1918; Adami, *The War Story of the C.A.M.C., 1914-15*, viii.

20 LAC, RG 9, III, v. 3604, file 24-4-0, pt. II, Lt. Col ADMS to AMD, 14 November 1917.

21 LAC, RG 9, III, v. 3604, file 24-4-0, pt. II, Memo to S-G. J.T. Fotheringham, 10 April 1918.

22 Veronica Strong-Boag, "Canada's Women Doctors: Feminism Constrained," in S.E.D. Shortt (ed.), *Medicine in Canadian Society* (Montreal: McGill-Queen's University Press, 1981) 235.

23 LAC, RG 9, III, v. 3604, file 24-4-0, pt. II, The Surgeon-General, DMS, to Secretary, Royal College of Surgeons, 8 February 1918.

24 James R. Wright and Harry W.V. Letts, "Morton E Hall: Conservator of the Canadian War Museum in London, England during the Great War and Alberta's Second Pathologist," *Journal of Medical Biography* (June 2019) 1–10.

25 Arthur Keith and M.E. Hall, "Specimens of Gunshot Injuries of the Long Bones, to Show the Type of Fracture Produced: Contained in the Army Medical Collection Now on Exhibition in the Museum of the Royal College of Surgeons of England," *British Journal of Surgery* 7 (1919) 149.

26 Snell, *The CAMC*, 92–93, 114. Dr. Hall returned to Edmonton in November 1919 to take over the laboratories at the Royal Alexandra Hospital, where he was engaged in much profitable medical research, including blood transfusions, and he practised and taught for another thirty years.

27 LAC, RG 9, III, v. 3604, file 24-4-0, pt. II, Maude Abbott to Lt-Col J.G. Adami, 15 February 1918.

28 Ibid., Maude Abbott to Lt-Col J.G. Adami, 15 February 1918; Ibid., Captain A.B. Chandler, CAMC, to Director General of Medical Services, 12 March 1918; Ibid., Maude Abbott to Lt-Col J.G. Adami, 15 February 1918.

29 LAC, RG 9, III, v. 3604, file 24-4-0, pt. II, Captain Chandler, Proposal for Work in England and France (ca. March 1918); Ibid., Memorandum upon the Present Position with References to Museum Specimens, 25 September 1918.

30 LAC, RG 9, III, v. 3604, file 24-4-0, pt. II, Insurance on CAMC exhibit, 24 February 1918; LAC, RG 9, v.3754, Major F. Lessore to Colonel J.G. Adami, 8 May 1919.

31 "Canadian National War Museum," *CMAJ* 9.10 (October 1919) 947–48; John Pateman, *The Ontario Military Hospital, Orpington, Kent* (Lincolnshire: The Pateran Press, 2012) 43–44; LAC, RG 9, III, v. 3604, file 24-4-0, pt. II, Analysis of source of origin, 18.3.1918.

32 *Hamilton Spectator*, 1 June 1918, 4. I wish to thank Kelly Bucci of the Hamilton Public Library for her assistance in locating this story.

33 "Report of the Museum and Laboratory Section," *CMAJ* 8.7 (July 1918) 649.

34 Ibid.

35 Ibid.

36 LAC, RG 9, III, v. 3604, file 24-4-0, pt. II, "Canadian Army Medical Corps Museum," 31 July 1918.

37 LAC, RG 9, III, v. 3604, file 24-4-0, pt. 1, Memo, 28 September 1917. For the influence of Beaverbrook, see LAC, RG 9, III, v. 3604, file 24-4-0, pt. II, AMDS to AMD, Memo, 18 April 1918.

38 LAC, RG 9, III, v. 3604, file 24-4-0, pt. II, Notes by Colonel Adami on interview with Major L. Wilson, Director of Museum Unit, AEF, 16 April 1916.

39 LAC, RG 9, v. 3754, Office of DMS, On the Medical History of the War, written by J.G. Adami, n.d. [ca. 1918]; LAC, RG 9, III, v. 3604, file 24-4-0, pt. II, Memorandum on proposed establishment of a National Medical Museum.

40 LAC, RG 9, III, v. 3604, file 24-4-0, pt. II, Memorandum on proposed establishment of a National Medical Museum; LAC, RG 9, III, v. 3604, file 24-4-0, pt. II, Adami to Colonel T.R. Elliott, 27 July 1918.

41 Fetherstonaugh, *No. 3 Hospital (McGill)*, 243.

42 Gunn and Dutton, *Historical Records of Number 8 Canadian Field Ambulance 1915–1919*, 148.

43 LAC, RG 9, III, v. 3604, file 24-4-0, pt. II, Memo re: collection of Specimens . . . for National War Museum [ca. April 1918].

44 LAC, RG 9, III, v. 3604, file 24-4-0, pt. II, Memo re: collection of Specimens . . . for National War Museum [ca. April 1918]; LAC, RG 9, III, v. 3604, file 24-4-0, pt. II, Canadian Specimens, July 1918; "Wax Models for the National War Museum," *CMAJ* 9.10 (1919) 937; also see Samuel J.M.M. Alberti, "Wax Bodies: Art and Anatomy in Victorian Museums," *Museum History Journal* 2 (2009) 7–36.

45 LAC, RG 9, III, v. 3604, file 24-4-0, pt. II, undated document.

46 Service Number 90230.

47 J. Castell Hopkins, *Canadian Annual Review of Politics and Public Affairs, 1915* (Ottawa, 1916) 181; J.G. Adami, *The War Story of the C.A.M.C., 1914–15*, introduction [written by Sir Robert Borden].

48 LAC, RG 9, III, v. 3604, file 24-4-0, pt. I, Colonel ADMS to Lt-Gen Sir R.E.W. Turner, 13 August 1918.

49 "Canadian Medical War Collection," *British Medical Journal* (17 August 1918) 169.

CHAPTER 14

1 J. Alexander (Sandy) Bain, *A War Diary of a Canadian Signaller: My Experiences in the Great War, 1914–1918* (Moncton: J.D. Bain, 1986) 99.

2   For Haig and Passchendaele, see Gary Sheffield, *Douglas Haig: From the Somme to Victory* (London: Aurum Press, 2016).

3   Nicholson, *Seventy Years of Service*, 102.

4   Mitchell and Smith, *Medical Services*, 43.

5   Quoted in Tim Cook, *Passchendaele: Canada's Brutal Victory* (The Legion: Special Issue Publication, 2017) 31.

6   WD, No. 8 Canadian Field Ambulance, November 1917, Appendix 1.

7   Glenn R. Iriam, *In the Trenches 1914–1918* (Self-published, 2011) 186.

8   Mitchell and Smith, *Medical Services*, 170–71.

9   Jeffrey Booth (ed.), *Opened by Censor: A Collection of Letters Home from World War I Veterans from Elgin County* (Aylmer, Ontario: Aylmer Express Ltd., 2008) 173.

10 Morrison (ed.), *Hell upon Earth*, 138.

11 Norman Miles Guiou, *Transfusion: A Canadian Surgeon's Story in War and in Peace* (Yarmouth: Stoneycroft Pub., 1985) 24.

12 CWM, 58A 2. 7.7, George McFarland, memoirs, 26 October 1917.

13 Gunn and Dutton, *Historical Records of Number 8 Canadian Field Ambulance 1915–1919*, 82.

14 Canadian Bank of Commerce, *Letters from the Front*, 244.

15 Reginald H Roy (ed.), *The Journal of Private Fraser, 1914–1918: Canadian Expeditionary Force* (Victoria: Sono Nis Press, 1985) 315.

16 N.M. Christie (ed.), *Letters of Agar Adamson 1914–1918* (Nepean: CEF Books, 1997) 309.

17 Morrison, *Hell upon Earth*, 133.

18 Cook, *No Place to Run*, 140–41.

19 LAC, RG 9, v. 3751, personal diary of Major G.S. Strathy, several entries in early November 1917.

20 CWM, 19920187-002, Herbert Heckford Burrell, diary, 31 October 1917.

21 Morrison, *Hell upon Earth*, 138.

22 11th Canadian Field Ambulance. *Diary of the Eleventh: Being a Record of the Xlth Canadian Field Ambulance (Western Universities) Feb. 1916–May 1919* (Winnipeg, 1919) 83.

23 Gunn and Dutton, *Historical Records of Number 8*, 73.

24 CWM, 20120021-004, Lt. Col. R.P. Wright, diary, 9 November 1917.

25 Gabriel and Metz, *A History of Military Medicine*, volume II, 240.

26 Melanie Morin-Pelletier, "'At Peace with the Germans, but at War with the Germs': Canadian Nurse Veterans after the First World War," in Tim Cook and J.L. Granatstein (eds.), *Canada 1919: A Nation Shaped by War* (Vancouver: UBC Press, 2020) 196.

27 Will Bird, *Ghosts Have Warm Hands* (Ottawa: CEF Books, 1997) 59–61.

28 Gunn and Dutton, *Historical Records of Number 8*, 73.

29 Cook, *Shock Troops*, 365.

30 CLIP, Gordon Morrisette, letter, 10 November 1917.

CHAPTER 15

1 CLIP, Herbert Laurier Irwin, letter, 20 February 1918.

2 Noyes, *Stretcher-Bearers*, 177.

3 LAC, RG 24, v. 1842, file 10-44, Statement of the CEF in Canada and Overseas.

4 Patrice Dutil and David Mackenzie, *Embattled Nation: Canada's Wartime Election of 1917* (Toronto: Dundurn Press, 2017).

5 Debbie Marshall, *Give Your Other Vote to the Sister: A Woman's Journey into the Great War* (Calgary: University of Calgary Press, 2007).

6 Tim Cook, "From Destruction to Construction: The Khaki University of Canada, 1917–1919," *Journal of Canadian Studies* 37.1 (Spring 2002) 109–43.

7 Heather Moran, "Stretcher Bearers and Surgeons" (Ph.D. thesis: Western University, 2008) 221.

8 LAC, RG 9, III B-2, v. 3752, file 3-3-2-1, George Adami personal diary, interview with Captain C.S. McKee, 12 December 1917.

9 LAC, MG 30 E 505, William Howard Curtis, letter, 2 June 1915.

10 On suicide, see Patricia Prestwich, "Suicide and French Soldiers of the First World War: Differing Perspectives, 1914–1939," in John Weaver and David Wright (eds.), *Histories of Suicide: International Perspectives on Self-Destruction in the Modern World* (Toronto: University of Toronto Press, 2008) 135–55; Matthew Barrett, "Absolutely Incapable of 'Carrying On': Shell Shock, Suicide, and the Death of Lieutenant Colonel Sam Sharpe," *Canadian Military History* 25.1 (2016) 1–31.

11 See Mark Humphries, "Wilfully and With Intent: Self-Inflicted Wounds and the Negotiation of Power in the Trenches," *Social History* 47.94 (2014) 369–97.

12 See Mark Harrison, "The Medicalization of War—The Militarization of Medicine," in *Social History of Medicine* 9.2 (1996) 267–76.

13 CLIP, Private J.G. Sproule, letter, 7 July 1916.

14 LAC, RG 9, III-B-1, v. 2246, file A-5-30, pt. III, case of Pte. E.A. Stonebridge, 887132.

15 LAC, RG 9, III, v. 878, file A-63-3, pt. 19, The case of Pte. J.E. Vienneau, [ca. 5 April 1918].

16 War Office, *Report of the War Office Committee of Enquiry into "Shell Shock"* (London: HMSO, 1922) 140–41.

17 See Humphries, *A Weary Road*.

18 LAC, RG 9, III, v.4105, file 1, DDMS circular, 2 October 1917; see Cook, *No Place to Run*, 157–62.

19 Directorate of History and Heritage, Ottawa, Edwin Pye papers, 74/672/-II-57a, Self-Inflicted Injuries, 11; LAC, RG 24, v. 6992, file: chapter VII, v. 2, Notes on Self-Inflicted Injuries.

20 Black, *I Want One Volunteer*, 28–29.

21 Teresa Iacobelli, *Death or Deliverance: Canadian Courts Martial in the Great War* (Vancouver: UBC Press, 2013) 4–5.

22 LAC, Sir Andrew Macphail papers, volume 2, diary, 29 October 1916.

23 Aaron Pegram, *Surviving the Great War: Australian Prisoners of War on the Western Front, 1916–18* (Cambridge: Cambridge University Press, 2020) 36.

24 Hyatt and Poole, *Battle for Life*, 40.

25 Canadian Bank of Commerce, *Letters from the Front*, 268–69.

26 Nicholson, *Seventy Years of Service*, 103.

27 L. Bruce Robertson, "Further Observations on the Results of Blood Transfusion in War Surgery," *British Medical Journal* 2.2969 (1917) 679–83.

28 Canadian Bank of Commerce, *Letters from the Front*, 291–92.

29 CWM, Military History Research Centre, 19950037-014, Katherine Maud MacDonald, scrapbook.

30 Macphail, *The Medical Services*, 238.

31 J.H. Becker, *Silhouettes of the Great War: Memoir of J.H. Becker, 1915–1919* (Ottawa: CEF Books, 2001) 173.

32 Macphail, *The Medical Services*, 234.

33 Nicholson, *Seventy Years of Service*, 107.

34 See William F. Stewart, "'The Most Vivifying Influence': Operation Delta in Preparing the Canadian Corps for the Hundred Days," *Canadian Military History* 27.2 (2018) 1–34.

35 CWM, 20000148-001, Frederick Robinson, letter, 1 June 1918.

36 Overseas Military Forces of Canada, *Report of the Ministry* (London: OMFC, 1919) 383.

37 Arthur Lapointe, *Soldier of Quebec (1916–1919)* (Montreal: Garnad, 1931) 100.

38 LAC, RG 9, III-B-2, v. 3613, file 25-3-7, J.A. Amyot, "Influenza amongst Canadian Troops in England," 14 October 1918.

39 Fetherstonaugh, *No. 3 Hospital (McGill)*, 198.

40 CLIP, Cecil Moody, letter to Budsie, 29 June 1918.

41 Jack Sheldon, "German Defeat and the Myth of the 'Stab in the Back,'" in Peter Liddle (ed.), *Britain and Victory in the Great War* (Barnsley: Pen and Sword, 2018) 42; and Robert Foley, "From Victory to Defeat: The German Army in 1918," in Ashley Ekins (ed.), *1918 Year of Victory: The End of the*

Great War and the Shaping of History (Auckland: Exisle Publishing Ltd., 2010) 83.

42 Erich Ludendorff, *Ludendorff's Own Story, August 1914–November 1918* (Freeport 1971 reprint of 1920 edition) 277.

43 L. McLeod Gould, *From B.C. To Baisieux: 102nd Canadian Infantry Battalion* (Victoria: Thos R. Cusack Presses, 1919) 88.

CHAPTER 16

1   LAC, RG 24, v. 1844, file 11-5, Casualties [Hundred Days].

2   MHRC, CBC Radio Flanders Fields transcripts, episode 14, 8.

3   Brian Douglas Tennyson (ed.), *Merry Hell: The Story of the 25th Battalion (Nova Scotia Regiment)* (Toronto: University of Toronto Press, 2012) 209.

4   Guiou, *Transfusion*, 51–52.

5   Noyes, *Stretcher Bearers,* 215.

6   CWM, 20020024-003, Badeu to Whitmore, 16 August 1918.

7   A.E. Snell, *The CAMC with the Canadian Corps during the Last Hundred Days of the Great War* (Ottawa: F.A. Cland, 1924) 41.

8   Clifton J. Cate and Charles C. Cate, *Notes: A Soldiers Memoir of World War* (self-published, 2005) 50.

9   LAC, RG 24, v. 1844, 11-5, Amiens.

10 Canadian War Museum (CWM), Sir Arthur Currie papers, 58A 1.60.3, Extract from G.H.Q. Summary of Information, 26 August 1918; Dean Chappelle, "The Canadian Attack at Amiens, 8-11 August 1918," *Canadian Military History* 2.2 (1993) 89–101.

11 J.L. Granatstein, *The Greatest Victory: Canada's One Hundred Days, 1918* (Don Mills: Oxford University Press, 2014) 32.

12 Noyes, *Stretcher Bearers*, 213–14.

13 James Robert Johnston, *Riding into War: The Memoir of a Horse Transport Driver, 1916–1919* (Fredericton: Goose Lane, 2004) 80.

14 Nicholson, *Canadian Expeditionary Force*, 414.

15 Victor N. Swanston, *Who Said War Is Hell!* (self-published, 1983) 51.

16 Noyes, *Stretcher Bearers*, 111.

17 CWM, MHRC, 20060105-001, First World War Diaries of Private Andrew Robert Coulter, August 1918.

18 Percy Climo (ed.), *Let Us Remember: Lively Letters from World War One* (Colborne: P.L. Climo, 1990) 285.

19 Tennyson (ed.), *Merry Hell*, 213.

20 LAC, RG 24, v. 1844, 11-5, Amiens; on prisoners, see Canadian War Museum, Sir Arthur Currie papers, 58A 1 60.3, Special Order [by Currie], 12 August 1918.

ENDNOTES

21 LAC, RG 24, v. 1844, 11-5, Amiens.

22 Snell, *The CAMC with the Canadian Corps*, 64.

23 Daniel Dancocks, *Spearhead to Victory: Canada and the Great War* (Edmonton: Hurtig, 1987) 91.

24 LAC, RG 9, III-C-10, v. 4546, War Diary of the ADMS, 3rd Canadian Division, "Battle East of Arras, 26th to 28th, 1918."

25 Snell, *The CAMC with the Canadian Corps*, 113.

26 CWM, 20060105-001, Andrew Coulter, diary, 27 August 1918.

27 LAC, RG 9, III-D-1, v. 4677, folder 9, file 4, Medical Arrangements for Operations, Canadian Corps, 26 August to 7 September 1918.

28 Ibid.

29 I would like to thank Dr. Bill Stewart for sharing his expertise on the battle, with some information here drawn from his forthcoming book on the Second Battle of Arras.

30 Deborah Cowley (ed.), *Georges Vanier, Soldier: The Wartime Letters and Diaries, 1915–1919* (Toronto: Dundurn Press, 2000) 252–53.

31 Nicholson, *Canadian Expeditionary Force*, 432. Nicholson gives a figure of 254 officers and 5,547 for the 2nd and 3rd Divisions, but this does not include those units attached to the Canadian Corps.

32 LAC, MG 30 E100, Sir Arthur Currie papers, diary, 29 August 1918.

33 Lynch, *Princess Patricia's Canadian Light Infantry, 1917–1919*, 166.

34 Daniel Dancocks, *Gallant Canadians: The Story of the Tenth Canadian Infantry Battalion, 1914–1919* (Calgary: Calgary Highlanders Regimental Funds Foundation, 1990) 191.

35 Dancocks, *Spearhead to Victory*, 111.

36 Granatstein, *The Greatest Victory, 103;* London Gazette, no. 31067, 14 December 1918.

37 London Gazette, no. 31067, 14 December 1918.

38 LAC, RG 9, III-D-1, v. 4677, 9/4, Medical Arrangements for Operations, Canadian Corps, 26 August to 7 September 1918.

39 Ibid.

40 Canadian Bank of Commerce, *Letters from the Front*, 297.

41 LAC, MG 30 E100, Sir Arthur Currie papers, v.2, file M-R, Currie to Morrison, 11 September 1918; WD, 4th Division, Report on the Scarpe Operations; Bill Rawling, *Surviving Trench Warfare: Technology and the Canadian Corps, 1914–1918* (Toronto: University of Toronto Press, 1992) 220.

42 Dancocks, *Spearhead*, 120.

43 Patrick Dennis, *Reluctant Warriors: Canadian Conscripts and the Great War* (Vancouver: UBC Press, 2017).

44 LAC, MG 30 E113, "Back to Blighty," George V. Bell, memoir, 113. See Jordan Chase, "Unwilling to Continue, Ordered to Advance: An Examination of the Contributing Factors Toward, and Manifestation of, War Wariness in the Canadian Corps during the Hundred Days Campaign of the First World War" (Master's thesis: University of Calgary, 2013).

45 Niall Ferguson, *The Pity of War* (New York: Basic Books, 1999) 350–57.

46 Harrison, *The Medical War*, 119; Gunn and Dutton, *Historical Records of Number 8 Canadian Field Ambulance 1915–1919*, 107–108.

47 For enemy defences, see Major-General Sir W. Hastings Anderson, "The Crossing of the Canal du Nord," *Canadian Defence Quarterly* 2.1 (October 1924) 65.

48 CLIP, T.C. Lapp, letter, 20 September 1918.

49 LAC, MG 30 E100, Sir Arthur Currie papers, v.1, file A to F, Currie to Borden, 26 November 1918.

50 LAC, RG 24, v. 1844, file 11-5, Casualties [Hundred Days]: There were 11,822 at Amiens from 8 August to 20 August, while other records from 22 August to 11 October reveal 30,806 casualties.

51 LAC, RG 9, III, v. 4810, file Medical Arrangements, Records of Canadian Medical Services during Last Hundred Days; LAC, RG 9, III, v. 3893, Medical Arrangements during the Second Battle of Amiens, August 8th to 20th, 4.

52 At Amiens, Currie's 1919 report gave these figures: 2,259 killed and missing in action vs. 9,103 wounded, for a ratio of 1 to 4. See Overseas Military Forces of Canada, *Report of the Ministry, Overseas Military Forces of Canada, 1918* (London: H.M. Stationery Office, 1919) 141, 168.

53 LAC, MG 30 E100, Sir Arthur Currie papers, v.2, file M-R, Currie to Miller, 4 October 1918.

CHAPTER 17

1 Canadian Bank of Commerce, *Letters from the Front*, 301.

2 Snell, *The CAMC with the Canadian Corps*, 170.

3 Report of the Ministry, *Overseas Military Forces of Canada 1918* (London: OMFC, 1919) 169.

4 J. Arthur Maguire, *Four Years of the War as Seen by a Buck Private* (self-published, 2004) 53.

5 Derek Grout, *Thunder in the Skies: A Canadian Gunner in the Great War* (Toronto: Dundurn, 2015) 399.

6 J.F.B. Livesay, *Canada's Hundred Days: With the Canadian Corps from Amiens to Mons, Aug. 8–Nov. 11, 1918* (Toronto: T. Allen, 1919) 337.

7 CWM, MHRC, CBC, Flanders' Fields, episode 15, page 23.

8 CLIP, letter, Charles Willoughby, letter, 16 September 1918.

9 Gunn and Dutton, *Historical Records of Number 8 Canadian Field Ambulance 1915–1919*, 156–57.

10 LAC, RG 9, v. 4750, 3rd Canadian Division Report of Operations, 22 October to 11 November 1918.

11 Morrison, *Hell upon Earth*, 160.

12 LAC, personnel file, Sapper H.E. Cook, 2010571. Cook voluntarily enlisted and was not conscripted.

13 Eileen Pettigrew, *Silent Enemy: Canada and the Deadly Flu of 1918* (Regina: Western Producer Prairie Books, 1983) 5.

14 Alfred W. Crosby, *America's Forgotten Pandemic* (Cambridge: Cambridge University Press, 2012) 37–40.

15 Mark Osborne Humphries, *The Last Plague: Spanish Influenza and the Politics of Public Health in Canada* (Toronto: University of Toronto Press, 2013) 60–62.

16 Humphries, *The Last Plague*, 89.

17 Howard Phillips, "Influenza Pandemic," *1914–1918-online. International Encyclopedia of the First World War*, Berlin 2014-10-08. DOI: 10.15463/ie1418.10148.

18 Mark Humphries, "The Horror at Home: The Canadian Military and the 'Great' Influenza Pandemic of 1918," *Journal of the Canadian Historical Association* 16.1 (2005) 250–55.

19 Macphail, *The Medical Services*, 267.

20 J. Castell Hopkins, *Canadian Annual Review of Public Affairs, 1918* (Toronto: Canadian Annual Review, 1919) 574–75.

21 Mark Osborne Humphries, "In Death's Shadow: The 1918–19 Influenza Pandemic and War in Canada," in Tim Cook and J.L. Granatstein (eds.), *Canada 1919: A Nation Shaped by War* (Vancouver: UBC Press, 2020) 138.

22 CWM, 19980129-003, Clarence McCann collection, letter, 18 November 1918.

23 Clint, *Our Bit*, 112–13.

24 CLIP, Jeannette Bridges, letter, 30 October 1918.

25 Macphail, *The Medical Services*, 266.

26 Lieutenant-Colonel H.C. Parsons, "Official Report on Influenza Epidemic, 1918," *CMAJ* 9 (1919) 351.

27 Magda Fahrni and Esyllt W. Jones (eds.), *Epidemic Encounters: Influenza, Society and Culture in Canada, 1918–20* (Vancouver: UBC Press, 2012) 4.

28 Mary-Ellen Kelm, "British Columbia First Nations and the Influenza Pandemic of 1918–19," *BC Studies* 122 (1999) 23–47.

29 For an overview, see John M. Barry, *The Great Influenza: The Epic Story of the Deadliest Plague in History* (New York: Viking, 2004).

30 T.H. Whitelaw, "The Practical Aspects of Quarantine for Influenzas," *CMAJ* 9.12 (1919) 1070.

31 See Captain E.A. Robertson, "Clinical Notes on the Influenza Epidemic Occurring in the Quebec Garrison," *CMAJ* 9.2 (1919) 158; Janice P. Dickin McGinnis, "The Impact of Epidemic Influenza: Canada, 1918–1919," in S.E.D. Shortt (ed.), *Medicine in Canadian Society: Historical Perspectives* (Montreal: McGill-Queen's University Press, 1981) 457.

32 Vincent Massey, *What's Past Is Prologue: The Memoirs of the Right Honourable Vincent Massey* (Toronto: Macmillan, 1963) 52.

33 The Bank of Commerce, *Letters from the Front*, 308.

34 LAC, RG 24, v. 1844, file 11-5, Casualties [Hundred Days].

35 John Swettenham, *To Seize the Victory: The Canadian Corps in World War I* (Toronto: The Ryerson, Press, 1965) 238.

36 Daniel Dancocks, *Sir Arthur Currie: A Biography* (Toronto: Methuen, 1985) 174.

37 Percy Leland Kingsley, *The First World War as I Saw It* (self-published, 1972) 79.

38 Chase, "Unwilling to Continue," 74.

39 LAC, RG 9, III, v. 1830, Prophylactic Measures against Venereal Disease, 31 January 1919; Snell, *The CAMC with the Canadian Corps*, 208.

40 LAC, MG 30 E15, W.A. Griesbach papers, v. 3, file 16(a), Book of Wisdom III, G.166-11, 1st Brigade to all BNs, 26 December 1918.

41 LAC, RG 9, III-B-1, v. 1830, Circular to 3rd Canadian Division, 3 December 1918.

42 See Lyndsay Rosenthal, "New Battlegrounds: Treating VD in Belgium and Germany, 1918-19," in Tim Cook and J.L. Granatstein (eds.), *Canada 1919: A Nation Shaped by War* (Vancouver: UBC Press, 2020) 57–71.

43 LAC, RG 9-III-D-3, v. 5025, War Diary, ADMS 1st Canadian Division, 29 December 1918.

44 LAC, RG 9, III-B-1, v. 1830, Lieutenant-General Arthur Currie memorandum, 21 March 1919.

45 Clint, *Our Bit*, 128–30.

46 For other failures in the BEF, Michael Bresalier, "Fighting Flu: Military Pathologies, Vaccines, and the Conflicted Identity of the 1918–19 Influenza Pandemic," *Journal of the History of Medicine and Allied Sciences* 68 (2013): 87–128.

47 Desmond Morton, "Kicking and Complaining: Demobilization Riots in the Canadian Expeditionary Force, 1918–19," *Canadian Historical Review* 61.3 (1980) 334–60.

48 CLIP, John Hudgins, letter, 9 March 1919.

49 John W.S. McCullough, "Sanitation in War," *CMAJ* 9.9 (September 1919) 790.

50 McCullough, "Sanitation in War," 790.

51 Grout, *Thunder in the Skies*, 412–13.

CHAPTER 18

1 Overseas Military Forces of Canada, *Report of the Ministry* (London: OMFC, 1919) 394.

2 Macphail, *The Medical Services*, 6, 242.

3 G.A. Anderson, "Presidential Address, Alberta Medical Association," *CMAJ* 10.3 (1920) 217.

4 Colonel A. Primross, "War Activities in Medicine and Surgery," *CMAJ* 9.9 (1919) 2.

5 Primross, "War Activities in Medicine and Surgery," 10.

6 Colonel E.J. Williams, "Return of the Army Medical Officer," *CMAJ* 9.9 (1919) 221.

7 See Michael Bliss, *Banting: A Biography* (Toronto, McClelland & Stewart, 1984).

8 Sir W.G. Macpherson (ed.) *Medical Services Pathology* (London: His Majesty's Stationery Office, 1923) 33.

9 George Armstrong, "Influence of War on Surgery," *CMAJ* 9.9 (1919) 396.

10 William Hutchinson, "A Study of Four Hundred and Fifty Cases of Wounds of the Chest, with Special Reference to a New Method of Treatment for Infected Hæmothorax," *CMAJ* 8.11 (1918) 972.

11 J.A. Gunn, "Lessons from War Surgery," *CMAJ* 10.4 (1920) 357.

12 Bruce Robertson, "Blood Transfusion in Severe Burns in Infants and Young Children," *CMAJ* 11.10 (1921) 744–51.

13 See Kim Pelis, "Taking Credit: The Canadian Army Medical Corps and the British Conversion to Blood Transfusion in WW1," *Journal of the History of Medicine and Allied Sciences* 56.3 (2001) 238–77.

14 Captain A.H. Pirie, "Shrapnel Balls: Their X-Ray Characteristics, Compared with Bullets and Other Foreign Bodies," *CMAJ* 7.9 (1917) 750.

15 Katherine McCuaig, *The Weariness, the Fever, and the Fret: The Campaign against Tuberculosis in Canada, 1900–1950* (Montreal: McGill-Queen's University Press, 1999) 24, 40, 61, 67–68.

16 See Alyse Waugh, "'Once a Soldier: Always a Man': The Military Hospitals Commission and Society, 1915–1928" (Master's thesis: Carleton University, 2011).

17 Dave McIntosh, "Where We've Been," *Legion* (January 1986) 10.

18 Cited in Robert Tait McKenzie, *Reclaiming the Maimed: A Handbook of Physical Therapy* (New York: The MacMillan Company, 1918). I thank Dr. Dennis Pitt for bringing this to my attention.

19 See Suzanne Evans, "Coming in the Front Door: A History of Three Canadian Physiotherapists Therapists through Two World Wars," *Canadian Military History* 19.2 (2010) 55–62.

20 John Pateman, *The Ontario Military Hospital, Orpington, Kent* (Lincolnshire: The Pateran Press, 2012) 17.

21 See Fulton Risdon, "Plastic Surgery of the Head and Neck," *CMAJ* 12.11 (1922) 797–98.

22 Macphail, *The Medical Services*, 114.

23 "Canadian National War Museum," *CMAJ* 9.10 (October 1919) 947–48; "Wax Models for the National War Museum," *CMAJ* 9.10 (October 1919) 937.

24 Tom Brown, "Shell Shock and the Canadian Expeditionary Force, 1914–18: Canadian Psychiatry in the Great War," in Charles Roland (ed.), *Health, Disease and Medicine: Essays in Canadian History* (Toronto: Hannah Institute, 1983) 308.

25 F.H. Mackay, "Some Aspects of the Psychoneuroses," *CMAJ* 13.7 (1923) 495.

26 See Kandace Bogaert, "Dealing with the Wounded: The Evolution of Care on the Home Front to 1919," in Tim Cook and J.L. Granatstein (eds.), *Canada 1919: A Nation Shaped by War* (Vancouver: UBC Press, 2020) 117–34.

27 Freeman and Nielsen, *Far from Home*, 233.

28 For some of the legacies, including those learned imperfectly, see Terry Copp and Mark Osborne Humphries, *Combat Stress in the 20th Century: The Commonwealth Perspective* (Kingston, ON: Canadian Defence Academy Press, 2010); Martin Stone, "Shellshock and the Psychologists," in W.F. Bynum et al. (eds.), *The Anatomy of Madness: Essays in the History of Psychiatry, volume 1* (London, 1985) 242–71.

29 LAC, RG 9, III, v. 3618, Adami to Todd, 15 June 1917; Colonel J.G. Adami, "The Policy of the Ostrich," *CMAJ* 9.4 (1919) 289–301.

30 On pension battles, see Desmond Morton and Glenn T. Wright, *Winning the Second Battle: Canadian Veterans and the Return to Civilian Life, 1915–1930* (Toronto: University of Toronto Press, 1989).

31 Colonel George Adami, "Medicine and the War," *CMAJ* 10.10 (1920) 899–900; H.W. Hill, "The Future Function of Modern Medicine," *CMAJ* 11.6 (1921) 445; and Cassel, *The Secret Plague*, 155. For postwar reforms, see Renisa Mawani, "Regulating the 'Respectable' Classes: Venereal Disease, Gender, and Public Health Initiatives in Canada, 1914–35," in John McLaren et al. (eds.), *Regulating Lives: Historical Essays on the State, Society, the Individual, and the Law* (Vancouver: University of British Columbia Press, 2002) 170–95.

32 Van Bergen, *Before My Helpless Sight*, 166.

33 Using Macphail's statistics in *The Medical Services*, 242: 395,084 disease cases vs. 144,606 battle casualties. He also gives battle deaths as 51,678 vs. 4,960 deaths from disease.

34 Fred Bagnall, *Not Mentioned in Dispatches: The Memoir of Fred Bagnall, 14th Battalion, Canadian Expeditionary Force* (Ottawa: CEF Books, 2005) 83.

35 G.A. Anderson, "Presidential Address, Alberta Medical Association," *CMAJ* 10.3 (1920) 218.

36 G.D. Shortreed, "Abstract of Presidential Address,' *CMAJ* v. 10 (1923); also see John W.S. McCullough, "Sanitation in War: An Address in Public Health," *CMAJ* 9.9 (September 1919) 792.

37 Humphries, *The Last Plague*, 109.

38 T. Glen Hamilton, "Presidential Address Delivered at the Annual Meeting of the Manitoba Medical Association," *CMAJ* 13.3 (1923) 151.

39 T.H. Whitelaw, "Presidential Address," *CMAJ* 6.11 (November 1916) 964–65.

40 "Compulsory Inoculation," *CMAJ* 5.3 (March 1915) 220–21.

41 Ibid.

42 Angus McLaren, *Our Own Master Race: Eugenics in Canada, 1885–1945* (Toronto: McClelland & Stewart Inc., 1990); Erika Dyck, *Facing Eugenics: Reproduction, Sterilization, and the Politics of Choice* (Toronto: University of Toronto Press, 2013).

43 See Mariana Valverde, *The Age of Light, Soap, and Water: Moral Reform in English Canada, 1885–1925* (Toronto: McClelland & Stewart, 1991).

44 G. Stewart Cameron, "Annual Address of the President, Ontario Medical Association," *CMAJ* 9.7 (July 1919) 585.

45 Cynthia Comacchio, *Nations Are Built of Babies: Saving Ontario's Mothers and Children, 1900 to 1940* (Montreal: McGill-Queen's University Press, 1993) 54; "A Federal Department of Public Health," *CMAJ* 7.4 (April 1917) 545–46.

46 P.H. Bryce, "The Scope of a Federal Department of Health," *CMAJ* 10.1 (1920) 8–9.

47 P.H. Bryce, "The Scope of a Federal Department of Health," *CMAJ* 10.1 (1920) 6, 9.

48 P.H. Bryce, *The Story of a National Crime: An Appeal for Justice to the Indians of Canada* (1922).

49 Senate Debates, v. 1 (1919) 288.

50 See Heather A. MacDougall, *Activists and Advocates: Toronto's Health Department, 1883–1983* (Toronto: Dundurn, 1990).

51 Morton and Wright, *Winning the Second Battle*, 9–10, 25.

52 Macphail, *The Medical Services*, 396–97.

53 CWM, Military History Research Centre, 20140473-001, scrapbook.

54 Matthew Barrett, "Absolutely Incapable of 'Carrying On': Shell Shock, Suicide, and the Death of Lieutenant Colonel Sam Sharpe," *Canadian Military History* 25.1 (2016) 19.

55 Morin-Pelletier, "'At Peace with the Germans, but at War with the Germs,'" 190.

56 Suzanne Kingsmill, *Francis Scrimger: Beyond the Call of Duty* (Toronto: Dundurn Press, 1991) 67.

57 Guiou, *Transfusion*, 30.

58 T.H. Whitelaw, "Presidential Address," *CMAJ* 6.11 (November 1916) 965.

CHAPTER 19

1 CWM, 20040015-005, Lawrence Rogers collection, letter to wife, 16 and 30 April 1916.

2 See Tim Cook and Natascha Morrison, "Longing and Loss from Canada's Great War," *Canadian Military History* 16.1 (2012) 53–60.

3 Garrett, "Tribute to the Fallen," 146.

4 Jay Doucet, Gregory Haley, and Vivian McAlister, "Massacre of Canadian Army Medical Corps Personnel after the Sinking of *HMHS Llandovery Castle* and the Evolution of Modern War Crime Jurisprudence," *Canadian Journal of Surgery* 61.3 (June 2018) 155–57.

5 William Philpott, *War of Attrition: Fighting the First World War* (New York: The Overlook Press, 2014) 344. Also see Antoine Prost, "War Losses," *1914–1918-online. International Encyclopedia of the First World War*.

6 Reid, *Medicine in the First World War Europe*, 31.

7 Nicholson, *Canadian Expeditionary Force*, 548.

8 Nicholson, *Canadian Expeditionary Force*, 548. This figure includes Canadians killed in France and Belgium, as prisoners of war, in Britain and Canada, and in other theatres of war such as Siberia, North Russia, Palestine, Bermuda, St. Lucia, and while travelling at sea. This last category is different from those who died while in uniform serving in the Royal Canadian Navy. William Johnston et al., *The Seabound Coast. The Official History of the Royal Canadian Navy, 1867–1939, volume I* (Toronto: Dundurn, 2010) 723–24. See S.F. Wise, *Canadian Airmen and the First World War, volume 1* (Toronto: University of Toronto Press, 1980) 645.

9 For the Newfoundlanders, see G.W.L. Nicholson, *The Fighting Newfoundlander: A History of the Royal Newfoundland Regiment* (Carleton Library Series, Montreal, 2006) 508–9.

10 See Cook, *Shock Troops*, 618.

11 Nicholson, *Canadian Expeditionary Force*, 548; Macphail, *The Medical Services*, 242.

12 On Canadian gas casualties, see Cook, *No Place to Run*, 230.

13 Nicholson, *Seventy Years of Service*, 112.

14 Dianne Dodd, "Canadian Military Nurse Deaths in the First World War," *Canadian Bulletin of Medical History* 34.2 (Fall 2017) 327.

15 Macphail, *The Medical Services*, 245.

16 See Adami, *The War Story of the C.A.M.C., 1914–15*, 46.

17 John W.S. McCullough, "Sanitation in War," *CMAJ* 9.9 (September 1919) 793.

18 Magda Fahrni and Esyllt W. Jones, *Epidemic Encounters: Influenza, Society, and Culture in Canada, 1918–1920* (Vancouver: UBC Press, 2012) 4.

19 Nicholson, *Seventy Years of Service*, 114.

20 Dodd, "Canadian Military Nurse Deaths," 327.

21 See Kathryn McPherson, "Carving Out a Past: The Canadian Nurses' Association War Memorial," *Histoire sociale/Social History* 29 (November 1996) 417–29.

22 "Solemn Notes," *Ottawa Journal*, 24 August 1926.

23 Fetherstonaugh, *No. 3 Canadian General Hospital*, preface; for this genre of writing, see Tim Cook, "Literary Memorials: The Great War Regimental Histories, 1919–1939," *Journal of the Canadian Historical Association* 13.1 (2002) 167–90.

24 Cameron, *No. 1 Canadian General Hospital*, introduction.

25 Gunn and Dutton, *Historical Records of Number 8 Canadian Field Ambulance, 1915–1919*, 164.

26 Boyd, *With a Field Ambulance at Ypres*, 1916.

27 Noyes, *Stretcher Bearers*.

28 CWM, 19740213-009, autograph book.

29 Toman, *Sister Soldiers of the Great War*, 7.

30 Clint, *Our Bit*, 56.

31 Mann, *Margaret Macdonald*, 184.

32 Ibid., 165–68.

33 Ibid., 161.

34 See Mélanie Morin-Pelletier, *Briser les ailes de l'ange: les infirmières militaires canadiennes (1914–1918)* (Montréal: Athéna éditions, 2006); Christina Bates et al. (eds.), *On All Frontiers: Four Centuries of Canadian Nursing* (Ottawa: University of Ottawa Press, 2005); and other works cited in this book, especially Mann and Toman.

35 United States Army Surgeon General's Office, *The Medical and Surgical History of the War of the Rebellion*, 6 vols. (Washington: US Government Printing Office, 1870–88).

36 Mitchell and Smith, *Medical Services*, xi.

37 LAC, RG 9, III, v. 3604, file 24-3-4 to 24-3-12, Adami to Wyatt, 22 September 1917; Ibid., Birkett to Adami, 27 July 1917.

38 Colonel J.G. Adami, *The War Story of the C.A.M.C., 1914–1915* (Toronto: The Canadian War Records Office, 1918) viii.

39 Arthur Evans Snell, *The C.A.M.C. with the Canadian Corps during the Last Hundred Days of the Great War* (Ottawa: F.A. Acland, Printer to the King, 1924) introduction.

40 Snell, *The C.A.M.C. with the Canadian Corps*, 1.

41 Tim Travers, "Allies in Conflict: The British and Canadian Official Historians and the Real Story of Second Ypres (1915)," *Journal of Contemporary History* 24 (1989) 301–25; Wes Gustavson, "'Fairly Well Known and Need Not Be Discussed': Colonel A.F. Duguid and the Canadian Official History of the First World War," *Canadian Military History* 10.2 (2001) 41–54.

42 Tim Cook, *Clio's Warriors: Canadian Historians and the Writing of the World Wars* (Vancouver: UBC Press, 2006) 41–92.

43 A.F. Duguid, *Official History of the Canadian Forces in the Great War, 1914–1919, volume 1: From the Outbreak of War to the Formation of the Canadian Corps, August 1914–September 1915* (Ottawa: King's Printer, 1938).

44 J.F.B. Livesay, "Canada's Black Watch, 1914–1918," *Ottawa Evening Journal*, 13 February 1932.

45 Ian Ross Robertson, *Sir Andrew Macphail: The Life and Legacy of a Canadian Man of Letters* (Montreal: McGill-Queen's University Press, 2008) 184.

46 Sir Andrew Macphail, "John McCrae: An Essay in Character," *In Flanders Fields and Other Poems* (1919).

47 Godefroy, *Bruce*, 99.

48 Macphail, *The Medical Services*, 8.

49 David Campbell, "Politics, Polemics, and the Boundaries of Personal Experience: Sir Andrew Macphail as Official Historian," 81st Annual Meeting of the Canadian Historical Association, 28 May 2002.

50 Macphail, *The Medical Services*, 188–89.

51 Robertson, *Sir Andrew Macphail*, 210.

52 DHH, unprocessed registry files, box 58, file 10-4, pt. 1, MacBrien to Minister, 22 February 1922; and Macphail to MacBrien, 30 January 1923; Ibid., box 58, file 10-4, pt. 2, Macphail and Medical History, MacBrien to Private Secretary, Minister of National Defence, 18 January 1924.

53 For the disclaimer, see RG 24, v. 1739, file DHS 3-17A, Neal to Duguid, 23 July 1924. For the reviews, see RG 24, v. 1872, file 13, History of the Canadian Forces Medical Services, Reviews, Remarks and Comments Culled from

Various Sources; and "General Sam Hughes Would Roll Over in His Grave," *The Lethbridge Herald*, 25 July 1925.

54 LAC, RG 24, C-6-i, v. 1872, file 13, collection of reviews, remarks, and comments on Macphail's official history, compiled by the Historical Section, Department of National Defence.

55 Ibid.

56 Macphail, *The Medical Services*, 169–70.

57 "MacPhail's Book," *Charlottetown Guardian*, 31 August 1925.

58 For a previous assessment of Macphail's *The Medical Services*, harsher due to the context of placing Macphail's work within the larger corpus of historical writing, see Cook, *Clio's Warriors*, 55.

CHAPTER 20

1 David Crane, *Empires of the Dead: How One Man's Vision Led to the Creation of WWI's War Graves* (London: Collins, 2013).

2 "Report on Material Received for the Canadian National War Museum from the Royal College of Surgeons, London," *CMAJ* 9.10 (1919) 949–50.

3 LAC, RG 9, III, v. 3604, file 24-4-0, pt. II, Hall to Birkett, [received 21 July 1919].

4 "Report on Material Received for the Canadian National War Museum from the Royal College of Surgeons, London," 949–50.

5 LAC, RG 9, III, v. 3604, file 24-4-0, pt. II, List of Articles from Museum of Surgical Records, Packed to be Sent to Canada, n.d. [early 1919]; "Report on Material Received for the Canadian National War Museum from the Royal College of Surgeons, London," 949.

6 Alberti, "The 'Regiment of Skeletons," 116; Keith and Hall, "Bones Showing the Effects of Gunshot Injuries, in the Army Medical Collection Now on Exhibition in the Museum of the Royal College of Surgeons of England," 537.

7 Sir W.G. Macpherson (ed.), *Medical Services Pathology* (London: His Majesty's Stationery Office, 1923) 575.

8 Major-General Sir W.G. Macpherson, *Medical Services, General History*, volume I (London: His Majesty's Stationery Office, 1921) x.

9 LAC, RG 9, III, v. 3604, file 24-4-0, pt. II, Collection and Preservation of Pathological Specimens, 6 February 1919. This document was circulated to all hospitals overseas and in Canada, urging doctors to contribute pathological samples. The records are silent on whether a body parts program occurred in Canada.

10 LAC, RG 9, III, v. 3604, file 24-4-0, pt. I, Adami to Elliot, 27 July 1918.

11 For the 181 figure, see LAC, RG 9, III, v. 3604, file 24-4-0, pt. II, Memorandum upon the Present Position with References to Museum specimens, 25 September 1918.

12 "Canadian Collection of Medical War Specimens," *The Lancet*, 17 August 1918, 215; "A National Collection of War Specimens," *The Lancet*, 19 July 1919, 120; Alberti, "The Regiment of Skeletons," 128; James R. Wright Jr., Samuel J.M.M. Alberti, Christopher Lyons, and Richard S. Fraser, "Maude Abbott and the Origin and Mysterious Disappearance of the Canadian Medical War Museum," *Archives of Pathology & Laboratory Medicine* 142.10 (2018) 1294.

13 LAC, RG 9, III, v. 3604, file 24-4-0, pt. 1, Canadian Specimens, Box No. 10, n.d. [ca. July 1918].

14 MacRae's regimental number was 442532.

15 LAC, RG 9, III, v. 3604, file 24-4-0, pt. II, Hall to Birkett [received 21 July 1919]; "Report on Material Received for the Canadian National War Museum from the Royal College of Surgeons, London," 949–50.

16 No Newfoundlanders have been found in the archival records, although the pathological samples would have been sent and kept at the Royal College of Surgeons and not likely to be sent to Montreal since Newfoundland was a separate dominion.

17 All citations from "Symposium on Pathological Specimens from France, Canadian Army Medical Services, through the Pathological Museum McGill University," *CMAJ* 10.8 (1920) 773–84. For other updates to the medical community by Abbott, see "Report of Meeting of the American and Canadian Section of the International Association of Medical Museums," *CMAJ* 9.8 (1919) 753; "Progress Report upon Preparation of Material for Army Medical Department of Canadian War Museum," *CMAJ* 10.3 (1920) 285–86.

18 Primross, "War Activities in Medicine and Surgery," 6.

19 Edward Peter Soye, "Canadian War Trophies: Arthur Doughty and German Aircraft Allocated to Canada after the First World War" (Master's thesis: Royal Military College of Canada, 2009); and Maria Tippett, *Art at the Service of War: Canada, Art and the Great War* (Toronto: University of Toronto Press, 2013).

20 Laura Brandon, "'A Unique and Important Asset'? The Transfer of the War Art Collections from the National Gallery of Canada to the Canadian War Museum," *Material History Review* 42 (1995) 67–74.

21 Tim Cook, "Canada's Great War on Film: *Lest We Forget* (1935)," *Canadian Military History* 14.3 (Summer 2005) 5–20.

22 Maude Abbott, "The Preparation of the Canadian Army Medical Museum, and Its Descriptive Catalogue in Collaboration with Experts," *Bulletin of the International Association of Medical Museums* 8 (1923) 34–39.

23 LAC, RG 9, III, v. 3604, file 24-4-0, pt. II, Fotheringham [Surgeon-General, A/DGMS] to Director of Medical Services, OMFC, 16 October 1917; Wright Jr. et al., "Maude Abbott and the Origin and Mysterious Disappearance of the Canadian Medical War Museum," 1296.

24 "Symposium on Pathological Specimens from France, Canadian Army Medical Services, through the Pathological Museum McGill University," 773–84.

25 See *Catalogue of Exhibits from the Canadian Medical War Museum* [microform, presented at the Medical School, McGill University by American College of Surgeons. Congress (10th: 1920: Montréal, Quebec)].

26 "Canadian National War Museum," *CMAJ* 9.10 (October 1919) 947–48; and LAC, RG 9, III, v. 3604, file 24-4-0, pt. II, List of Cases and Contents from 16th Canadian General (Ont) Hospital, 29 July 1919.

27 Wright Jr. et al., "Maude Abbott and the Origin and Mysterious Disappearance of the Canadian Medical War Museum," 1294.

28 On postwar memory, see Vance, *Death So Noble*; Alan Bowker: *A Time Such as There Never Was Before: Canada after the Great War* (Toronto: Dundurn Press, 2014); Cook, *Vimy: The Battle and the Legend*.

29 Macphail, *The Medical Services*, 305–9.

30 LAC, RG 2, v. 1,278, Order in Council 1921–2042. Calculated through Bank of Canada Inflation Calculator.

31 McGill University Archives, Canadian Army Medical Corps War Museum, RG 4, C.A.M.C. War Museum Fund, 16 September 1938; and Ibid., RG 4, C.A.M.C. War Museum Fund, Report on Conference of Descriptive Catalogue, [ca. 21 April 1921].

32 Surprisingly, Adami has no DCB entry, but his memoirs were published after his death. Marie Adami, *J. George Adami: A Memoir* (1930).

33 McGill University Archives, Army Medical Museum, RG 2, Dean, Faculty of Medicine to Principal F. Cyril James, 24 June 1947; and see RG 4, C.A.M.C. War Museum Fund, Report on Conference of Descriptive Catalogue [ca. 21 April 1921].

34 McGill University Archives, Canadian Army Medical Corps War Museum, RG 4, C.A.M.C. War Museum Fund, 16 September 1938.

35 Wright Jr. et al., "Maude Abbott and the Origin and Mysterious Disappearance of the Canadian Medical War Museum," 1297; McGill University Archives, Army Medical Museum, RG 2, Dean, Faculty of Medicine to Principal F. Cyril James, 11 September 1947.

36 For the sad state of the Canadian armed forces in the interwar period, see J.L. Granatstein, *Canada's Army: Waging War and Keeping the Peace*, 3rd ed. (Toronto: University of Toronto Press, 2021).

37 Arthur Keith, *An Autobiography* (London: Watts, 1950) 381.

38 McGill University Archives, Army Medical Museum, Acc No. R.G. 2, RG 2, Dean, Faculty of Medicine to Principal F. Cyril James, 24 June 1947; Ibid., James to DG, Medical Services, 18 August 1947; Ibid., Dean, Faculty of Medicine to Principal, 3 November 1947.

39 DHH, Kardex file 325.009 (D728), Pathological Museum, 3 May 1955. I would like to thank Dr. John Macfarlane and archivist Emilie Vandal for making this file available during the COVID crisis.

40 Ibid., Memorandum on Army Museum, Camp Borden, n.d. [ca. 1952].

41 Ibid., Army Medical Pathological Museum, 2 March 1955.

42 Ibid., "New Specimens for Army Medical Pathological Museum, Camp Bore, Ont."

43 Ibid., Pathological Museum, 3 May 1955.

44 There were also a few cases of families bringing bodies of loved ones home early in the war or, later, of engaging in illegal grave robbing.

ACKNOWLEDGMENTS

All books have their own history. This one began in 1997, when I was converting my master's thesis into my first book, *No Place to Run*. As part of the research, I further explored the RG 9 medical records and Macphail's official history, which piqued my interest in war and medicine. A few years later, while completing my doctoral dissertation on the writing of the two world wars, which became my second book, *Clio's Warriors* (2006), I studied Macphail's history intensely, taking note of the intriguing pages on the medical museum. At the time, I was more interested in how Macphail researched and wrote *The Medical Services*, and in the controversies surrounding his book, but I again explored another aspect of the medical war. My two-volume history of the Great War, *At the Sharp End* (2007) and *Shock Troops* (2008), had chapters that presented the medical experience, and they were written with significant research into the private and official archival records. Along the way, I researched and wrote other academic articles and books. With each research project taking me in a new direction, I nonetheless would take some time to explore another aspect of the medical war. The story of the medical museum and the body parts program was revealed to me again in 2010, this time with my co-curator, Dr. Andrew Burtch, when we curated *War and Medicine*, a major exhibition at the Canadian War Museum. That exhibition featured pathological museum pieces of soldiers' body parts from a German museum, and I began to search in earnest for the Canadian records at Library and Archives Canada. The files were obscurely named, however, and they escaped my first sustained round of searching. I put the research aside as I had a personal fight with cancer that spanned several years, although I continued to write during that time, with one friend noting that my output of books, articles, and book reviews offered new insight into the phrase "publish or perish." In 2015, I returned to Library and Archives Canada for additional research and eventually found the missing pathology files, documents that had never been accessed by any other researcher. My own research, along with others', allowed me to piece together the final story of the missing body parts, and I realized it could only be properly told if it was situated within a larger history of the Canadian medical services. I wrote this book during the coronavirus pandemic of 2020–2022, drawing on two decades of research and pouncing on the archives when the doors periodically opened in between lockdowns. This recounting of the research process is necessarily brief, but it shows some of the intellectual journey that informed this work, as well as the historical detective work that was also part of the writing process. If all books have their own history, all books also reflect the life and times of the author. This one is no different.

I have many to thank who assisted me in my intellectual development as a historian over twenty-five years. My colleagues at the Canadian War Museum are an astonishing group of scholars with tremendous drive and expertise. For this book, I will single out three colleagues in particular: Dr. Melanie Morin-Pelletier, an expert on First World War nursing; Dr. Andrew Burtch, co-curator of the *War and Medicine* exhibition; and Dr. Peter Macleod, who commented on the chapters. Other historians also offered insight in their close reading of individual chapters, and my thanks go to Dr. Bill Stewart, Dr. John Macfarlane, Dr. Sharon Cook, and Sarah Cook. Special thanks are offered to Dr. John Macfarlane of the Directorate of History and Heritage and Christopher Lyons of McGill University, both of whom facilitated access to important archival files during the lockdown. They and many others made this book better, as did researcher Eric Story, who lent his expertise in the search for important articles in *CMAJ*, and I remain grateful that I am a Fellow of the Laurier Centre for the Study of Canada.

My editor at Penguin Random House Canada, Diane Turbide, had faith in this book and championed it. We worked on nine books together, and she brought her formidable skills to bear on each one. Diane retired during the pandemic and her colleague, Nick Garrison, took over the book, asking good questions and, like Diane, giving me the freedom to shape the message and structure. I thank them both, along with Shona Cook, my hardworking and cheerful publicist at Penguin. My long-time literary agent, Rick Broadhead, continued to work his magic, and Tara Tovell provided her skilful expertise in line and copy editing, with this our tenth book together. Tara's patience and talent in working with authors is astonishing and I'm lucky to have worked with her for over fifteen years.

A special thanks also goes out to Ray Reipas and Adrienne Blazo, who gave my family access to their cottage in the summers of 2020 and 2021. Not only was it grand for our kids to play water sports, being whipped around Kawagama Lake by our in-laws, Graham, Sam, Calla, and Redden Shantz, but I had an astonishingly productive period of writing by the water. I am also grateful to have received a City of Ottawa writers' grant and a

Canada Council grant, and I thank those cultural institutions for championing writers. As a historian, there are some stories you look for, while others find you. This was history that I had to tell.

I wish to thank the many doctors and nurses who worked together in saving my life from cancer. While I am many years in remission now, I went through multiple rounds of treatment—radiation, chemotherapy, and stem cell transplants—before the cancer was destroyed. I was told more than once that I was facing my last battle, with no more fallback positions. During all the time I spent at the Ottawa Hospital, I was surprised and more than a little interested to discover how many doctors read military history and understand its importance in the advancement of medical procedures, treatments, and discussions around ethical issues.

I thank my many friends in Manor Park, across Ottawa, in Canada, and around the world, as well as my many readers. I think often of my father, Dr. Terry Cook, who passed away in 2014, and who would have liked this book. My mother, Dr. Sharon Cook, read chapters and offered expert advice, and has always given so much to me and my brother, Graham; I am grateful and awed by her ability to balance the challenges of life and live it to the fullest. For my family, this book did not weigh as heavily as some, although I think the periodic updates on rotting feet, blood transfusions, battlefield surgery, and stolen body parts attracted more attention than some of my previous works. I hope that Paige, Emma, and Chloe read it with interest someday, and that they know how much Sarah and I find inspiration in their lives. And to Sarah, who heard much about this book and offered sage advice throughout the research and writing, I offer my love. I'm a better person because of you.

CREDITS

The Author has been collecting images from multiple sources for two decades. All of the images here are his own unless otherwise stated.

Page 3: Library and Archives Canada (LAC), PA-002044

Page 5: LAC, PA-003192

Page 13: CEF official photograph, O-913

Page 49: Adami, J.G. *War Story of the Canadian Army Medical Corps* (London: Canadian War Records Office, 1918), Northern Sector of Ypres Saliant map.

Page 58: LAC, C-019919

Page 65: CEF official photograph, O-736

Page 72: LAC, 3192141

Page 75: "Silent Thoughts." Cartoon. *The Iodine Chronicle*, no. 6, 1918.

Page 79: "Canada No.9" Cartoon. *The Iodine Chronicle*, 1918.

Page 85: CEF official photograph, O.2553

Page 87: CEF official photograph, O-2076

Page 88: CEF official photograph, O-1519

Page 110: CEF official photograph, O.802

Page 114: "A White Man." Illustration. *Canada in Khaki*, vol. 3, 1918.

Page 120: LAC, PA-000625

Page 122: CEF official photograph, O-1002

Page 124: CEF official photograph, O-756

Page 125: "The A.D.S" Sketch. *NYD*, Christmas, 1917.

Page 127: CEF official photograph, O-924

Page 154: "Dr. John George Adami." Photograph. From McGill University, Osler Library.

Page 183: LAC, PA-000324

Page 188: CEF official photograph, O-814

Page 191: "What's wrong, chum, shell-shock." Cartoon. *The Listening Post*, no. 29.

Page 203: LAC, 3405107

Page 208: "The Canuck." Drawing. *Canada in Khaki*, vol. 3.

Page 221: "Water, water everywhere, but not a drop to drink!" Cartoon. *Canada in Khaki*, vol. 1.

Page 225: "What's the matter, Bill—inoculation?" Cartoon. *Canada in Khaki*, vol. 1.

Page 227: CEF official photograph, O-1691

Page 233: CEF official photograph, O-811

Page 235: CEF official photograph, O-1768

Page 236: CEF official photograph, O-2214

Page 246: CEF official photograph, O-1467b

Page 248: Cartoon. *The Splint Record*, vol. 2.

Page 263: LAC, PA 149313

Page 268: CEF official photograph, O-1080

Page 271: CEF official photograph, OM-0353

Page 275: CEF official photograph, O-1970

Page 279: CEF official photograph, O.1637

Page 288: CEF official photograph, O-4456

Page 291: Macpherson, Sir W.G. ed., *Medical Services, Pathology*, vol. 1 (London: H.M. Stationery Office, 1923), plate 10.

Page 292: Macpherson, Sir W.G. ed., *Medical Services, Surgery*, vol. 1 (London: H.M. Stationery Office, 1921), plate 3.

Page 305: LAC, C-150801

Page 317: CEF official photograph, O-3758

Page 319: CEF official photograph, O-2201

Page 322: CEF official photograph, O-2211

Page 324: CEF official photograph, O-2202

Page 333: CEF official photograph, EM 0381c

Page 342: CEF official photograph, O.1469e

Page 345: LAC, a003747

Page 357: CEF official photograph, O-3231

Page 359: CEF official photograph, O-3027

CREDITS

Page 362: CEF official photograph, O-3242
Page 370: CEF official photograph, O-2999
Page 372: CEF official photograph, O-3316
Page 379: CEF official photograph, O-3582
Page 389: CEF official photograph, O-3641
Page 424: CEF official photograph, O-0880
Page 447: *The British Journal of Surgery* no. 7 (1919): 309, fig. 282, 283.
Page 449: *The British Journal of Surgery* no. 6 (1918): 549, fig. 460, 461.
Page 452: *The British Journal of Surgery* no. 8 (1920): 118, fig. 67.
Page 466: CEF official photograph, O-3214

INDEX

Note: Page numbers in italic refer to photographs

NUMBERED UNITS

1st Artillery Brigade, 48
1st Battalion, 40, 124, 369
1st Battalion, London Regiment, 448
1st Canadian Division, 73, 104, 180,
    233, 274, 281
1st Canadian Field Ambulance, 325
1st Canadian Infantry Brigade, 49
1st Canadian Mounted Rifles, 228, 321
2nd Battalion, 105, 253, 378, 448
2nd Canadian Division, 109, 233, 274
2nd Canadian Infantry Brigade, 49
2nd Canadian Mounted Rifles, 231
3rd Battalion, 47, 54
3rd Canadian Division, 109, 180, 233
3rd Canadian Field Artillery, 55
3rd Canadian Infantry Brigade, 49
4th Brigade, Canadian Field Artillery,
    378
4th Battalion, 125, 354
4th Canadian Division, 233, 274
4th Canadian Mounted Rifles, 317
5th Battalion, 43, 356, 389
5th Canadian Field Ambulance, 122
5th Canadian Machine Gun Company,
    261
5th Canadian Mounted Rifles, 421
6th Canadian Field Ambulance, 355
7th Battalion, 27, 33, 47, 275, 277, 325
8th Battalion, 51, 325
10th Battalion, 46, 325, 367

12th Battery, Canadian Field Artillery,
    358
13th Battalion, 44
14th Battalion, 53, 411
15th Battalion, 51, 217
16th Battalion, 46
19th Battalion, 83, 378
20th Battalion, 325
21st Battalion, 309
22nd Battalion, 126, 350, 365, 366
23rd Battery, Canadian Field Artillery,
    396
24th Battalion, 365
25th Battalion, 287, 340
26th Battalion, 316
28th Battalion, 117, 289
28th British Division, 43
31st Battalion, 180, 318, 390
37th Battery, Canadian Field Artillery,
    218
41st Battery, Canadian Field Artillery,
    174, 331
42nd Battalion, 327
45th Algerian Division, 43, 44
46th Battalion, 231, 338
47th Battalion, 320
50th Battalion, 72, 174, 277, 321
52nd Battalion, 252
54th Battalion, 367
58th Battalion, 145, 350
75th Battalion, 359

78th Battalion, 151
87th Battalion, 338, 368
87th French Territorial, 44
102nd Battalion, 352
116th Battalion, 361, 416
182nd Siege Battery, Royal Garrison
    Artillery, 306
First British Army, 363, 388
No. 1 Canadian Clearing Station, 42,
    219, 287
No. 1 Canadian Field Ambulance,
    76–77, 249
No. 1 Canadian General Hospital, 34,
    64, 101, 160, 162, 201, 283,
    345–46, 448
No. 1 Canadian Stationary Hospital, 42,
    135, 198, 199
No. 1 Casualty Clearing Station, 51
No. 1 Southern General Hospital, 239
No. 2 Canadian Field Ambulance, 49
No. 2 Canadian General Hospital, 103
No. 2 Casualty Clearing Station, 326
No. 2 Military Hospital, 249
No. 2 Stationary Hospital, 37
No. 3 Canadian Field Ambulance, 49,
    50, 343, 357
No. 3 Canadian General Hospital, 54,
    130, 134, 146, 147, 165, 166,
    249, 250, 264–65, 296, 304,
    403, 450, 451
No. 3 Canadian Stationary Hospital,
    188, 195, 198, 200, 341–42,
    346–47
No. 4 Canadian Field Ambulance, 123
No. 4 Canadian General Hospital, 201,
    214
No. 4 Stationary Hospital, 257
No. 5 Canadian General Hospital, 201
No. 6 Canadian Field Ambulance, 127,
    235
No. 6 Canadian General Hospital, 242
No. 7 Canadian General Hospital, 198
No. 8 Canadian Field Ambulance, 280,
    304, 317, 328, 351, 364, 433
No. 9 Canadian Field Ambulance, 232

No. 10 Canadian Stationary Hospital,
    31, 298, 434
Ontario Military Hospital, 249–50,
    258–59, 301, 334, 455
Queen Mary's Hospital, 255
Royal Irish Rifles, 305
Royal Victoria Hospital, 30, 402, 418

A
Abbott, Maude, 295, 301
    as assistant curator at medical
        museum, 154–55
    and body parts collection, 300, 455,
        457, 461
    career, 299, 461–62
    and catalogue of pathology collection,
        458, 460
    death, 463
    and gender discrimination, 299
    and symposium on specimens, 450,
        451
    treatment of pathological samples,
        300, 301, 454
Adami, John George, 154, 287
    Aitken as inspiration, 167, 168
    and body parts collection, 155,
        157–58, 159, 160, 163, 165,
        169–70, 294, 294–95, 447, 464
    collection of artifacts, 296–97, 304,
        306
    desire for medical museum, 160,
        166–67, 168–69, 295–96,
        297–99, 303, 307
    as medical historian, 157
    post-war life, 459
    on preventive medicine, 227
    publication of Canadian Army
        Medical Corps history, 436
    reputation of, 154, 155
    responsibilities of, 155–57
    on vaccination for soldiers, 26
    on venereal disease, 99, 395, 408
Adamson, Agar, 278, 319–20
Adie, W.J., 185
advance aid posts, 123–24, 124

INDEX

Aitken, Sir Max (Lord Beaverbrook),
    167–68, 296, 298, 452–53
Alderson, E.A.H., 49
American College of Surgeons, 454, 457
Ames, Thaddeus Hoyt, 190–91
amputations
    caused by infection, 139, 147
    caused by trench foot, 293
    as last resort, 130
    of limbs, 73, 125, 139, 147, 201, 245,
        261, 346, 366
    number of, 147
    number surviving, 415
    quadruple, 415–16
    rate of, 143
    treatment for survivors, 259
Amyot, John A., 204, 226
anaesthesia, 138–39
Anderson, G.A., 398, 411
Andrews, Alfred, 142
Archibald, Edward, 134, 142, 143, 451
Armistice Day, 429. See also
    Remembrance Day
Armstrong, George E., 13, 131, 149,
    204, 265, 402
Armstrong, J.A., 258
Armstrong, John, 55
Army Medical Collection of War
    Specimens, 290–96
Army Medical Museum, 166–67
Army Medical Pathological Museum,
    464
Arthrell, William Gerald, 287–88
Asser, W., 448
Atkins, George, 207
Auld, F.M., 161
autograph books, 252–53, 433
autopsies, 153

B
Babbit, Pearl, 434
Babtie, Sir William, 210
bacteria, as cause of infection, 18
Bagnall, Fred, 411
Bain, John Alexander, 309

Ball, William, 218
Banting, Frederick, 401–2
Barrey, Clair, 277
Barrie, H.J., 463
Battle of Amiens, 353–62
Battle of First Ypres, 35, 37, 42–44
Battle of Hill 70, 274–78, 275, 309
Battle of Mount Sorrel, 103–4, 162
Battle of Passchendaele, 273–74,
    310–26, 335–36
Battle of Second Ypres, 1, 44–47, 49,
    49–50, 51–53, 113, 119, 167, 178
Battle of St. Eloi, 178–79
Battle of the Somme, 103–12, 113–19,
    123–28, 180, 215, 217
Battle of Verdun, 270
Battle of Vimy Ridge, 228–36
Battles of Canal du Nord and Cambrai,
    371–73
Bazin, Alfred Turner, 451
Beaverbrook, Lord. See Aitken, Sir Max
    (Lord Beaverbrook)
Becker, Harold, 359
Becker, John Harold, 347
Becket, R., 306
Bell, George, 52, 76, 124, 369
Bell, Percy G., 50, 67, 142
Best, Charles, 401–2
Biddle, George, 390
Bird, Will, 327
Black, Ernest, 69, 174, 339
Black Canadians, 114
bleeding, as treatment, 283–84
Blighty, 133, 146, 175–76, 176, 247–48,
    314, 324, 367
blindness, 416
    from mustard gas, 271, 272, 273,
        278–79, 280, 282–83, 320
    and syphilis, 91
    treatment for, 282
Blue, Edison, 237
body parts
    in Abbott's care, 300, 301, 458, 460,
        461, 462
    Adami's pressure to collect, 161–62

American collection of, 163
bones, 165, 169–70, 447, 449, 451, 455
brain, 162, 288
Canadian, in London exhibition, 291, 293, 294, 295
cataloguing of, 450, 462
challenge of transferring, 161
clearing stations as collectors of, 158
collecting, 156–57, 161, 305–6
collections of, 162–64
conservation of specimens, 464
destruction of collection, 464, 465, 466
display of, 160, 290, 291, 292–93
distribution of, 446–48
documentation of, 446
educational use of, 154–55, 156, 159–60, 162, 164–65, 290, 445–46, 461
gun shot wounds to, 451
hearts, 160–61, 292, 452
information about deceased soldier, 162, 164
lungs, 161, 162, 291, 293, 306, 448–49, 455
moving of collection, 463–64
need for, 159–60, 289
number of bodies from, 468
number of specimens, 446, 447, 449, 465
organization of, 164
organs, 293
ownership issues, 165, 295, 297, 298, 304
preparation of, 161
public display of, 302–3
purpose of preserving, 465
quantities of gathered, 304
sent to Canada, 300–302
skeletal, 293
spinal cord, 448
spine, 152
storage of, 297–98
symposium on specimens, 450–51, 455, 456

trachea, 306
vascular system, 293
bomber strikes, 344–45, 345–47
Books of Remembrance, 426
Borden, Sir Robert, 16, 98, 99, 200, 210, 215, 305, 306–8, 458
Bowness, Elmer, 251
Boyd, William, 50–51, 140, 204, 433. See also With a Field Ambulance at Ypres
Boyer, George F., 417
Bridges, Jeannette, 384
British Expeditionary Force, 339
British Journal of Surgery, 300
British Medical History Committee, 156
bronchitis and broncho-pneumonia, 34
brothels, 100
Brown, Charles, 125
Bruce, Constance, 199
Bruce, Herbert A., 202, 205, 206, 208, 209, 210, 211, 439, 442
Bryce, J.A., 318
Bryce, Peter Henderson, 413–14
Buckley, Douglas George, 83
Bulletin of the Canadian Army Medical Corps, 290–91, 334
burials, 287–89
Burns, H.L., 19
Burrell, Herbert, 228, 229–31, 321, 322
buses, use of at Second Battle of Arras, 365
Byng, Sir Julian, 274, 431

C
The C.A.M.C. with the Canadian Corps during the Last Hundred Days of the Great War (Snell), 437
Cameron, G. Stewart, 413
Cameron, Kenneth, 101
Campbell, George Alexander, 451, 454
Campbell, Roland, 127
Camp Borden, 465
Canada in Flanders (Aitken), 167
Canada in Khaki, 114
Canadian Army Dental Corps, 257

Canadian Army Hydrological Corps and
   Advisers on Sanitation, 223
Canadian Army Medical Corps (CAMC)
   Adami as medical historian, 157
   and British medical services, 155–56
   British support for, 210
   Bruce book on, 439, 442
   Bruce report on, 205–7, 208, 209,
      210–11, 439, 442
   cases of self-inflicted wounds, 339
   casualties in, 127, 362
   clinic for facial wounds, 258–59
   cutting back of, 429
   demobilization of, 397–98
   effect of liberation on, 379, 380
   equipment, 29
   establishment of, 16
   granted title of "Royal," 454
   growth of, 202–3
   improvements in, 211–12, 214
   investigation of, 202–3
   losses in, 427
   Macphail book on, 439–43, 460.
      See also The Medical Services
   makeup of in 1914, 7, 27–28, 29
   medical examinations on drafts, 207
   memorials to, 423
   and museum issue, 460
   removal of Bruce as acting com-
      mander, 211
   and Royal Army Medical Corps, 204
   staffing of, 17
   success of, 427
   support for specimen collection, 165
Canadian Corps
   aftermath of Somme battle, 217
   casualties in, 180, 187, 284, 354, 373,
      377
   Currie appointed as commander, 274
   and end of war, 388–89
   makeup of, 88
   seeking revenge, 353
   size of, 91, 107, 215
   success of, 352, 361
   water intake, 221

Canadian Expeditionary Force (CEF),
   6–7, 16, 17, 241–42, 399, 425, 426
Canadian Field Artillery, 48, 55, 174,
   218, 312, 331, 358, 378, 396
Canadian Hospital News, 249
Canadian Lancet, 441
Canadian Legion, 404, 416
Canadian Machine Gun Corp, 180
Canadian Medical Association, 302
Canadian Medical Association Journal
   (CMAJ), 11, 27, 74, 92, 95, 134,
   222, 257, 281, 292, 294–95, 299,
   303, 334, 406, 407, 412, 438, 457
Canadian Military Medical Service
   Memorial, 431
Canadian Patriotic Fund, 394
Canadian War Museum, 303, 423
Canadian War Record Office, 298
Cantilie, Mary Stuart, 436
casualties. See also deaths
   at Amiens, 354, 358, 360, 362, 373
   at Arras, 366, 368, 373
   battle compared to non-battle, 227
   of bomber strikes, 345–47
   in Canadian Corps, 373, 377
   at Canal du Nord and Cambrai, 373
   causes, 73, 240, 284
   in CEF, 426
   at First Ypres, 35–36
   at Hill 70, 277, 278, 309
   in Hundred Days campaign, 389
   improvement in numbers, 374
   lessened by mud, 314
   medical officers, 127
   at Mount Sorrel, 103, 180
   in Operation Michael, 341
   at Passchendaele, 312, 314, 319, 320,
      325, 326, 329, 331
   post-war, 426
   at Second Ypres, 46, 55
   at the Somme, 103, 126, 127, 217
   suffered by Canadian Corps, 354
   total in war, 424, 425
   treated by CAMC, 398
   treated by No. 3 General Hospital, 265

at Vimy Ridge, 217, 227, 237, 238
on the Western Front, 332
in the Great War, 6, 7–8, 426–27
Cate, Clifton, 358
cemeteries, 423, 424, 445
Chandler, Arthur Butler, 301
Charlottetown Guardian, 442
Charrett, Alfred, 305–6
chlorine gas, 44
    compared to mustard gas, 272
    effect of, 45–46, 48, 52, 56
    effect on morale, 267
    in lung specimens, 158
    recovery from effects, 56
    release of, 44, 51–52
Christianson, Ethelbert "Curley,"
    415–16
Churchill, Winston, 195–96
Chute, Arthur Hunt, 34–35
City of Cairo, 383
Civil War (U.S.), 3, 21, 166, 436
Clarke, Charles Edward, 105
clearing stations, 106
    at Battle of Amiens, 358
    challenges of moving, 341
    deaths at, 144
    directed to collect body parts, 158
    equipment in, 107, 131
    lack of written history, 432–33
    operating rooms at, 326
    position in battles, 356, 363
    purpose, 131
    rest areas in for shell shock, 190
    stress on, 341
    surgery at, 51, 126, 326, 327
    transport to, 125
    triage at, 144
Clements, Robert, 285, 361
Clements, William J., 206
Clint, Mabel, 201, 384, 392, 434–35
Clostridium perfringens, 137–38
cocaine, 236, 282
Commonwealth War Graves
    Commission, 423, 465
Connoy, Jim, 232

conscription, 215, 333
convalescent hospitals, 247–48, 250–51
Cook, Harold Edward, 380
corpses, 69–70, 169. *See also* body parts
Corrigall, D.J., 87
Coulter, Andrew, 361
Cramm, Richard, 196
creeping barrage, 108–9
Crimean War, 4, 224
Currie, Sir Arthur
    and Battle of Amiens, 361
    and Battle of Canal du Nord, 371–72
    and Battle of Passchendaele, 315
    and body parts issue, 461
    casualties report, 373
    and Hill 70, 274–75
    and LC Operation, 353
    and Mount Sorrel battle, 180
    ordered to Passchendaele, 310
    praise for Canadian Corps, 389
    reputation, 274, 275
    and Second Battle of Arras, 365, 366,
        369
    success of corps, 352
    and Vimy Ridge, 331
Curtis, William, 335

D
Davies, Isabel, 326–27
Davis, Ernest, 23
deaths. *See also* casualties
    causes, 56–57, 284
    rate of, 265
    of veterans, post-war, 404
death sentences, 339–40
demobilization, 397–400, 433
dentistry, 24, 257–58
Department of Health, 388, 413–14
Department of National Defence, 441,
    458, 461, 462, 464
Department of Soldiers' Civil
    Re-establishment, 415
Department of Veterans Affairs, 264
desertion, 339, 340
diabetes, 19, 401–2

diaries, 433
Dillon, Frederick, 188
diphtheria, 18, 19
disease. *See also* sexually transmitted
    disease; *specific diseases*
    compared to battle wounds, 408–11
    deadliness of, 67–68
    death from in Civil War, 3
    and latrines, 68–69
    in Mediterranean hospitals, 199–200
    and sanitation, 68, 199, 223, 224
Distinguished Conduct Medal, 126,
    232, 392
Distinguished Service Order, 328, 417
doctors. *See also* medical officers
    activities at Valcartier, 21–25
    assessing fitness for combat, 262–63
    education of, 18
    effect of battlefield injuries on, 4–5, 6
    and emergency medicine improvements,
        218–19
    fees, 19, 20–21
    health inspections by, 23–24
    and hierarchy challenges, 30
    moral dilemmas, 74, 77, 119, 144,
        190–91, 467
    practices in early 20th century, 19, 20
    as professionals, 18
    ranks of, 30
    request to for body parts, 156
    responsibilities undertaken by,
        37–38
    shortage in Canada, 211–14, 212
    status in community, 20, 21
Dominion Orthopaedic Hospital, 406
Doughty, Sir Arthur, 298
Draycott, W.L.M., 218
dressing stations, 105, 106, 123, 232,
    233, 363. *See also* medical stations
Drocourt-Quéant Line, 363, 366, 369
Duguid, A.F., 437, 438, 441
Duncan, H.A., 46, 47
Dutton, E.E., 433
Dyment, Walter H., 126
dysentery, 197, 199, 200, 223–24

E

education, 334, 335
87th French Territorial, 44
Elder, J.M., 130
executions, 339–40

F

Fargey, James, 80
feet, 72
    amputation of, 73, 147, 201
    diseases and conditions of,
        72–73
field ambulances, *106, 125*
    in Battle of Amiens, 356
    damage to, 357
    deaths in, 144
    demobilization of, 433
    equipment, 124–25
    makeup of, 28
    priority given to, 105
    purpose, 28
    rest areas in for shell shock, 190
    at Second Battle of Arras, 364
    staffing of, 105
    as support for doctors, 107
    triage at, 123
Finley, Enid, 406
Finley, Frederick Gault, 34
firing squads, 339–40
fitness levels, for returning to combat,
    262–63
Foch, Ferdinand, 363
Forbes, A. Mackenzie, 64
Ford, James, 107
Forster, W.B., 70
The Forty-Niner, 176
Foster, Gilbert L., 48–49, 203, 214
Foster, Sir George, 210
Fotheringham, John Taylor, 28, 177,
    458
Fowlds, Helen, 417
Fraser, Donald, 318–19
Freud, Sigmund, 81
frostbite, 201

G

Gallipoli campaign, 196–98
Gamble, Laura, 200
Gamester, Arthur, 250–51
gangrene, 73, 137, 138, 139, 140, 142, 244, 245, 326
gas. *See also* chlorine gas; mustard gas; phosgene gas
    casualties from, 278
    categories of, 269
    effects of, 269–70, 272, 278–80, 284–85
    gas masks as protection, 268
    reaction to terror of, 339
    treatment for attacks by, 283
gas gangrene, 137–38, 244–45
Gass, Clarence, 368
George V, King, 454
Gibson, Ethel May, 151, 152
Gibson, George, 23, 27, 47, 151–52
Gibson, James Herbert, 247
Gillespie, Bob, 396
Gillies, Harold, 257, 406
gonorrhea, 90–91. *See also* sexually transmitted disease
Goose, Bert, 50
Gorssline, R.M., 454
Gould, L. McLeod, 352
Granville Canadian Special Hospital, 249
Guiou, Norman, 120, 317, 343–44, 355–56, 419
Gunn, John Alexander, 137, 149, 204, 304, 379–80, 403
Gunn, John Nisbet, 280, 328, 433

H

Haig, Sir Douglas, 108, 187, 273, 274, 310, 353, 423
Halifax Explosion, 243
Halifax Memorial, 423
Hall, Morton, 299–300, 446
Hamilton, John, 463
Hamilton, T. Glen, 412
Hart, William Malloch, 43, 54, 55

Haywood, A.K., 54–55
headstones, 152, 288, 306, 346, 423, 465
Helmer, Alexis, 58
Hemmings, William, 180–81
Hickson, Arthur, 189
Hindenburg Line, 363, 368
Hingston, Donald, 136
histories
    of CAMC, 436
    of Great War, 436
    by Macphail, 439–43
    medical, 438
    of No. 8 Canadian Field Ambulance, 433
    planned, 437–38
    of units, 431–32
Hitler, Adolf, 463
Hoerner, Sophie, 181, 239
Holmes, R.J., 368
Horne, Robert A., 182–83
hospitals
    admissions at, 342–43
    attacks on, 345, 345–47
    base, 130
    convalescence in, 248–51, 264
    cooperation among, 204–5
    locations of, 130–31
    opening of new, 214
    organization of, 130–31
    sanitation in, 199
    sent to Mediterranean, 198–99
    staffing of overseas, 30–31
hospital ships, 347–49
hospital trains, 242
Hudgins, Jack, 392
Hughes, Peter A., 33, 113
Hughes, Sir Sam, 16, 26, 167, 202, 203, 209–10, 257, 440–41, 460
humour, 249–50
Hundred Days campaign, 354–74.
    See also Battle of Amiens; Battles of Canal du Nord and Cambrai; Second Battle of Arras
Hunter, John, 157

Hutcheson, Bellenden, 368
Hutchinson, John William, 402–3
Hutson, F.R., 136
hygiene, 225–26
hypothermia, 201, 374

I

Imperial War Graves Commission, 426,
    450. *See also* Commonwealth War
    Graves Commission
Imperial War Museum, 459
Indigenous children, deaths, 414
infections. *See also* gangrene
    deaths from, 260, 261
    innovations in controlling, 402
    treatment, 245–47
"In Flanders Field" (McCrae), 58–59,
    168, 419, *430*, 439, 454
influenza, 34, 350–51, 380–88, 392,
    411, 428–29
injuries and wounds. *See also* amputa-
    tions
    to abdomen, 142, 143
    to arteries, 111–12
    burden of caring for, 265
    burns, 129–30
    causes, 111, 129, 132–36, 145,
        292–93, 294, 337–39, 448
    to chest, 142, 143
    counting of, 424
    death from, post-war, 404
    death rate, 265
    displayed at exhibition, 292–93
    facial, 255–57, *256*, 406
    gut, 326
    to the head, 140–42, 255, 287
    and infection, 130, 136, 137–38,
        139, 146–47
    investigation of, 337
    to the leg, 145–46, 233–34
    loss of eye, 142
    to lungs, 283
    models of, 304–5
    from mustard gas, 282–83
    necessitating return to Canada, 264

recovery from, 239, 240–41
rehabilitation from, 243
self-inflicted, 336–37, 338, 339
survival from, 120–21
survivors of post-war, 404
to thorax, 143
to torso, 143
treatments for, 115, 118–19, 139, 283
types of, 50, 66, 314, 337–38, 373
at Vimy Ridge, 230–31
wound stripe to indicate, 263
innovations
    Carrell-Dakin solution, 246
    medical, 233, 402–3
    motivated by gas attacks, 279–80,
        283–84
    in transportation of wounded, 233,
        234, 242
inoculation, 25–26, 27, 224–25, 225,
    412, 419
insulin, 401–2
The Iodine Chronicle, 75, 77, 249
Irwin, Herbert, 331
Ivey, Pauline, 341

J

Jack, Richard, 45
Jackson, T. Stanley, 182
Jaggard, Jessie Brown, 200
Johns Hopkins Medical School, 153
Johnson, James Robert, 360
Johnson, William, 55
Jones, C.B.J., 218
Jones, Guy Carleton, 27, 29, 198,
    202–3, *203*, 205, 209, 210
Junger, Ernst, 424

K

Keene, Louis, 110
Keith, Arthur, 157, 159, 164–65, 299,
    300, 307, 463
Kemp, A.E., 211
Kentner, Robert, 231–32
Keogh, Sir Alfred, 198, 290, 402
Kerr, Wilfred, 312

Khaki University, 334, *390*
King, William Lyon Mackenzie, 459
Kingsley, Percy, 389–90
Kirk, James, 109–10
Koch, Robert, 18

L
Landsteiner, Karl, 343
Lapointe, Arthur, 350
Lapp, Thomas Clarke, 371
latrines, 68–69
LC Operation, 353–54
Lee-Enfield rifle, 132, 268
Lest We Forget (film), 453
lice, 70–71, 223, 226, 240
The Listening Post, 76, 80, *191*
Lister, Joseph, 18
Llandovery Castle, 347–48, *348,*
   353, 423
Loffler, Frederick, 18
Lougheed, James, 414
Lower, Arthur R.M., 407
Ludendorff, Erich, 351
lungs. *See also* body parts
   mustard gas damage to, 306
Lunt, Albert George, 354
Lynch, John, 267, 366–67

M
MacAdams, Roberta, 334
Macdonald, George, 253
MacDonald, Katherine Maud, 346
Macdonald, Margaret, 29, 203, 209,
   431, 435
MacEwen, John C., 320
Macfarlane, Joseph Harrison, 232–33
MacHaffie, Lloyd Philips, 304, 305,
   446–47Mack, Andie, 23
Mack, Thomas, 445
Mackay, F.H., 407
MacKinnon, Archie, 145
Macklin, Wilfred H.S., 378
Maclean's, 442
Macleod, J.J.R., 402
MacNutt, Edgar, 380

Macphail, Sir Andrew, 7–8, 67, 165–66,
   183, 184, 293, 340, 426, 438–39,
   440–41, 457, 460. *See also The
   Medical Services*
Macpherson, Sir William Grant, 436
MacRae, Peter, 448
Maguire, J. Arthur, 378
Maheux, Frank, 93
malaria, 197
malingerers, 74–78, *75–77*
Malloch, Thomas Archibald, 142, 244
Manion, Robert James, 21, 81, 190, 267
Manning, Frederic, 158
Massey, Vincent, 388
Matheson, J.C., 46
McCann, Clarence, 384
McCrae, John, 20–21, 42, 48, 53,
   57–59, *58,* 155, *168,* 178, 204,
   305, 418, 419, 430, 439, 454, 466
McCullough, Georgina Beach, 253,
   433–34
McCullough, John W.S., 2, 427–28
McDonald, H.F., 53–54
McDonald, William, 322–23
McFarland, George, 317
McGill, Harold W., 63, 64, 180
McGill College, Faculty of Medicine,
   153, 154, 159
The McGilliken, 249
McGill Medical Journal, 462
McGill Medical Museum, 154–55, 299,
   304
McGill University, 30, 299, 446, 450
McKenzie, Robert Tait, 405
McLean, David, 217
McNaughton, Andrew, 45
McPherson, Cleopatra, 415medical edu-
   cation, 18–19
medical museum
   Abbott hired at, 154–55
   body parts as basis for, 291
   desire for, 160, 166–67, 168–69,
      295–96, 297–99, 303, 307,
      451–52, 454, 457–59
   rejection of plan, 466

medical officers. *See also* doctors; nurses
  bravery of, 54–55
  casualties among, 127, 427
  challenges of, 61, 62
  and collection of body parts, 161, 445
  compassion of, 192–93
  cooperation among, 204–5
  and demobilization, 399–400
  diagnosing shell shock, 176–78
  and firing squads, 339–40
  at Hill 70, 277
  for infantry battalions, 47–48
  inspection for venereal disease, 94–95
  and malingerers, 74–76, 77–78
  mortality of, 80
  praise for, 64
  responsibilities of, 61–62, 74, 80–81,
    86–87
  soldiers' view of, 80
  as source of comfort, 67
  training of, 28
  treatment of influenza, 393
  treatment of venereal disease, 92–93,
    393–95
medical samples. *See* body parts
medical schools, need for corpses, 154
medical services
  emotional support of, 370–71
  evolution of, 328
  history of, 439–43
  integration with military, 350
  and planning operations, 312
The Medical Services (Macphail), 8,
    439–43, 457
medical units
  and CEF expansion, 241–42
  difficulties of retreating, 341, 342
  number of patients treated, 398
  position of, 49
  post-war in England, 397
medicines, 78–79, 79. *See also*
    morphine; rum
Meighen, Arthur, 458
mementos and talismans, 240
memoirs, 434–35

memorials, erection of, 429
Menin Gate, 422–23, 465
meningitis, 34–35, 37, 222
Military Cross, 55, 190, 401
Military Hospital Commission, 264
Military Medal, 275, 422
Military School of Orthopaedic Surgery
    and Physiotherapy, 406
Millar, William, 252
Mills, Gertrude, 253
Mockler, Edward, 40
Montreal General Hospital, 30
Moody, Arnott Grier, 377
Moody, Cecil, 351
morale, 67, 175–76, 187, 267, 315,
    370–71
morphine, 116, 236, 280
Morris, Harry, 260–61
Morrisette, Gordon J., 329
Moshier, Heber Havelock, 300
Munroe, H.E., 132
museums. *See also* medical museum
  desire for medical section in, 295, 297
  Hunterian Museum, 157
  ideas for, 295–96
  lack of support for medical, 462
  military, 459–60
  of pathology, 153, 299
  proposed medical war, 307
  war, 160, 295–96, 303
  for war memorabilia, 452–53
mustard gas, 271–73, 276, 277, 279–83,
    281, 284, 294, 306, 314, 320

N
Nasmith, George, 26, 35, 178, 223
National Gallery, 453
Newfoundland, casualties, 425
Newfoundland Regiment, 196
Nicholas II, Czar, 15
Nicholson, G.W.L., 425
1914 Star, 37
No Man's Land, 219
  clearing wounded from, 120–21,
    289, 374

conditions on, 8, 41, 107, 110, 111,
    117
corpses in, 70, 128
deaths in, 57
soldiers' experience in, 84, 86, 226,
    229–30
wounded left in, 364
Noyes, Frederick W., 122, 331, 356,
    433
nurses
    ability to vote, 333
    admiration for, 252, 253
    as anesthesiologists, 139
    autograph books, 252–53, 433
    average age, 29
    casualties among, 200, 427
    documenting of service, 435
    emotional cost of job, 4–5, 242–43
    honouring of, 431
    importance of, 200–201
    memorial to, 432
    nationality, 29
    numbers on surgical teams, 417
    patients' relationships with, 252
    in post-war world, 417–18
    preparation for Vimy Ridge battle,
        228–29
    ranks of, 30
    recruitment of, 29
    responsibilities undertaken by, 37–38
    treatment of infections, 246–47

O
Ontario Medical Association, 303
Ontario Military Hospital, 249–50,
    258–59, 301, 334, 455
Operation Michael, 340–41
Ormsby, George, 175
O'Rourke, James, 275–76
Osler, William, 18, 153–54, 156, 210
Our Bit: Memoirs of War Service by a
    Canadian Nursing Sister (Clint),
    434–35
Overseas Ministry of Canadian Forces
    (OMFC), 211

Ower, John James, 160, 162, 448
oxygen treatment, 280

P
Paine, Annie, 261
pain relief, 66, 112, 116, 236, 280,
    282–83
pandemics, 12
Paynter, Elizabeth, 260
Pearson, Lester "Mike," 201–2
Peat, Gilbert, 281
Peat, Harold, 47
pensions, 408, 415
Perley, George, 211
Peters, C.S., 450–51
Petrie, H.V., 342
phosgene gas, 269–71, 272
photographs of war effort, 453
physiotherapy, 405–6
Piper, A.E., 253
Pirie, Alexander Howard, 147, 403–4
poison gas. See chlorine gas; gas;
    mustard gas; phosgene gas
Politics and the C.A.M.C. (Bruce), 439.
    See also Herbert A. Bruce
Polson, Archibald John, 261–62
poppies, 429, 430
postcards, 22, 88, 90, 254
Pottle, Frederick, 139–40Primross,
    Alexander, 398, 399, 452
Princess Patricia's Canadian Light
    Infantry, 218, 267, 278, 318,
    366–67
Princess Patricia's Red Cross Hospital, 261
The Principles and Practice of Medicine
    (Osler), 18
prisoners of war, 120–21, 231–32, 364
prosthetics, 148, 257, 259, 404, 405,
    410, 415
prostitutes, 89
Public Archives of Canada, 453
public health, desire for improved,
    411–13
Pullen, W.J., 306
pyrexia of unknown origin (PUO), 71

INDEX

Q

Queen's University, 30–31, 198, 251

R

racial barriers, 114
radiology, 403–4. *See also* X-ray
rails/railways, 234, 363–64
Rankin, Allan Coats, 71, 223
rats, 69–70
Red Cross, 249
Reed, Marjorie, 329
Reid, A.P., 345, 346
Reilly, Margaret, 252–53
Remembrance Day, 429, 443, 453.
    See also Armistice Day
respirators, 268, 268–69
rest and restoration, 86–93
Rhea, Laurence Joseph, 165, 166, 451
Riel, Louis, 29
riots, by Canadian soldiers, 392
RMS *Lusitania*, 347
Robertson, Gordon, 226
Robertson, Lawrence Bruce, 343, 403
Robison, Frederick, 350
Roentgen, Wilhelm, 18
Rogers, Lawrence, 171, 220, 421–22, 422
Ross, Arthur Edward, 311–12
Ross, Stanley Graham, 235
Ross rifle, 52
Roy, Joseph Napoleon, 257
Royal Army Medical Corps (RAMC),
    155–56, 188, 204, 209, 213, 250,
    343, 402, 436
Royal Canadian Army Medical Corps.
    See Canadian Army Medical Corps
    (CAMC)
Royal Canadian Army Medical Corps
    School, 463
Royal Canadian Navy, 425
Royal Canadian Regiment, 320
Royal College of Surgeons, 9, 157, 158,
    159, 160, 163–64, 165, 167, 290,
    291, 295, 298, 299, 300, 306, 307,
    334, 446, 449, 457, 463Royal Red
    Cross Medal, Second Class, 434

Royal Victoria Hospital, 30, 402, 418
Ruddock, Henry, 117–18
rum, 66, 67, 69, 78–79, 112, 116, 118,
    236, 280, 313, 327, 370
Russel, Colin, 173
Russia, 340
Ryan, Edward, 182

S

Salisbury Plain, 32–35
Salvation Army, 390–91
sandbags, in trenches, 84
sanitation
    baths and showers, 225–26
    benefits and importance of, 221, 222,
        408, 411
    and flies, 70
    improvements in, 21–22
    and latrines, 68–69
    in Mediterranean hospitals, 199
    to prevent disease, 68
    resources for, 222–23
    in trenches, 41
    of water fouled by Germans, 379
Savage, Charles, 69, 109, 175, 224,
    243–44
Scott, Frederick, 51, 281
Scrimger, Alexander Canon, 418
Scrimger, Francis, 53–54, 418, 451
Second Battle of Arras, 363–69
sexually transmitted disease, 89–101,
    391, 408. *See also* gonorrhea;
    syphilis; venereal disease
sex workers, 89
Sharpe, Samuel, 416–17
Shelford, Arthut, 367
shell shock, 191
    attitudes to, 173, 174, 181, 183–84,
        406–7
    causes, 171, 172–73, 182
    defined, 184
    diagnosing, 176–78, 183–84, 186–87
    experienced by doctors, 321
    experiences of, 174–75, 178
    faking of, 176, 179

losses due to, 180
medical policy regarding, 338
numbers treated for, 192
from Passchendaele battle, 327–28
punishment for, 186–87
renaming of, 187, 338
resulting in suicide, 416–17
signs of, 171–72, 181
treatment, 176–77, 178, 181–82, 185–90
shrapnel, 111, 134, 244
"Sketches of a Tommy's Life," 78
Skidmore, James Walter, 144
smallpox epidemic, 20, 25
Smith, A.E., 361
Snell, Arthur Evans, 436–37, 454, 461. *See also The C.A.M.C. with the Canadian Corps during the Last Hundred Days of the Great War*
sodium bicarbonate, 282
"soldiers' heart," 160–61
South African War, 20, 21, 29, 48, 66, 93, 136–37, 202
specimens. *See* body parts
Sproston, Joseph, 367
Sproule, J.G., 337
Stonebridge, E.A., 338
Strathy, George S., 77–78, 284, 320–21
The Stretcher, 249–50
stretcher-bearers, 65, 106, *118*, 124
and battlefield clearing, 48, 54, 315, 316–18
in Battle of Amiens, 355, 359–60
carrying the wounded, 121–22, *122*
equipment, 112, 116
German prisoners as, 231
at Hill 70, 277
identification of, 113
increasing numbers at Passchendaele, 315
medals awarded to, 126–27
nickname for, 53
numbers of, 113
at Passchendaele, *319, 321, 322*

preparation for Vimy Ridge battle, 228–29
pressures on, 53
procedures of, 115–16
rescue of wounded, 8
in Second Battle of Arras, 365
at the Somme, 113–15
treatment of, 219–20
Stretcher Bearers at the Double (Noyes), 433
surgery. *See also* amputations
advances in, 145–46, 148–49
at clearing stations, 51, 326, 327
conditions for, 107, 138–39
dental, 257–58
facial, 255–57, *258*, 258–59, 305, 406
for head injuries, 140–42
impossibility of, 119
outdoors at clearing station, *359*
planning for procedures, 136–37
for shell fragment removal, 139–40
survival rates, 107, 143, 148–49
use of X-rays, 147
Swanston, Victor, 360
symposium on specimens, 450–51, 455
syphilis, 19, 91, 97–98, 300. *See also* sexually transmitted disease

T
tetanus, 137
Textbook of Pathology (Adami and McCrae), 155
The War Story of the C.A.M.C., 1914–1915 (Adami), 436
Thomas splint, 146, 233
Todd, Roderick Anderson, 249
tramways, 277
transfusions, 343–44, 366, 403
trench cough, 226
trench fever, 71
trench foot, 72, *72*, 73, 293, 314
tuberculosis, 18, 19–20, 207, 404, 449
Turner, Richard, 214
typhoid, 21, 224

INDEX

U

U-boats, 347–49
universities, staffing of overseas
    hospitals, 30–31
University Magazine, 438

V

vaccination. *See* inoculation
Vanier, Georges, 126, 366
venereal disease, 89–91, 393, 407–9,
    409. *See also* sexually transmitted
    disease
veterans, 404, 408, 426
Victoria Cross, 54, 126, 202, 210, 275,
    276, 368, 418, 451
Victory Bond, *168, 348, 400*
Vidler, Arnold G.A., 388
Vienneau, J.E., 338
Vimy Memorial, 423, 465
Vimy Ridge, 9, 217, 218, 332
Voluntary Aid Detachment workers
    (VADs), 239–40, 384–85, *385*

W

Walker, Frank, 219–20
Walker, James Stewart, 56
war art, 453
war artifacts, 296–97, 298, 304, 452–53
warfare, changes in, 350
water
    chlorine treatment of, 69
    daily consumption, 221
    lack of in Mediterranean hospitals,
        199
    lack of potable, 221
    supply of at Passchendaele, 313
    supply of at Vimy, 221
Watson, Ralph, 5, 66, 112
Watt, Walter Langmuir, 1
weapons, 104, 108, 109, 111, 129, 132,
    228
whale oil, 73
Wheeler, Victor, 72, 174, 277–78
Whitelaw, Dr. T.H., 222, 387
Whitmore, Thomas Hazel, 356–57
Wilhelm II, Kaiser, 15
Williams, Claude, 169, 226
Williams, E.J., 111, 135
Williams, John, 314–15
Willoughby, Charles, 107, 379
Wilson-Simmie, Katharine, 195, 201,
    255
Winnipeg General Strike, 395
Winterbottom, Sydney Amyas, 236–37
With a Field Ambulance at Ypres (Boyd),
    433
women
    as ambulance drivers, 342
    diseased, as enemy, *94, 99*
    wooing of, 88–89
Wright, Henry Pulteney, 184
Wright, Robert Pierce, 325

X

X-ray, 18, 147, 403–4

Y

Yealland, Lewis, 185
YMCA, 390–91
Young, Elsworth, 340
Young, Francis, 368

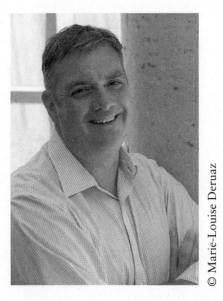

© Marie-Louise Deruaz

TIM COOK is Chief Historian and Director of Research at the Canadian War Museum. His bestselling books have won multiple awards, including three Ottawa Book Awards for Literary Non-Fiction and two C.P. Stacey Awards for the best book in Canadian military history. In 2008 he won the J.W. Dafoe Book Prize for *At the Sharp End* and again in 2018 for *Vimy: The Battle and the Legend*. *Shock Troops* won the 2009 Charles Taylor Prize for Literary Non-Fiction. Cook is a frequent commentator in the media, and a member of the Royal Society of Canada and the Order of Canada.